Nursing in Australia

Graduate nurses are expected to 'hit the ground running', taking on complex care challenges in a stressful and fast-paced environment. This comprehensive yet accessible textbook provides expert guidance for students and commencing nurses on the contexts for their practice.

Part 1 presents a pragmatic insight into the intersection, tensions and complexities of practice and professional issues for Australian nurses. It outlines the nature of nursing roles and professional codes of conduct, national health priority areas and legal and ethical issues including the growing use of health informatics. There is an examination of the diverse career paths available in nursing, a focus on nurses' mental health and well-being and a special examination of Aboriginal and Torres Strait Islander health issues. Part 2 unpacks key issues across a range of clinical contexts that will be a key resource for clinical practicums. Contexts covered include acute care, community nursing, paediatric nursing, mental health nursing and aged care. Part 3 examines the professional and practice issues of nursing in diverse, distinctive and emergent practice areas including aesthetic nursing, military nursing and international nursing with case studies and vignettes highlighting common issues and challenges.

Drawing on the expertise of a wide range of Australian clinical and academic nursing professionals, this text is a key reference for all nursing undergraduates seeking to enter successfully into the profession.

Nathan J. Wilson is an Associate Professor in the School of Nursing and Midwifery at Western Sydney University. Nathan is a registered nurse with over 30 years' experience in working with people with intellectual and developmental disabilities and their families as a nurse, manager, clinical specialist, clinical educator, applied researcher and independent consultant. Nathan's applied research is focussed on enhancing the health, wellbeing and social participation of people with intellectual and developmental disability, with an underlying emphasis on chronic illness, men's health, masculinity, participation and social inclusion. He has published over 90 scientific papers about disability and regularly presents his findings at national and international conferences.

Peter Lewis is a Senior Lecturer and Director of Academic Workforce at the School of Nursing and Midwifery at the Western Sydney University. Peter has more than 20 years' experience as a registered nurse in paediatrics with a focus on chronic illness and disability. His current research interest is in the nursing care of people with intellectual disability.

Leanne Hunt is a Senior Lecturer in Nursing and Deputy Director, Clinical Education (Nursing), in the School of Nursing and Midwifery at the Western Sydney University and Registered Nurse at Liverpool Hospital Intensive Care Unit. Leanne began nursing in 1992 as an RN progressing to CNC (trauma) and NUM 1. Leanne worked in the Kingdom of Saudi Arabia in paediatric cardiothoracic intensive care for 2 years. She has 10 years of education and research experience and is the current chair of the Critical Care Research in Collaboration & Evidence Translation (CCRICET) research group. Leanne is also an affiliate member of the Centre for Applied Nursing Research (CANR), Centre for Oral Health Outcomes & Research Translation (COHORT) and the Ingham Institute of Applied Medical Research. Leanne's research interests include clinical practice experience, critical care and nursing education.

Lisa Whitehead is a Professor of Nursing Research and Associate Dean Research, School of Nursing and Midwifery at Edith Cowan University. Lisa's research centres on improving health outcomes for people living with chronic conditions, self-management interventions and working with families to support the management of chronic conditions. Engagement with clinicians and conducting research in real world settings underpin all of her research activities with the goal of implementing evidence-based change into practice.

Nursing in Australia

Contemporary Professional
and Practice Insights

Edited by Nathan J. Wilson, Peter Lewis,
Leanne Hunt and Lisa Whitehead

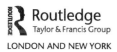
Routledge
Taylor & Francis Group

LONDON AND NEW YORK

First published 2021
by Routledge
2 Park Square, Milton Park, Abingdon, Oxon OX14 4RN

and by Routledge
52 Vanderbilt Avenue, New York, NY 10017

Routledge is an imprint of the Taylor & Francis Group, an informa business

© 2021 selection and editorial matter, Nathan J. Wilson, Peter Lewis, Leanne Hunt and Lisa Whitehead; individual chapters, the contributors

The right of Nathan J. Wilson, Peter Lewis, Leanne Hunt and Lisa Whitehead to be identified as the authors of the editorial material, and of the authors for their individual chapters, has been asserted in accordance with sections 77 and 78 of the Copyright, Designs and Patents Act 1988.

British Library Cataloguing-in-Publication Data
A catalogue record for this book is available from the British Library

Library of Congress Cataloging-in-Publication Data
Names: Wilson, Nathan, editor.
Title: Nursing in Australia: nurse education, divisions, and professional
    standards/edited by Nathan J. Wilson, Peter Lewis, Leanne Hunt and Lisa Whitehead.
Description: Milton Park, Abingdon, Oxon; New York, NY: Routledge, 2021. |
    Includes bibliographical references and index. |
Identifiers: LCCN 2020029450 (print) | LCCN 2020029451 (ebook) |
    ISBN 9780367637859 (hardback) | ISBN 9780367643881 (paperback) |
    ISBN 9781003120698 (ebook)
Subjects: LCSH: Nursing—Vocational guidance. | Nursing—Australia. |
    Nursing—Study and teaching.
Classification: LCC RT82 .N8654 2021 (print) | LCC RT82 (ebook) |
    DDC 610.7306/9—dc23
LC record available at https://lccn.loc.gov/2020029450
LC ebook record available at https://lccn.loc.gov/2020029451

ISBN: 978-0-367-63785-9 (hbk)
ISBN: 978-0-367-64388-1 (pbk)
ISBN: 978-1-003-12069-8 (ebk)

Typeset in Times New Roman
by KnowledgeWorks Global Ltd.

Contents

Illustrations

Figures

Tables

Boxes

Contributors

Nathaniel Alexander is an Associate Chief Nursing & Midwifery Information Officer for SLHD. Mr Alexander also holds adjunct appointments at the School of Nursing & Midwifery, Western Sydney University and the Faculty of Science at Charles Sturt University. Mr Alexander is an experienced nurse and lawyer and has a strong interest in the use of artificial intelligence in ways that improves outcome for patients and families as well as supporting new and existing clinical workflows for staff.

Debra Anderson is the Assistant Dean Research in the Faculty of Health and the Director and Founder of the Women's Wellness Research Program at the University of Technology Sydney. Previously she held positions as the Head, School of Nursing and Midwifery at Griffith University and the Director of Research at the School of Nursing, Queensland University of Technology. She has a distinguished international reputation as a scholar and leader in the field of women's health research and is a collaborator on the Australian Longitudinal Study on Women's Health and a chief investigator on the InterLACE consortium.

Jen Bichel-Findlay is a Faculty of Health Honorary Associate at the University of Technology Sydney, previously being the inaugural Director of Digital Health and Innovation in the Faculty. She holds voluntary positions in the International Medical Informatics Association, Health Information and Management Systems Society, and is a Director for the Australasian Institute of Digital Health and current Chair of its Nursing and Midwifery Community of Practice.

Deborah Brooke has been a paediatric nurse and registered midwife for more than twenty years. She is currently a Clinical Nurse Specialist in the area of Medical Assessment at the Children's Hospital at Westmead, Sydney, Australia.

Janie Brown is a Registered Nurse, a Senior Lecturer at Curtin University and a Senior Research Fellow at St John of God Midland Hospital, Perth. Janie has a PhD and a Master of Education (Adult) and had many years of experience as a Cardiothoracic ICU RN and educator, before moving to the university sector. She has been building a portfolio of research in acute-care nursing and nursing workforce issues.

Didy Button has a strong interest in educating nursing students to enable them to provide the highest quality evidenced-based nursing care. Her PhD research was in electronic learning and how e-Learning is impacting on you as students and the educators working with you.

Bernadette Cameron is the working Director of Albercam Enterprises Pty Ltd since 1997 and is known as *'The Corporate Nurse'*. Her qualifications include a Bachelor of Nursing Degree (BN); Post Graduate Diploma of Occupational Health and Safety and a Masters of Occupational & Environmental Health and Safety. She is an OSH Consultant specialising in Corporate Health & Safety Systems Management and Workplace Health Ownership.

Christine Chisengantambu-Winters is a Lecturer in School of Nursing, Midwifery and Paramedicine at Australian Catholic University, North Sydney, Australia.

Robin Curran has been in direct clinical care and management roles within the cosmetic/ dermatology area for the past 10 years. Robin has developed her skill and expertise in dermal conditions & treatments in private dermatology clinics. Robin has been involved in several research projects within the emerging field of cosmetic nursing and the current chairperson of the cosmetic nurse focus-group within the Australian College of Nursing. Robin is also a guest clinical trainer and speaker within the dermatology and cosmetic field. Robin is currently studying the Masters of Nurse Practitioner through Queensland University of Technology and will graduate in 2021.

Lynette Cusack is an Associate Professor in the Adelaide Nursing School, The University of Adelaide.

Linda Deravin is the Course Director for the School of Nursing, Midwifery and Indigenous Health at Charles Sturt University. Throughout her nursing career Linda has worked as a clinician, educator and senior nurse and health manager in a variety of settings in both the public and private sector. She has research interests in Indigenous health, chronic care and nursing workforce issues. Linda is also a Fellow of the Australasian College of Health Service Managers.

Kathleen Dixon is a registered nurse and holds qualifications in education, health management and a PhD. She is a senior lecturer in the School of Nursing and Midwifery and has held many senior governance roles in the School including Deputy Dean, Director Workforce, Associate Head of School and Head of both postgraduate and undergraduate programs in nursing. Kathleen has a broad range of research interests including enhancing academic literacy skills, examining issues for sessional teaching staff, evaluating diabetes education, clinical judgement in nursing and spirituality. Kathleen has expertise in qualitative research with a particular interest in critical discourse analysis and Foucauldian approach to methodology, she is currently supervising PhD, Masters Honours and BN Honours students.

Paul L. Donohoe is a registered nurse with expertise is both paediatric and adult perioperative nursing. He has post-graduate certificates in anaesthetic and post-anaesthetic nursing and has worked in multiple clinical and management roles, across multiple locations in Australia and New Zealand. Paul currently lives in Christchurch, New Zealand, and works at St Georges Hospital, Christchurch in the perioperative suite.

Mahnaz Fanaian is an academic with 20 years experiences working in Universities of NSW, Wollongong, and ACU in research & teaching, after finishing her Master degree in cardiac nursing and her PhD in Public Health & Nutrition. Her area of interests and expertise are Cardiovascular Disease, Diabetes, Public Health, Mental Health and Primary Health Care. Currently she is teaching undergraduate subjects in Nursing and Master degrees in public Health, health management and Nursing. She has been involved in supervising Master & PhD students in Public Health, mental Health and Health management.

Murray Fisher is a senior academic at the Susan Wakil School of Nursing and Midwifery, University of Sydney and is a Scholar in Residence at Royal Rehab. Murray's research examines nursing's contribution to patient rehabilitation outcomes. Research projects include: neurogenic bowel care practices for people with SCI; fall prevention in TBI rehabilitation; person-centred rehabilitation outcomes; and patient deterioration in rehabilitation settings.

Mandie Jane Foster is a Lecturer and research scholar at Edith Cowan University, School of Nursing and Midwifery, Joondalup, Perth, Australia. She teaches child and adolescent health for post-graduate students and into the Master of Nursing paediatric program, providing a child and family nursing lens to advanced paediatric education. Her research focuses on child and family centred care and the experiences, perceptions and needs of children, parents, families and staff within various healthcare settings globally.

Cathrine Fowler holds the Tresillian Chair in Child and Family Health and is a member of the School of Nursing and Midwifery at the University of Technology Sydney. Cathrine is a child and family health nurse who has extensive experience in the provision of professional, parent and community education. Her research and clinical focus are on working with families with complex and multiple vulnerabilities and child and family health nursing professional issues.

Iain Graham is the Emeritus Professor of Health Development in the School of Health and Human Sciences at Southern Cross University, New South Wales. He retired as the Dean and Head of School and Director of Clinical Services at Southern Cross, at the end of 2019 after a clinical and academic career spanning 40 years working in the U.K., the U.S.A. and Europe.

Marika Guggisberg is a Senior Lecturer at CQUniversity in Perth, Western Australia. After being awarded her PhD from the University of Western Australia, she has completed her Postdoctoral Fellowship at Curtin University, where she stayed on to teach into the postgraduate Sexology program and supervise research students until 2016. Her research interests are in Domestic and Family Violence victimisation and perpetration, particularly in relation to sexual violence. This includes new and emerging types of sexual and other forms of abuse and violence that affect children, young people, their families and the whole community. She is the author of numerous articles and book chapters as well as editor of several books.

Suzanne E Hadlow is currently Acting CNC Trauma/Surgery, previously Clinical Nurse Educator Operating Suite. She holds a Bachelor of Nursing Professional Honours Perioperative (UTAS), an Operating Room Certificate (RNSH), and a Cert IV T & A. Suzanne is also a Laser Safety Officer and is Chair of Laser Safety Committee. Her current research interests include Surgical Plume and COVID-19.

Elizabeth J Halcomb is Professor of Primary Health Care Nursing at the University of Wollongong, Australia. Professor Halcomb leads a strong research program in primary health care nursing, with particular emphasis on nursing in general practice, chronic disease and nursing workforce issues.

Virginia Howie is a Registered Nurse, lecturer, and a parent of a child with intellectual disability. As a nurse academic, Virginia has become a strong advocate for people with intellectual developmental disability through her teaching, research and doctoral studies. Virginia teaches Inclusive Practice for Nursing to first year UG nurses at CQUniversity, which introduces students to concepts that promote inclusivity for marginalised groups in Australian society.

Leanne Hunt is a Senior Lecturer in Nursing and Deputy Director, Clinical Education (Nursing), in the School of Nursing and Midwifery at the Western Sydney University and Registered Nurse at Liverpool Hospital Intensive Care Unit. Leanne began nursing in 1992 as an RN progressing to CNC (trauma) and NUM 1. Leanne worked in the Kingdom of Saudi Arabia in paediatric cardiothoracic intensive care for 2 years. She has 10 years of education and research experience and is the current chair of the Critical Care Research in Collaboration & Evidence Translation (CCRICET) research group. Leanne is also an affiliate member of the Centre for Applied Nursing Research (CANR), Centre for Oral Health Outcomes & Research Translation (COHORT) and the Ingham Institute of Applied Medical Research. Leanne's research interests include clinical practice experience, critical care and nursing education.

Sharyn Hunter has an extensive clinical background regarding older people. Her current role is a Senior Lecturer in the School of Nursing and Midwifery at the University of Newcastle, Australia. She has a passionate interest in the preparation of students for nursing older people and has received awards for her teaching from the University of Newcastle and the Australian Learning and Teaching Council. She has published an undergraduate textbook for nurses about health promotion of older people. Sharyn's research focusses on the education of health professionals about health and illness in the older person and exploring ways to support the wellness of older people. She is currently involved in projects about health promotion and older people, healthy ageing, and dementia care.

Deborah Ireson is an Academic and Research scholar at Edith Cowan University, School of Nursing and Midwifery, Bunbury, Western Australia. She coordinates the program child and adolescent health for undergraduate nursing students and teaches dual degree nursing/midwifery students, coordinating the antenatal and postnatal care units. She also teaches post graduate Master of Nursing and Master of Midwifery students. Her research interests focus on primary health care, child/youth health, neonates and midwifery practice.

Terrie Ivanhoe has worked for many years as a nurse across a variety of areas including CCU, ED, Management and Education. Wishing to advance her knowledge and skills in remote practice and primary health care, Terrie completed a Masters in Remote Health Practice/Nurse Practitioner in 2005, which led to an affiliation with Flinders University for a number of years teaching and providing mentorship for remote area nurses. Over the last 10 years Terrie has been employed as a Nurse

Practitioner by Nganampa Health Council as the Coordinator of the Chronic Disease Program and Diabetic Educator.

Sarah Yeun-Sim Jeong is an Associate Professor and Master of Nursing Program Convenor at the School of Nursing & Midwifery, University of Newcastle, Australia. Sarah's research includes clinical teaching and learning, Gerontological Nursing, Advance Care Planning, End-of-life Care, Dementia, Problem-Based Learning and internationalisation of nursing. She has been involved in the development of nursing curricula applying the concept and principles of problem based learning in Australia, China, Japan and Korea.

Amanda Johnson is the Dean of the School of Nursing and Midwifery at the University of Newcastle. Her research interests include aged care and palliation.

Rhys Jones is a registered Mental Health Nurse who works in Western Australia. He teaches part time at Murdoch University in the School of Health Professions. He holds a Bachelor of Nursing from Edith Cowan University and a Juris Doctor from Murdoch University in Western Australia.

Gladis Kabil is a lecturer and researcher at the School of Nursing and Midwifery, Western Sydney University, New South Wales, Australia. She is also currently practising as a registered nurse in the emergency department at a major trauma centre in Western Sydney. She teaches various medical surgical nursing related units across her undergraduate curriculum. She is currently undertaking her higher degree research. Her research focusses on management of sepsis in emergency departments with particular focus on intravenous fluid management.

Deborah Kirk is an Associate Dean (Postgraduate) in the School of Nursing and Midwifery at Edith Cowan University, Western Australia. She has practiced for more than 21 years as an oncology nurse practitioner in various settings and has extensive experience managing chronic disease. Her current work is expanding cancer/palliative nursing and nurse practitioner education at home and in parts of sub-Saharan Africa. Additionally, she has developed and expanded a mobile application for cancer resources for community resources locally in Alabama to help fill a gap identified in the clinical setting.

Richard Lakeman is a mental health nurse presently employed by Queensland Health, with particular research focus on suicide, migrant mental health and recovery.

Sue Lenthall is an associate Professor and Director at Katherine Campus, Flinders University, and has worked extensively as a remote area nurse in remote communities in Queensland and central Australia for over 20 years. Sue is also a Fellow at CRANAplus. Her research interests include Remote Health, Remote Area Nursing, Occupational Stress, and Aboriginal Health.

Peter Lewis is a Senior Lecturer and Director of Academic Workforce at the School of Nursing and Midwifery at the Western Sydney University. Peter has more than 20 years' experience as a registered nurse in paediatrics with a focus on chronic illness and disability. His current research interest is in the nursing care of people with intellectual disability.

Irene Mayo is a Lecturer in Nursing and Deputy Clinical Coordinator. Irene holds a Bachelor of Nursing (First Class Honours), Graduate Certificate in Anaesthetics and Recovery Nursing, and a Masters in Clinical Science.

Kylie McCullough is a Lecturer in Primary Health Care and Aboriginal and Torres Strait Islander people's health and wellness in the School of Nursing and Midwifery at Edith Cowan University. Her research focus is the work of nurses in rural and remote Australia.

Glenda McDonald is a Research Officer at the Centre for Nursing and Midwifery Research, Nepean Blue Mountains Local Health District, NSW, Australia. She is currently working on a collaborative research project of Aboriginal and non-Aboriginal researchers exploring the experiences of Aboriginal and Torres Strait Islander carers during the end-of-life phase. Her program of research relates to resilience at individual, organisational and community levels. Glenda's research aims are to enhance health, wellbeing and resilience outcomes through improved health service delivery.

Larissa McIntyre is a conjoint Lecturer at the School of Nursing and Midwifery at the University of Newcastle, Australia.

Faye McMillan is an Associate Professor and a Wiradjuri yinaa (woman), who was awarded 2019 NSW Aboriginal Woman of the Year. Faye was a founding member of Indigenous Allied Health Australia (IAHA) and is a member of a number of boards of directors. Faye is the Director of the Djirruwang Program – Bachelor of Health Science (Mental Health) at Charles Sturt University. In 2014 Faye was recognised in the Australian Financial Review and Westpac 100 Women of Influence. Her research interests are in Nation Building, Indigenous women in leadership roles; her Doctorate focused these two areas of research into her thesis as well as Mental Health. Faye seeks to use her own lived experiences to share with others with the hope that it could make a difference and to appreciate the transformative opportunities that education can provide.

Christine Minty-Walker is a Lecturer at the School of Nursing and Midwifery at Western Sydney University.

Sheila Mortimer-Jones is a Senior Lecturer at the School of Nursing and Midwifery at Edith Cowan University. Sheila registered as a Mental Health Nurse in England in 1994. She has a first-class honours degree in Biomedical Science and a PhD in Molecular Biology.

Evalotte Mörelius is a specialist in Paediatric and Neonatal Nursing and holds a joint position as Professor of Nursing (Children and Young People) at Edith Cowan University (ECU) and Perth Children's Hospital (PCH) in Perth WA. Her professorial position is partly supported by Perth Children's Hospital Foundation. Evalotte is the PI of the Stress Research Program and leader of the Stress Interest Group (STING). Her main research interest is stress within the family and parent-infant interaction and closeness in neonatal intensive care.

Claire Newman is a Senior Research Officer for Justice Health and Forensic Mental Health Network, NSW Health. Claire is a Registered Nurse and has worked in correctional health and/or forensic mental health for 16 years. Claire has a Master of Nursing (Hons) degree and is a current PhD Candidate at the University of Technology Sydney.

Lucy Nuzum is a Nurse Educator at Gold Coast Health, and Lecturer at Southern Cross University.

Elissa J O'Keefe is an Adjunct Associate Professor at the University of Canberra, and the Managing Director of Bravura Education. Her research interests include cosmetics, women's health, sexual health, and advanced nursing practice.

Kim Oliver is a Lecturer at the School of Nursing and Midwifery at Edith Cowan University. Her research interests include workplace stress, drug and alcohol use amongst young people, and workforce stressors.

Andrew Ormsby is the current Director Air Force Health, in the Royal Australian Air Force. He began his nursing career at the Repatriation General Hospital, Daw Park in Adelaide in 1985 and embarked on a 30 year military nursing career in 1990. He has undertaken a variety of roles at the clinical, flight nursing, training, staff officer, command and director levels within the Royal Australian Air Force. Operationally he deployed to Rwanda in 1994 and East Timor in 1999 and again in 2005. His primary research interest is in spirituality and spiritual nursing care in the Australian military nursing context.

Yvonne Parry is a Senior Lecturer at Flinders University, in the College of Nursing and Health Sciences. Dr Parry's work exists at the important intersection between nursing, primary health, public health, and community health services for vulnerable children and populations. Yvonne is actively involved in providing evidence-based, research informed undergraduate and postgraduate nursing and health topics, courses and programs. As a long standing, inter-disciplinary educator, she ensures health and population vulnerability are ensconced in all her teaching work at university and in the community.

Blake Peck has a Doctorate of Philosophy with a focus on developing new ways of understanding experience in qualitative research. Blake has previously published research exploring the experiences of fathers with chronically ill children living in rural areas of Victoria, he has a keen interest in understanding the experiences of children and families experiencing illness, and his works tends to take a rural focus. He is currently undertaking research seeking to find better ways to reduce the burden of childhood injuries on children and families in rural areas.

Julie Pryor is a Director of Research and Innovation at Royal Rehab and is a Clinical Associate Professor with the Susan Wakil School of Nursing and Midwifery at the University of Sydney.

Diane Russ is a Lecturer in Mental Health Nursing, School of Health & Human Sciences at Southern Cross University. Currently she is a Master of Research student. She has previous experience in Acute and Community Adult Mental Health and was a clinical educator and facilitator for student nurses. Current interests are the student nurse's placement experience.

Charrlotte Seib holds four tertiary qualifications in Nursing and a PhD in Public Health and Social Epidemiology, conducted as part of a legislative review commissioned by the Queensland Government. She has over 11 years of experience as a nurse researcher with expertise in women's health, chronic disease self-management, epidemiology and health statistics. Her research aims to understand the socio-cultural and environmental factors that impact on morbidity in women and seeks to build upon an individual's resources to mitigate these risk factors. Charrlotte leads a program of research broadly focusses on understanding the factors that impact on women's health and wellbeing across the lifespan. Her recent work utilizes a range of complex statistical approaches to explore how exposure to stress across the life course is associated with distinct health trajectories in women as they age.

Sharon-Ann Shunker is a Clinical Nurse Consultant in the Intensive Care Unit at Liverpool Hospital, NSW. She is also a Casual lecturer in the Australian College of Nursing at the University of Sydney. Her research interests include physical Activity and mobility of the ICU patient, ICU Patient Diaries, Delirium Prevention and Management, CRRT and Mechanical Ventilation.

Andrew Smith has experience in Aged Care, Perioperative, Community Health Nursing and Health Promotion and had a Masters in Public Health. He is passionate about social justice and empowerment, and in student retention and success at university. He is the program coordinator of the Bachelor of Nursing program at Federation University, Mt Helen Campus. Andrew has an interest in Rural Health issues and farm family health (especially farm men) – With a particular focus on how rural nurses work with and address health promotion challenges with this population group (health literacy). He also has an interest in Health professional knowledge and skills related to Health literacy.

Linda Starr is an associate Professor in the College of nursing and health sciences at Flinders University and a consultant educator providing health law and ethics education for nurses, midwives and other health professionals. Her research focuses on health law, regulation of the professions and forensics with a particular interest in elder abuse from bedside to courtroom.

Kathryn Steirn is a Lecturer at the Australian Catholic University, School of Nursing and Midwifery and Paramedicine, North Sydney, NSW, Australia. She teaches across acute care nursing theory and clinical units for undergraduate students. She has a clinical practice Masters and specialises in Critical care nursing. She currently works as a Registered Nurse in Intensive care.

Deborah Stockton has specialised in the field of child and family health nursing, with positions including Clinical Nurse Consultant and Director of Clinical Services. As Director Clinical Service Integration with Tresillian Family Care Centres, Deborah leads service development initiatives through collaboration and cross-sector partnerships. Deborah is an Adjunct Lecturer with Charles Sturt University and is a PhD candidate (UTS), with her area of research focusing on rural service development and the adaptation of service models for diverse settings.

Kylie Stothers is a mother of two children and a Jawoyn woman who was born and raised in Katherine, NT. Kylie comes from a large extended family with strong ties in Katherine and surrounding communities. Kylie is the Director of Workforce Development at Indigenous Allied Health Australia (IAHA) and is a social worker who has worked throughout the Northern Territory for over 20 years. She previously worked for the Centre for Remote Health/Flinders University NT at the Katherine site and has worked in the areas of Aboriginal Community Controlled Health Services, hospitals and NGO's. Kylie is passionate about education, health and issues that relate to remote and rural Australia. Her interests' areas are in health workforce, culturally safe and responsive practice, working with children and families, health promotion, child protection, remote health practice and contributing to supporting and growing our next generation of health professionals.

Daniel Terry has a Doctorate of Philosophy in health workforce in rural contexts. As an Academic with Federation University Australia and has extensive post-doctoral research experience on rural health, rural workforce, and chronic-ill health. With a background in community health nursing, his current research interest are nursing student career trajectory, rural health employment and profession longevity, while he has a keen interest in grit and communities of practice.

Sheeba Thomas is a lecturer at School of Nursing, Midwifery and Paramedicine, Australian Catholic University, North Sydney, Australia. She has experience in Intensive Care nursing and teaches acute care, Medical-Surgical nursing-related units across the undergraduate nursing curriculum.

Gail Tomsic is a Registered Nurse who has over 30 years nursing experience with qualifications in the following specialty areas, community paediatric nursing, hospital in the home, child & family health, paediatrics, lactation and infant feeding, and nursing management. Gail has practiced in a wide variety of settings including hospital paediatric units, parentcraft residential unit, and in the community setting providing home nursing to post-acute, acute and chronic children discharged from hospital to home. Gail has worked in senior nursing positions for the past 25 years as a Clinical Nurse Consultant (CNC) in a Grade 2 and a grade 3 level and as a Nurse Unit Manager.

Stephen Van Vorst is a Senior Lecturer in Mental Health Nursing at Southern Cross University, Queensland.

Stephanie Wheeler is a Registered Nurse, public health practitioner and field epidemiologist with extensive experience working in cross-cultural contexts. She is passionate about emergency preparedness and response and equity in global health, and currently works in developing field epidemiology capacity in Pacific Island Countries.

Lisa Whitehead is a Professor of Nursing Research and Associate Dean Research, School of Nursing and Midwifery at Edith Cowan University. Lisa's research centres on improving health outcomes for people living with chronic conditions, self-management interventions and working with families to support the management of chronic conditions. Engagement with clinicians and conducting research in real world settings underpin all of her research activities with the goal of implementing evidence-based change into practice.

Nathan J. Wilson is an Associate Professor in the School of Nursing and Midwifery at Western Sydney University. Nathan is a registered nurse with over 30 years' experience in working with people with intellectual and developmental disabilities and their families as a nurse, manager, clinical specialist, clinical educator, applied researcher and independent consultant. Nathan's applied research is focussed on enhancing the health, wellbeing and social participation of people with intellectual and developmental disability, with an underlying emphasis on chronic illness, men's health, masculinity, participation and social inclusion. He has published over 90 scientific papers about disability and regularly presents his findings at national and international conferences.

Preface

Becoming an Australian nurse

Nurses do wonderful work every day across Australia, and the nursing profession is, we would argue, the most rewarding of all the health professions. Becoming a nurse and gaining access to the rewards that the profession offers can be challenging. Entering the profession requires several years of university study after which new graduate nurses must take time to find their practice niche. Navigating career choices is not always straightforward. Once nurses enter practice, the tensions and complexities of being a practicing nurse within the Australian health system present their own sets of problems and challenges, many of which could not have been anticipated while studying nursing. Undergraduate nursing degrees might give insight into the culture and the system of health care, introduce the idea of evidence-based practice, and push students to think critically. However, there are limitations to this and there is only so much that new graduates will know at the end of their undergraduate education. To use an analogy, the knowledge passed on during an undergraduate degree represents the bricks in a well-built wall, but the mortar between the bricks, that holds it all together, go unnoticed and without comment. The mortar remains implicit. This book provides an insight into the 'mortar' by revealing and making explicit some of the hidden rules and unspoken understandings operating within the Australian health care system.

This nursing textbook, is unashamedly about the topic of contemporary nursing practice in Australia, and attempts to reveal and explain some of the complexity of nursing work undertaken in the Australian health care system that cannot be comprehensively replicated during university education. The practice environment is necessarily represented simplistically at undergraduate level to enable nursing students to develop a level of knowledge sufficient for them to begin practice as registered nurses. This textbook is therefore designed to see undergraduate and novice practitioners through their entire degree program and help navigate the transition from tertiary education to the nursing workforce by providing the opportunity to identify and understand some of the complexities that they will have to work with on a daily basis.

The Australian Nursing and Midwifery Accreditation Council (ANMAC) requires that graduate nurses understand contemporary trends in nursing and healthcare, including those related to recent major reforms in Australian health services, health service costs, service delivery contexts and inter-sectorial collaboration. This textbook offers insights into these trends using meaningful examples and vignettes to give student nurses an appreciation of the practical realities that they might find puzzling or confusing as graduate nurses. Description and explanation of these trends is therefore accessible, rather than a densely theoretical, thus providing a pathway to integrate theory and practice within the Australian context. ANMAC is not prescriptive about how an undergraduate course should be structured, however it does emphasise the inclusion of a discrete subject on Aboriginal and Torres Strait Islander health as well as broad content about nursing informatics. This text conforms to that prescription by including a discrete chapter that focuses on Aboriginal and Torres Strait Islander health, as well as a chapter about nursing informatics.

This is not a text that covers the fundamentals of nursing. The fundamentals of nursing are comprehensively covered in other texts. The goal of this text is to promote a critical understanding of the Australian nursing context. For example, the funding model for health care in Australia is complicated because health care is funded by two different government departments – one federally based and one state based – and that both public and private funding schemes operate within the one system. The regulation of the work force is also achieved by two different, but complementary, authorities. Nurses are registered to practice by the Australian Health Practitioners Registering Authority but their practice is overseen, and transgressions of the conditions of registration are sanctioned, by the Nurses and Midwives Board of Australia. Finally, it is not easy to understand the relationship between the tertiary education sector, which is responsible for educating and preparing students for registration and nursing practice, and the tertiary health care sector which is the largest employer of these nursing graduates, or how the systems of education and health integrate for the nursing profession. While novice nurses might know these points at a theoretical level, they cannot understand the implications of at a practical level without having them revealed.

Part One of this textbook offers a pragmatic insight into the intersection, tensions and complexities of practice and professional issues for Australian nurses. In addition to chapters about Aboriginal and Torres Strait Islander health and nursing informatics as previously noted, this section covers content about career pathways, tensions in the health care system and resilience and nursing. Part Two offers some critical insight into more traditional areas of nursing, providing concrete examples of current and future challenges for nurses working in a wide variety of well-known contexts. Part Three is unique in its coverage of diverse and distinctive areas of nursing practice. It highlights some of the emergent opportunities in non-traditional roles and contexts, making exploration of and comparison between these areas of nursing easier for nursing students and novice nurses. Contexts such as cosmetic surgery or overseas mission are becoming more popular career options for nurses, however pre-registration education remains necessarily based on biomedical categorisations of illness and disease and traditional, hospital-based nursing roles without highlighting alternative practice opportunities and career pathways.

We hope that you find in this textbook a pragmatic and accessible entry point into some of the 'messiness' of being a practicing nurse in Australia and that you will come to a deeper understanding of practice within the Australian health care system as a result of reading it.

Part I

Nursing in the Australian context

1   Nursing in Australia

Nurse education, divisions and professional standards

Peter Lewis, Nathan J. Wilson, Leanne Hunt and Lisa Whitehead

Chapter objectives

This chapter will provide the reader:

- Insight into the history and organisation of nursing education in Australia
- A description of the different divisions of nursing and the different roles undertaken by nurses in each division
- An overview of the regulation of nursing practice in Australia

Introduction

The nursing profession in Australia is regulated; nursing education is regulated by a system of accreditation and nursing practice by a system of registration. This dual regulation provides the structure for this chapter. In Part 1, we describe the accreditation of nurse education by the Australian Nursing and Midwifery Accreditation Council. This part explains how health care providers and consumers can be assured that the courses undertaken in order to enable a person to apply for nursing registration will actually qualify that person for registration. We then describe how nursing education came to be delivered in universities rather than in hospitals, as it was until the 1980s. In Part 2, we describe the registration process and what it means for nursing practice. Registration through the Nursing and Midwifery Board of Australia (NMBA) is required to enable nurses to practice legally; however, we also describe some of the associations that promote nursing as a profession apart from the legal requirements of registration.

Part 1: Nursing education

Accreditation of nurse education

Nursing education in Australia is regulated by a system of *accreditation*. This means that every single nursing course across Australia has to meet the same national accreditation standards in order to operate. The independent accrediting authority is the Australian Nursing and Midwifery Accreditation Council (ANMAC), which is primarily funded by the Australian Health Practitioner Regulation Agency (AHPRA). ANMAC develops the accreditation standards, they assess and determine if an education program meets those standards, and they also have a Migration Service where they are able to support nurses from overseas who are trying to immigrate to Australia by assessing their skills in comparison to the Australian standards. ANMAC has separate, published accreditation standards for both registered and enrolled nurses.

> Accreditation is a process where course content is validated against a set of standards that are developed by experts in the field

Enrolled nursing

Education relating to preregistration or preparation for practice is delivered to diploma level at a number of different institutions including, but not limited to, universities, colleges of Technical and Further Education (TAFE) and a variety of accredited, privately funded institutions. Students who are awarded a diploma can be recommended for entry onto the general register of nurses as an Enrolled Nurse (EN). As of December 2018, there were 63,081 ENs in Australia (NMBA, 2018). The most recent version of the EN accreditation standards was published in 2017 (ANMAC, 2017). These standards cover a range of issues, but mandate that students must have a minimum of 400 hours of clinical experience (not including simulation) and their studies/courses must include content on person-centred care, evidence-based care, analytical and reflective practice, legal and ethical issues, quality and safety, health informatics and technology and cultural safety. All courses must also have a discrete unit on Aboriginal and Torres Strait Islander people's health, history, wellness and culture.

Registered nursing

Education relating to preregistration or preparation for practice is delivered to degree level at universities and other accredited nongovernment institutions. Students who are awarded a Bachelor's degree can be recommended for entry onto the general register of nurses as a Registered Nurse (RN). As of December 2018, there were 294,390 RNs in Australia (NMBA, 2018). The latest version of the standards for RNs was published in 2012 (ANMAC, 2012). These, however, are currently under review, and the process of consultation is proposed to conclude in 2019. Similar to the EN accreditation standards, the RN accreditation standards mandate clinical hours; however, for RNs, the total is 800 hours (not including simulation). The academic content of accredited courses must cover knowledge and skills in critical thinking, analysis and problem solving, quality improvement methods, research, legal and ethical issues, and health informatics and health technology. Again, all courses must have a discreet unit on Aboriginal and Torres Strait Islander people's health, history, wellness and culture.

Registered nursing courses across Australia

Current projections suggest that with the changing demographic in Australia, there is going to be a major shortfall of nurses in the future (Department of Health, 2014). This means that the nurse education system and standards that govern this system will not only need to adapt to the changing demographic of Australia, but also to the increased numbers of nurses that will need to be trained.

There are a total of 35 different educational institutions teaching registered nursing across Australia with about 62,000 undergraduate students enrolled nationally. All of these courses have some generic content and do not differ significantly. For example, the need for a discrete unit on Aboriginal and Torres Strait Islander Health means that every course will have at least one unit of study exploring the health needs of this population group. For more information about these needs and the issues facing Aboriginal and Torres Strait Islander Australians, refer to Chapter 6. Nevertheless, the conceptual framework of each course is likely to differ between educational institutions. This degree of variation has the potential to give students greater choice, especially if they believe that one type of framework is a better match to their learning needs. For example, the curriculum at Western Sydney University is based on the principles of primary health with a dedicated unit of study about primary health care. The course also adopts a body-systems approach to many of the theoretical units, based on the National Health Priority Areas (Australian Institute of Health and Welfare, 1997), such as a focus on endocrine, respiratory and neurological issues in the one second year unit of study. By contrast, the University of South Australia adopts a more population-based approach, where units of study are focussed on subpopulations such as the health of older people, adults, infants, children and young people.

History of nurse education in Australia

Nursing education has not always been delivered in universities or even in educational institutions. A systematic method of nurse education was introduced to Sydney Hospital by 'Nightingale Nurse,' Lucy Osborn, who came to Australia with five others at the request of New South Wales (NSW) premier Sir Henry Parkes in 1868. Osborn established a nurse training school based on Nightingale's nursing principles upon her arrival (Russell, 1990). So, for almost 100 years, nurse education in Australia was predominantly based on an apprenticeship model, which was generally characterised by on-the-job training supplemented with theoretical instruction provided by 'nurse tutors' in a hospital setting. Entry into the profession under the apprenticeship model was therefore, by appointment to the position of student nurse at a hospital, or occasionally, at another type of health care facility (Russell, 1990).

The apprenticeship model began to change from the time of the Kelly Report in 1943, which was commissioned in response to shortage of nurses during the time of war and the problem of retaining nurses in the workforce. Amongst other things, the Kelly Report identified that hospital-based nurse education was compromised when the service needs of the hospital took precedence over the educational needs of the nurses. The Kelly Report recommended abandoning the apprenticeship model altogether in favour of 'a system of training based upon sound educational principles' (Committee for the Reorganisation of the Nursing Profession, 1943: 6). The concern of the commissioners was that nursing education under the apprenticeship model was simply not good at attracting and retaining young women in the nursing work force, especially at a time when better occupational opportunities were readily available.

There followed a large number of committees and commissions of inquiry into nurse education during the 1960s and 1970s. Some of these recommended that nursing education should be relocated into the advanced education system (Committee on the Future of Tertiary Education in Australia, 1964), because theory and practice frequently lacked correlation and were not well connected (Institute of Hospital Matrons of New South

Wales and the ACT 1967). The imperative for the employer was to prepare nurses as quickly as possible to execute their tasks on the ward. This had the result, according to the Matron's committee, of producing nurses '…who were restricted in outlook, resistant to change, and unable to cope confidently with the scientific and technical advances in medicine and the social problems of nurses' (Institute of Hospital Matrons of New South Wales and the ACT 1967). The Chittick report for the World Health Organisation was unstinting in its criticism of nurse training in NSW, when it observed that nursing students '…are cut off from any educational program that would enlarge their vision, develop their potential resources, and make them aware of the social, political, and cultural problems they face as citizens … Perhaps no other group of young people in modern society receives such a narrow, restricted, and unimaginative type of education' (Chittick, 1968: 10). Clearly, in light of these criticisms, the climate was ripe for a revolution in the delivery of preregistration education and preparation for RNs in Australia.

Transition out of hospitals

Prior to 1970, nursing was taught to diploma level over four years in hospitals whereas, during the 1970s, nursing was taught to diploma level over three years in hospitals. During the 1980s, the predominant educational qualification was a three-year diploma delivered at colleges of advanced education or universities (Lusk et al., 2001). Various pilot deliveries of the Diploma of Applied Science (Nursing) were offered in 1978. In NSW, diploma courses were offered by Cumberland College of Health Sciences and Riverina College of Advanced Education. In Victoria, they were offered by Lincoln College of Health Sciences and Preston Institute of Technology. In South Australia, one course was offered by Sturt College of Advanced Education and in Western Australia by the Western Australian Institute of Technology (Committee of Inquiry into Nurse Education and Training, 1978: 20–24). Although nurse education had been removed from the Health portfolios of the NSW state government and allocated to the Education portfolio in 1972 (Committee of Inquiry into Nurse Education and Training, 1978), not until 1993 were all courses for the preparation of RNs in Australia removed from hospitals and relocated to universities (Mason, 2013).

What has this transition achieved? Whereas once a student nurse was recruited to a hospital, which became the focus of her (or, from 1967, occasionally his) life–work, study, meals, accommodation–she or he now has the opportunity to pursue a diversity of personal and professional interests. Whereas once a student nurse's educational needs were subordinate to the needs of her or his employer–the hospital–they are now valued in themselves independently of such constraints. Whereas once a student nurse's education was confined to the services offered by her or his employer, she or he now has the benefit of exposure to different types of service and ways of delivering those services by attending a wide variety of clinical placements (Mannix et al., 2009). On 18 January 2019, Senator Bridget McKenzie announcedthe latest review in a long line of reviews of nursing education dating back nearly 80 years. We eagerly await the outcome and recommendations of this review and expect a continuation of a rich tradition of nursing education in this country.

Online resource

1 ANMAC: https://www.anmac.org.au/

Part 2: Nursing practice

Nursing is a practical occupation, the effective execution of which can have serious implications for the health and wellbeing of the people in the nurses' care. Nursing practice is regulated by a system of registration. The registering authority is the Nursing and Midwifery Board of Australia (NMBA), which approves the admission of individuals to the general register of health professionals in Australia to practice as either RNs or ENs. The NMBA is supported financially and administratively by the Australian Health Practitioner Regulation Agency (AHPRA). AHPRA is a national governing body that manages the registration of nurses and a number of other health care professionals. Assistants in Nursing (AINs) are not regulated by a system of registration and, therefore, do not have to apply for registration with the NMBA. Their practice will, therefore, not be discussed here.

The NMBA is constituted by national legislation, and its objectives are designed primarily to benefit the nursing workforce. These include aims to facilitate: workforce mobility for health practitioners; high-quality education and training of health practitioners; assessment of overseas-trained health practitioners; and development of a flexible, responsive and sustainable workforce. The use of the verb to 'facilitate' suggests that the NMBA plays an enabling role for nurses who wish to enter the nursing workforce and to practice nursing in Australia. These aims do not identify any specific role for the NMBA in the preparation of nurses for practice but for the support of nurses who have qualified to enter the occupation. The only aim that specifically applies to patients is the aim to protect public safety, which is really the rationale for the regulation of practice (NMBA, 2018).

The NMBA is also responsible for the development and implementation of a range of instruments designed to regulate the practice of those who have qualified for registration. First, they provide a mechanism of entry into the occupation by setting the criteria for registration of nurses and nursing students. Setting criteria for admission to the profession is one of the hall marks of professionalization of an occupation (Freidson, 1988). Second, for those who have been admitted to the occupation, the NMBA provides a number of standards against which a nurse's practice can be held accountable. These include the provision of standards for practice, and codes of conduct and ethics. Third, the NMBA provides mechanisms by which sanctions can be imposed on nurses who breach the standards. For example, the NMBA handles notifications of misconduct and complaints made against nurses, and it has the power to investigate complaints and convene disciplinary hearings in order to enforce the standards of practice and various codes that govern practice. The NMBA, therefore, has the power to set the standards for nurses' practice, monitor adherence to those standards and impose sanctions for any breaches of those standards (NMBA, 2018).

Standards for practice

Standards for Practice perform two functions. One is to define the differences between the roles and responsibilities of RNs and ENs. This means that nurses' daily activities should clearly fall within the scopes of practice provided in the relevant Standards for Practice. The other is to provide a framework within which the quality of practice can be assessed. Standards for Practice are necessarily constructed in a generic way in order to allow for adaptability to a variety of practice situations. This means that when a nurse is contemplating any specific activity on a daily basis, she or he will likely have to interpret what the Standards for Practice mean before deciding whether or not the activity is covered by them. Standards for Practice are reviewed every five years. The Standards for Practice can also be used to assess the capability of students, new graduates and nurses educated in countries other than Australia to practice safely and within the terms of their registration. In addition, they can be used to assess a nurse's capability to practice when returning to work after breaks in service.

The EN Standards for Practice are patient-centred and principle-based allowing for professional development in a range of settings. They are also clinically-focussed and reflect the role of the EN within the health sector. You can access the EN Standards for Practice by typing the web address given under the section below titled Online resource. Nine EN Standards for Practice exist and are divided into three domains that appear to be presented in order of priority: professional and collaborative practice; provision of care; and reflective and analytical practice. Perhaps the key consideration when interpreting the EN Standards for Practice is that the work of ENs must be undertaken in collaboration with and under the supervision of a RN. Although ENs remain accountable and responsible for their own clinical practice and they develop collaborative relationships with other members of the health care team and with patients and their families, their practice is defined, to a large extent, by the collaborative relationship that they develop with the RN. This is central to the fulfilment of their responsibilities of the first domain – professional and collaborative practice. The second domain focuses on the role of the EN in providing care. This is the central activity of the EN, and it includes assessment of patient needs, delivery of care and evaluation of the outcomes of care. The third domain relates to the EN's capability to develop and maintain essential knowledge of current, best, evidence-based practice for informing the care they deliver (NMBA, 2018).

The RN Standards for Practice provide a framework for nurses to undertake their clinical practice. The differences in Standards for Practice reflect the increased level of education and training, scope of practice and responsibilities for the RN over those of an EN. There are many similarities between the Standards for Practice for RNs and ENs that reflect the unique, yet symbiotic, roles that both RNs and ENs play within the health system, and the important roles each have in patient care. The important differences lie in the enhanced sophistication of the practice expected of RNs. For example, whereas ENs might be expected to 'reflect and analyse', RNs are expected to 'think critically' and analyse. Critical thinking is a sophisticated skill that needs to develop in supportive educational environments. ENs might be expected to engage in collaborative practice, whereas RNs might be expected to engage in therapeutic and professional relationships. The difference appears to lie in the degree of sophistication in ways of relating to others.

Online resource

1   Nursing and Midwifery Board of Australia. https://www.nursingmidwiferyboard. gov.au/

Nursing associations

There are over 20 national nursing and midwifery associations in Australia, with many more state-based organisations. These organisations do not oversee the registration of nurses and midwives, nor are they a union body such as the Australian Nursing and Midwifery Federation. However, many of these organisations offer speciality education and accreditation and hold registers of nurses and midwives certified in a speciality area. Specialty-focused organisations can be setting-specific (e.g. Australian Primary Health Care Nurses Association [APNA]), specific to disorders or conditions (e.g. Cancer Nurses Society of Australia [CNSA]), specific to a life stage (e.g. the Australian College of Children and Young People's Nurses), culturally specific (e.g. The Congress of Aboriginal and Torres Strait Islander Nurses and Midwives [CATSINaM]), or specific to registration category (e.g. Australian College of Nurse Practitioners).

The main nursing organisation in Australia is the Australian College of Nursing (ACN). The ACN seeks to represent and promote the participation of nurses in governmental and social policy decisions related to the nursing profession and health, both nationally and internationally (ACN, 2019). Where the specialty organisations speak for nurses and nursing specific to their specialty interests, goals, and purposes, nationally, the ACN, and internationally, the International College of Nurses (ICN), speak to the needs of, and advocate for, all nurses and the nursing profession independent of specialty area.

Unique to all organisations and professional bodies is the role of advocacy. Advocacy on behalf of the members takes the form of political advocacy, the distribution of information to members on key initiatives, changes and consultations and the dissemination of professional knowledge through publications and professional development. Political advocacy can take several forms, through membership of national committees, submissions in response to consultations and the production of position statements. These activities have the goals of generating greater nurse involvement in advancing health equity, influencing the cost and quality of care, enhancing health for all and the evolution of the nursing workforce.

Membership of a nursing organisation is optional; however, they play an important role in providing opportunities to create and promote a strong collective voice for nurses from the entire spectrum of experience from student through to nurse practitioners.

Summary

In this chapter, we have provided an overview of the regulation of nursing in Australia. Nursing education is regulated by a system of accreditation in which courses designed to prepare nurses for practice are evaluated by an external authority and verified for delivery. Nursing practice is regulated by a system of registration that recognises two broad levels of practice– Enrolled or Registered Nurse– in a variety of primary, secondary and tertiary health care contexts. It is worth reflecting on why nursing is organised in the way that it is in 2019 and on the historical factors that have shaped our occupation especially during the last 40 years.

Reflective questions

1 What was the focus of the nursing education that you have received?
2 How has your education prepared you for practice?
3 What are your primary roles and responsibilities as a nurse in (1) primary care, (2) Secondary care, or (3) tertiary health care?

References

Australian Institute of Health and Welfare and Commonwealth Department of Health and Family Services. (1997). *First report on National Health Priority Areas 1996*. AIHW Cat. No. PHE 1. Canberra: AIHW and DHFS.

ANMAC. (2012). *Registered nurse accreditation standards, 2012*. ANMAC, Canberra: ANMAC.

ANMAC. (2017). *Enrolled nurse accreditation standards, 2017*. ANMAC, Canberra: ANMAC.

Australian College of Nursing. *Advancing Nursing Leadership*. Retrieved 3rd July 2019. https://www.acn.edu.au/about-us/who-we-are-what-we-do

Chittick, R. (1968). *Assignment Report: April to June 1968*. World Health Organization, Manila.

Committee for the Reorganisation of the Nursing Profession. (1943). *First report of the Committee for Reorganisation of the Nursing Profession (in NSW)*. Government Printer, Sydney

Committee of Inquiry into Nurse Education and Training. (1978). *Nurse education and training: report of the Committee of Inquiry into Nurse Education and Training to the Tertiary Education Commission*. Australian Government Printing Service, Canberra.

Committee on the Future of Tertiary Education in Australia. (1964). *Tertiary education in Australia: report of the Committee on the Future of Tertiary Education in Australia to the Australian Universities Commission, volume II*. Commonwealth of Australia, Canberra.

Department of Health. (2014). *Australia's future health workforce: Nurses overview report*. Department of Health, Canberra: Commonwealth of Australia.

Freidson, E. (1988). *Profession of medicine: a study of the sociology of applied knowledge*. Chicago: University of Chicago Press.

Institute of Hospital Matrons of New South Wales and the ACT. (1967). *Report of the committee to consider all aspects of nursing: part 1, the general nurse in the hospital environment*. Institute of Hospital Matrons for New South Wales and the ACT, Sydney.

Lusk, B., Lynette Russell, R., Rodgers, J., & Wilson-Barnett, J. (2001). Preregistration nursing education in Australia, New Zealand, the United Kingdom, and the United States of America. *Journal of Nursing Education*, *40*(5), 197–202.

Lynette Russell, R. (1990). *From Nightingale to now: nurse education in Australia*. Sydney: W.B. Saunders.

Mannix, J., Wilkes, L., & Luck, L. (2009). Key stakeholders in clinical learning and teaching in Bachelor of Nursing programs: A discussion paper. *Contemporary Nurse*, *32*(1–2): 59–68.

Mason, J. (2013). *Review of Australian Government Health Workforce Programs*. Commonwealth of Australia, Canberra.

Nursing and Midwifery Board of Australia. (2018). *Code of Conduct for Nurses*. Retrieved 3rd July 2019. https://www.nursingmidwiferyboard.gov.au/Codes-Guidelines-Statements/Professional-standards.aspx

Nursing and Midwifery Board of Australia (NMBA) Registrant Data. Reporting period 1 October 2018–31 December 2018. Retrieved 25th May 2019.

2 Nursing and tensions within the Australian health care system

Yvonne Parry and Didy Button

Chapter objectives

This chapter will offer the reader:

- Insight into the systemic structures that impact on the practice of nursing in Australia.
- An outline of the Australian health care system and the key areas of governance, funding and tensions within the system.
- A description of contemporary contexts of nursing and the tensions between the system and nursing practice.
- An overview of the National Strategic Framework for Chronic Conditions and the health system and the future challenges to nursing meeting the changing health care needs of the population.

Introduction

As a registered nurse in Australia you will be employed in either the public or private sector of the health system. So, an understanding of the difference and implications of these systems for your patient's total care is important. This chapter will outline the complexity of the Australian health system, the roles of nurses within this system and the tensions for nurses in circumventing a system that often confuses new Registered Nurses.

Nurses represent the largest section of the health workforce and are required to work in a variety of roles both within and across different sectors of the health system that are likely to be differently funded. Nurses contribute to the foundational functioning of the healthcare system, by providing a variety of unique activities including health promotion, disease prevention and supporting patients and their carers through mental and physical illness (Dor et al., 2019).

Despite this, nurses remain underrepresented in the system of decision-making processes. Therefore, as the cornerstone of the health care system it is important that nurses in the future proactively pursue opportunities to participate in making decisions, which govern their work and the health care system.

Nurses and universal health care

Internationally, nurses provide the majority of health care service delivery as part of any Universal Health Care (UHC) system (Cashin, 2015). UHC is defined by the World

Health Organization (2018) as means of ensuring access to the appropriate health services required by people at their time of need that is of sufficient quality to assist in improving health outcomes, while also ensuring that health services do not expose the user to financial hardship. UHC has therefore 'become a major goal for health reform in many countries and a priority objective of WHO' (WHO, 2018 p. 6). Nurses are foundational to the provision and delivery of accessible, affordable and timely healthcare (WHO, 2015). Given that the provision of nursing services forms the cornerstone of health access and service delivery globally (Cashin, 2015; WHO, 2018), it raises the question as to why nurses are often excluded from the decision-making processes. The lack of nursing representation on boards, policy working parties and other groups that determine their roles and work practices within the health system blinds policy makers and governments to the effective use of nursing capacities, capabilities, resources and skills in addressing the complex needs of communities and patients (Cashin, 2015; WHO, 2018). This, therefore, impacts on the provision of UHC and affordability of healthcare. Thus, utilising nurses to their full education, knowledge, scope of practice and capacity has a myriad of benefits for the nurse, patient and health care system. This does, however, require nurses to be fully engaged in the leadership roles, and decision-making processes in the health service, service delivery and system wide processes.

Universal health care in Australia

Medicare is recognised as a form of UHC. The Australian Medicare health funding model provides healthcare for all through a variety of funding mechanisms, both public and private. The development of the UHC system in Australia sought to promote equity of access through the Medicare Benefits Scheme (MBS) and the Pharmaceutical Benefits Scheme (PBS) to assist in defraying health care costs (Parry, 2012). The Australian approach to the provision of UHC is the use of the 'Medicare levy', a 2% tax from every employee's income to provide healthcare for all Australians (ATO, 2019).

General Practitioners (GPs) and Surgeons (Medical Professionals) can charge the patient a 'gap' or 'out-of-pocket' fee. All medical professionals receive a rebate from the federal government for every patient visit – the Medicare Rebate. This is covered by the 2% Medicare Levy. The 'gap' or 'out-of-pocket' fee is at the discretion of the GP/Medical Professional and has the potential to undermine the UHC as it inhibits some people from accessing health care (Russell et al., 2019; WHO, 2018). For example, unemployed or pensioners may pay a 'gap' fee to attend their GP, therefore they may not attend in a timely fashion and use Emergency Department services instead.

Medicare was introduced in 1984 (Palmer, 2002) as an explicit ethical ideal to address health inequities (Parry, 2012). The health inequities were argued at the time as being structurally produced, and an unfair distribution of health (including access to healthcare) that infringed on the concept of health as a human right (Parry, 2012). Although Medicare was founded on the ideal of equitable health access, it does not enshrine health as a human right and as such leaves Medicare and the funding and delivery of health care services vulnerable to government discretion and interference. One example of this occurred in the 1990s. The decrease of Medicare bulk billing rates in Australia (the universal health care system) saw an increase in 'gap' or 'out-of-pocket' fees for individuals and their families (Parry, 2012). Where gap fees increase, Medicare no longer provides 'free' health care for those in need. GPs who charge gap fees limit access to their services. Therefore, the concept of UHC is not fully realised through Medicare.

It has been argued that MBS and PBS are based on outdated concepts of health service provision and practices that provide health care that is neither sustainable nor patient centred (Cashin, 2015). For example, a fee for service health care model, such as GP services, suits access to health care that is aligned with single instance service delivery, such as the treatment of an infectious disease, rather than chronic health conditions that require ongoing oversight by health practitioners. Using GP services long-term when gap fees are charged can be prohibitively costly for disadvantaged populations. Contemporary health care delivery must account for the multimodal impacts of social, environmental and psychological factors on health (Parry et al., 2016). Nursing as a discipline has sought to address this need through the introduction of expanded nursing roles. Nurse Practitioners (NPs) provide a patient centred hub for the delivery and organisation of multimodal care consistent with chronic health conditions (Woo et al., 2017). The NP is ideally situated to deliver cost effective care (Jennings et al., 2015). All NPs can provide combinations of nursing care, diagnostic activities and intervention-based treatments, including the use of medicines (Martin-Misner et al., 2015). For example, NPs who can prescribe medications have been shown to improve the care of patients with chronic respiratory conditions and extend periods between appointments and between exacerbations of their illness (Carey et al., 2014). They also provided the support required to decrease the burden of disease on the patient overall and therefore to decrease the cost to the taxpayer as the UHC funders. While Medicare provides UHC to all, the Australian system also has a private healthcare component for those with private health insurance.

Conversely, the private health care system is privately owned and operates on a for-profit (e.g. listed companies) or not-for-profit (e.g. charitable organisations) basis (AIHW, https://www.aihw.gov.au/reports-data/health-welfare-services/hospitals/overview). Patients with private health insurance can opt to access care from a private hospital. Funding for private patients in private hospital is also covered by the Medicare Rebate Scheme, which covers the costs of the surgery and some accommodation. Some Nurse Practitioners are also private providers and maintain their own clinics to provide service for people with chronic health conditions (e.g., diabetes). Nurses work in both the private and public health care sectors in a variety of roles.

The underutilisation of nurses within the system

The underuse of nurses across the system remains the foremost cause of health service and delivery inefficiency. A recent Productivity Commission (2017) report stated that increasing the use of nurses to their full potential remained the most cost-effective measure to achieve health system improvements. Additionally, the policy directives and decisions of the Council of Australian Governments Health Council (COAG)

COAG brings together Australian State and Federal Government Ministers to discuss Health policy nationally to determine the policy and strategic direction of the health system nationally.

sought to increase the cost-effective use of nurses throughout the healthcare system stating that this would be effective in addressing several of the Australian Health Ministers' Advisory Council's (2017) aspirational outcomes for Australians. These aspirations included *to receive consistent, holistic, and coordinated care across the health system to manage their chronic conditions* (AHMAC, 2017, p. 34). Therefore, government ministers, policy makers, system managers and services recognise that contemporary health systems need to directly address growing numbers of patients with complex, chronic and long-term health conditions in a cost-effective manner, and Nurses and NPs may be the answer (Parry et al., 2016). NPs are recognised for providing safe, cost effectively and appropriately providing care that directly meets these needs (Clifford et al., 2019). Part of the issue is the funding arrangements for NPs. Currently NPs are paid $30.00 for a 30-minute consultation. NPs in private practice pay room rental and other costs such as receptionists to provide services. The remuneration does not cover the cost of service provision. The use of NP has been proven to be cost effective and provide long-term benefits for patients with complex or chronic health needs. To expand the use of NPs within the health system, Medicare funding needs to be increased. Thus, Medicare funding mechanisms that improve access to diverse nursing services, such as Nurse Practitioner-led clinics and community nursing clinics, could provide cost-effective care along with decreased hospital use. Yet, the capacity of the system to provide such change seems limited when reviewing the role of nursing and the use of nurses to their full scope of practice. This is evidenced by the lack of nursing representation on hospital and local area management boards, and the reluctance of the AMA (2017) to acknowledge the evidence-base for safe, cost-effective care provided by nurses in autonomous settings and practice (Cashin et al., 2017).

The underuse of a highly skilled, effective and efficient workforce could potentially undermine the future sustainability and cost-effectiveness of the health system as a whole (Duffield, 2011). Internationally the provision of UHC could be undermined by the failure to fully utilise nurses. The WHO 'Global action plan for the prevention and control of non-communicable diseases 2013-2020' states that healthcare systems need to:

> Optimize the scope of nurses' practice to contribute to prevention and control of non-communicable diseases, including addressing barriers that contribute to ill-health and chronic health burdens (p42).

The public system funded by the Australian public through Medicare and the private system has both public and private funding mechanisms. The focus of the care provided by nurses is altered partly by the ethos of the organisation and the population it serves. For example, the private system mostly provides services for patients with single instance care, such as arthroscopies, which entail prompt services and short-term care. In contrast the public system provides the most complex and difficult care as the patients often require services not available or cost effective for private sector service provision.

Using the public and private health care systems in Australia

Health care provided by public hospitals is funded by state and territory governments. Access to GPs is funded by the federal government through the Medicare rebate scheme. The preference for ED services often occurs when access to other health services is limited or denied (Parry, 2012). As access to ED services is provided free to patients by the state governments in Australia and gap fees for GP services have increased and impacts directly on affordable health access (Parry, 2012). This scenario is believed to have also increased the use of ED services for primary care. Further, the limited access to GPs in some areas of outer metropolitan areas has caused a strain on the ED at some public hospitals (PHCIS, 2005). For example, The Northern Division of General Practice (in South Australia) acknowledges that the lack of GPs in the northern suburbs of Adelaide is 'serious' and 'places a serious strain on emergency services' (PHCIS, 2005, p. 2).

Thus, the Australian health care system has two points of entry for services. These points of entry are funded differently. As the GPs are paid through the Medicare Rebate Scheme for services by the federal government, and the ED services are provided by public hospitals funded by the state government, there is a cost shift from the federal government to the state. Therefore, the use of ED for primary care is not cost effective for the taxpayer and is a misuse of highly skilled nursing services. Additionally, the Medicare Australia Act requires state governments to provide free and timely care to citizens (Medicare Australia Act [Commonwealth of Australia] 1973 amended 2008). Conversely, the Medicare Act does not require GPs to provide free access or access with no co-payment and therefore GPs may and do charge a co-payment or gap fees directly to patients for services provided (Medicare Australia Act 1973 amended 2008). Furthermore, patients delay care due to cost often present to ED for more complex and exacerbated episodes of illness requiring complex multimodal care from nurses. This creates an additional cost for the state and workload for the nursing staff. The Medicare system in Australia aspires to achieve UHC and nurses play a pivotal role in improving access to services. The lack of access to GPs impacts on timely care and the acuteness of illness. Additionally, the mix of State and Federal funding for different services provides comprehensive but sometimes confusing access for the nurses, allied health professionals and patients. Nurses have a role to play in understanding these complexities and assisting patients in navigating the health care system comprising of GP (private primary care), public and private hospitals.

Nursing work in the public and private sectors

Nurses face different stressors and issues depending on whether they are employed in the public or private sector. Nurses in the public sector face issues related to the structure of the workplace and work force impacts their autonomy and subsequent levels of empathy and stress (Dor et al., 2019). Additionally, the public sector nursing directors and managers cope with high level of staff turnover and burnout as a result of working conditions that may devalue the work of nurses, often by other health professionals and the broader health system (Dor et al., 2019). Conversely, workplaces, such as the private or community sectors, that promote the autonomy (Carey et al., 2014), or professional development and specialty accreditation (Serafin et al., 2019) enhance nurses' job satisfaction and support more cost-effective health service delivery.

Nurses working in the Private sector report higher levels of collegiality and respectful interactions with nursing managers when compared to nurses working in the public sector (Brunetto et al., 2011). The public sector upline nurse managers have more power resulting in lower levels of nurse satisfaction (Brunetto et al., 2011). Additionally, Brunetto et al. (2011) found higher levels of nurses' autonomy, role ambiguity, poor communication and information sharing impact directly on job sat-isfaction and patient care outcomes (Brunetto et al., 2011). In conclusion many factors impact on nurses' job satisfaction, burnout and sense of autonomy illustrating the needs for inclusive nursing leadership and proactive management.

Primary care

Primary health care is federally funded through the MBS and PBS (Cashin, 2015). General practitioners are private providers of the majority of primary health care services in Australia (Parry, 2012). The Australian Medical Association (AMA) nego-tiates the remuneration and practice of GPs with the federal government on behalf of the medical profession (Cashin, 2015). The effective use of nurses in the primary health care sector is limited by policies, which restrict the funding available to health profes-sionals other than GPs through the Medicare system (Cashin, 2015).

The use of Nurse Practitioners in the provision of primary health care through the management of chronic health conditions has shown in Australia to promote person-centred and cost-effective care (Bonner et al., 2019).

The Australian Nursing and Midwifery Board defines the Nurse practitioners as having 'the capability to provide high levels of clinically focused nursing care in a variety of contexts in Australia. Nurse practitioners care for people and communities with prob-lems of varying complexity.

The nurse practitioner (NP) scope of practice is built on the platform of the registered nurse (RN) scope of practice and must meet the regulatory and professional requirements for Australia including the Registered nurse standards for practice and Code of conduct for nurses. The nurse practitioner has a high degree of systems literacy and can manage care across a variety of health systems to maximise outcomes; NPs engage in complex and critical thinking; integrate information and/or evidence; judiciously use clinical investigations; and skilfully and empathetically communicate with all involved in the care episode, including the person receiving care and their family and community, and health professional colleagues).

The use of NP in the primary healthcare setting is often not well understood by the general public, sometimes maligned by other autonomous health professionals, and not well reimbursed by Medicare. This causes tension for the NP as the lack of reim-bursement limits their autonomous scope of practice, thus the ability to effectively care for their patients and limits cost effective options for patients.

Tertiary care

Nurses need to identify and embrace the new and expanding roles available to them in the redesigning of health care systems that meet the needs of patients with complex conditions (IOM, 2011; WHO, 2015). For example, the work by Carey et al. (2014) out-lines the role of nurse prescribers in the acute care setting. The outcomes have high-lighted the improved efficiency in terms of patient flow and waiting times, treatment, person-centred care, and job satisfaction for nurses. Along with a decrease in ED admissions, condition exacerbations, inappropriate service use and non-compliance (Carey et al., 2014). Additionally, the nurses acknowledged an increase in their confidence, role responsibility and leadership in role expansion and change to address other chronic health conditions (Carey et al., 2014).

The advanced nursing practice (ANP) roles for Registered Nurses are continuing to develop in the current health delivery systems (https://www.nursingmidwiferyboard. gov.au/Codes-Guidelines-Statements/FAQ/fact-sheet-advanced-nursing-practice-and-specialty-areas.aspx). Experienced RNs who have specialty knowledge and skills can apply for recognition as ANP, for example an advanced practice RN in medical cardiology or respiratory nursing. In addition, many of these advanced practice nurses are undertaking further tertiary study at a Master level degree and becoming endorsed Nurse Practitioners (NP). An endorsed NP can apply for his or her own Medicare provider number for limited item reimbursement, can order specific diagnostic tests and prescribe medications from a formulary of medications specific to their area of endorsement (https://www.nursingmidwiferyboard.gov.au/Codes-Guidelines-Statements/Professional-standards/nurse-practitioner-standards-of-practice.aspx). These examples illustrates how nurses can practice within their full scope of practice, meet the needs of a contemporary health system, and proactively engage in leadership roles to prepare them to deliver patient-centred, equitable, safe and high-quality health care services.

Australian nurses within the acute care or tertiary sector have identified a range of barriers to in the uptake of leadership roles. These barriers can lead to higher rates of job dissatisfaction, attrition and nursing staff turnover (Hayes, Bonner & Pryor, 2010). It is consistently noted that for tertiary care and health system improvement that nurses and nurse leaders play an integral role in ensuring care is patient-centred, and better integrated into systems and services (IOM, 2011; WHO, 2015). Australian research by Opie et al. (2011) into job satisfaction between nurses working in acute care hospitals and those working remotely found that nurses working in remote areas (n=349) expressed higher levels of job satisfaction than nurses working in acute care hospitals (n=277). By comparison, nurses working in acute care hospitals had higher levels of psychological distress, emotional exhaustion and lower levels of job satisfaction than those working in remote areas (Opie et al., 2011). One of the factors highlighted by Opie et al's. (2011) research is the lack of input from acute care nurses in their work practices compared to the autonomy of nurses working remotely.

Another example, that highlights the lack of consultation with nurses was demonstrated in the development of the electronic health care records (EHR) (Jedwab et al., 2019). In Australia nursing professionals comprise the largest proportion of the health workforce (Australian Institute of Health & Welfare, 2018) where the EHRs are used extensively, so they are currently the highest users EHRs. Nursing care directly influences patient care outcomes in hospitals (Wickramasinghe et al., 2014). However, examinations of the benefits of EHR have often failed to capture impacts on nursing work and clinical workflows across many contexts (Narcisse et al., 2013). Early research in the area by Darbyshire in 2004 (2004) found the EHR that was offered at the time of the study was not fit for purpose as the Information technology (IT) was unable to capture 'real nursing'. Nursing feedback on the EHR system included; it(IT EHR) was difficult to use, it contained incompatibilities, was nonresponsive and irrelevant to patient care and meaningful clinical outcomes for nurse users (Zadvinskis et al., 2014). Genuine engagement by nurses in the development processes of IT and EHR systems that includes its implementation may well assist to 'proactively' anticipate system interactions, rather than repair them post-implementation (Kuziemsky et al., 2013).

The contemporary use of EHR in assisting care and health system functioning will be ineffectual if it fails to engage with the largest group of service providers, namely nurses. This again highlights the importance of nurses being a valued part of the team and enacting their autonomous health assessments to work within their full scope of practice.

Conclusion

This chapter explored a range of issues about the role of nurses within the UHC in Australia. It could be said that nursing exists within a 'perfect storm' of funding constraints, high personal, professional and community expectation, and limiting regulations and autonomy of practice models, constrains nursing to delivering care that does not entirely meet the needs of the unwell in Australia. Or permits nurses and NP to practice to their full remit within their scope of practice. The ability to meet the health and nursing needs of a future health service system in Australia is hamstrung by the lack of proactive productive findings, policy enactment failures and medico-centric focus of the current health system, which is costly and unsustainable. The future role/s of the nurse who specialise in community-based care or hospital and community nexus could meet the gap in current health delivery and access models. By exercising patient advocacy at advanced levels through board and governing bodies representation and to self-advocate to practice to their full potential and scope of practice to meet the needs of those population groups who remain under-serviced, with limited health access and miss managed within the current health system, nurses can change the health care system to meet consumer and community needs.

Online resources

1 Australian Institute of Health and Welfare Hospitals: https://www.aihw.gov.au/reports-data/health-welfare-services/hospitals/overview
2 Medicare Levy Australian Taxation Office: https://www.ato.gov.au/Individuals/Medicare-levy/
3 World Health Organisation — A vision for primary health care in the 21st century: towards universal health coverage and the Sustainable Development Goals: https://www.who.int/docs/default-source/primary-health/vision.pdf
4 Nurse Practitioner led care: https://www.transforminghealthcare.org.au/

References

Australian Commission on Safety & Quality in Health Care. (2017). Australia's health. 2018. Canberra: ACT: AIHW

Australian Government. (2009). Emergency Triage Education Kit. Ageing: Canberra Australian Government.

Australian Health Ministers' Advisory Council. (2017). *National Strategic Framework for Chronic Conditions.* Canberra: Australian Government.

Australian Institute of Health and Welfare [AIHW]. (2012). *Disability in Australia: Intellectual Disability* (Cat No: 4433.0.55.003). Canberra, Australia: AIHW.

Australian Medical Association [AMA]. (2017). Submission to the Nurse and Midwifery Board proposed prescribing models AMA submission – Registered nurse and midwife prescribing models. Canberra.

Australian Nursing Federation. (2009). Primary Health Care in Australia: A nursing and mid-wifery consensus view. Commonwealth Department of Health and Ageing.

Australian Taxation Office (ATO 2019). Medicare Levy. Australian Government. https://www.ato.gov.au/Individuals/Medicare-levy/

Brunetto, Y., Farr-Wharton, R., & Shacklock, K. (2011). Supervisor–nurse relationships, team-work, role ambiguity and well-being: Public versus private sector nurses. *Asia Pacific Journal of Human Resources, 49*(2), 143–164.

Bonner, A., Havas, K., Tam, V., Stone, V., Abel, J., Barnes, M., & Douglas, C. (2019). An inte-grated chronic disease nurse practitioner clinic: Service model description and patient pro-file. *Collegian, 26*(2019), 227–234.

Carey, N., Stenner, K., & Courtenay, M. (2014). An exploration of how nurse prescribing is being used for patients with respiratory conditions across the east of England. *BMC Health Services Research, 2014, 14*, 27. http://www.biomedcentral.com/1472-6963/14/27

Cashin, A. (2015). The challenge of nurse innovation in the Australian context of universal care. *Collegian, 22,* 318–324.

Cashin, A., Theophilos, T., & Green, R. (2017). The internationally present perpetual policy themes inhibiting development of the nurse practitioner role in the primary care context: An Australian-USA comparison. *Collegian, 24*, 303–312.

Clifford, S., Lutze, M., Maw, M., & Jennings, N. (2019). Establishing value from contemporary Nurse Practitioners' perceptions of the role: A preliminary study into purpose, support and priorities. *Collegian, 27*, 95–101 https://doi.org/10.1016/j.colegn.2019.05.006

Darbyshire, P. (2004). "'Rage against the machine?': nurses' and midwives' experiences of using Computerized Patient Information Systems for clinical information." *Journal of Clinical Nursing, 13*, 17–25.

Dor, A., Mashiach Eizenberg, M., & Halperin, O. (2019). Hospital nurses in comparison to community nurses: Motivation, empathy, and the mediating role of burnout. *Canadian Journal of Nursing Research, 51*(2), 72–83.

Duffield, C., Diers, D., O'Brien-Pallas, L., et al. Nursing staffing, nursing workload, the work environment and patient outcomes. *Appl Nurs Res* 2011;24:244–55. 10.1016/j.apnr.2009.12.004

Hayes, B., Bonner, A., & Pryor, J. (2010). Factors contributing to nurse job satisfaction in the acute hospital setting: a review of recent literature. *Journal of Nursing Management, 18*, 804–814.

Health Workforce Australia. (2014). Health Workforce Australia: Australia's Future Health Workforce – Nurses Detailed Report. Canberra

IOM (Institute of Medicine). (2011). *The Future of Nursing: Leading Change, Advancing Health.* Washington, DC: The National Academies Press.

Jedwab, R. M., Chalmers, C., Dobroff, N., & Redley, B. (2019). Measuring nursing benefits of an electronic medical record system: A scoping review. *Collegian,* ISSN 1322-7696, *https://doi.org/10.1016/j.colegn.2019.01.003.*

Jennings, N., Clifford, S., Fox, A.R., O'Connell, J., & Gardner, G. (2015). The impact of nurse practitioner care, satisfaction and waiting times in the emergency department: A systematic review. *International Journal of Nursing Studies, 52*, 421–435.

Kuziemsky, C., Nohr, C., Aarts, J., Jaspers, M., & Beuscart-Zephir, M-C. (2013). Context sen-sitive health informatics: Concepts, methods, and tools. *Studies in Health Technology and Informatics, 194*, 1–7.

Martin-Misner, R., Harbman, P., Donald, F., Reid, K., et al. (2015). Cost-effectiveness of Nurse Practitioners in Primary and Specialised Ambulatory care: Systematic review. *BMJ Open, 5*(6). https://bmjopen.bmj.com/content/5/6/e007167

Medicare Australia Act (Commonwealth of Australia), 1973, Medicare Australia Act Amendment 2008, Act no 41 1974 taking into account amendments up to Act no 42 2008. http://www.comlaw.gov.au/Dctails/C2008C00265 accessed 19th July 2010.

Narcisse, M.R., Kippenbrock, T. A., Odell, E., & Buron, B. (2013). Advanced Practice Nurses' Meaningful use of electronic health records. *Applied Nursing Research*, Volume 26, Issue 3, Pages 127–132, ISSN 0897-1897, https://doi.org/10.1016/j.apnr.2013.02.003.

Nursing and Midwifery Board of Australia [ANMB]. (2018). *Registrant data: Reporting period: 1 October 2018 – 31 December 2018*. Nursing and Midwifery Board of Australia & AHPRA.

Opie, T., Lenthall, S., Wakerman, J., Dollard, M., MacLeod, M., Knight, S., Rickard, G., & Dunn, S. (2011). Occupational stress in the Australian nursing workforce: a comparison between hospital-based nurses and nurses working in very remote communities. *JAN*, June - August Volume 28 Number 4.

Palmer, G. (2002). "Politics, Power and Health: From Medibank to Medicare; Flashback 1983" *New Doctor*. Volume 78, Autumn, pp. 28–32.

Parry, Y.K. (2012). Understanding the relationship between the social determinants of health (SDH), Paediatric Emergency Department use and the provision of primary care: a mixed methods analysis. Thesis Unpublished Flinders University.

Parry, Y.K., Hill, P., & Horsfall, S. (2018). Assessing levels of student nurse learning in community-based health placement with vulnerable families: Knowledge development for future clinical practice. *Nurse Education in Practice*, 10.1016/j.nepr.2018.06.015, 32, (14–20).

Parry, Y. K., Ullah, S., Raftos, J., & Willis, E. (2016). Deprivation and its impact on non-urgent Paediatric Emergency Department use: Are Nurse Practitioners the answer? Journal of Advanced Nursing, Volume 72, Issue 1, https://onlinelibrary.wiley.com/doi/abs/10.1111/jan.12810

Productivity Commission. (2017). *Integrated Care*, Shifting the Dial: 5 year Productivity Review, Supporting Paper No. 5, Canberra.

Public Health Information Development Unit (PHIDU), 2005, Population health profile of the Adelaide Northern Division of General Practice. Population Profile Series No. 87. *Public Health Information Development Unit* (PHIDU), Adelaide.

Russell, L., & Doggett, J. (2019). "A road map for tackling out-of-pocket health care costs" *Menzies Centre for Health Policy*. Centre for Policy Development: University of Sydney.

Serafin, L., Bjersa, K., & Doboszyńska, A. (2019). Nurse Job Satisfaction At A Surgical Ward –A Comparative Study Between Sweden And Poland. *Medycyna Pracy*, 70(2), 155–167.

WHO. (2015). Health workforce: Moving the nursing agenda forward. News and events HRH News release 2015, https://www.who.int/hrh/news/2015/global_nurse_conf-kor/en/

Wickramasinghe, N., Kent, B., Moghimi, F. H., Stien, M., Nguyen, L., Redley, B., & Botti, M. (2014). Using technology solutions to streamline healthcare processes for nursing: The case of an intelligent operational planning and support tool (IOPST) solution. In N. Wickramasinghe, L. Hakim, C. Gonzalez, & J. Tan (Eds.), *Lean thinking for healthcare: Healthcare delivery in the information age*. (pp. 405–430). New York, NY: Springer.

Woo, B.F.Y., Lee, J.X.Y., & Tam, W.W.S. (2017). The Impact of Advanced Practice Nursing Role on Quality of Care, Clinical Outcomes, Patient Satisfaction, and Cost in the Emergency and Critical Care Settings: A systematic review. *Human Resources for Health*, 15, 63.

World Health Organization [WHO]. (2013). *Global Action Plan for the Prevention and Control of Noncommunicable Diseases (NCDs) 2013–2020 [Internet]*. Geneva, Switzerland: WHO Press; 2013. 42, p. 103 Available from: http://apps.who.int/iris/bitstream/10665/94384/1/9789241506236_eng.pdf

World Health Organization [WHO]. (2018). *A vision for primary health care in the 21st century: towards universal health coverage and the Sustainable Development Goals*. Geneva: World Health Organization and the United Nations Children's Fund (UNICEF), 2018 (WHO/HIS/SDS/2018.X). Licence: CC BY-NC-SA 3.0 IGO. https://www.who.int/docs/default-source/primary-health/vision.pdf

Zadvinskis, I. M., Chipps, E., & Yen, P. Y. (2014). Exploring nurses' confirmed expectations regarding health IT: A phenomenological study, *International Journal of Medical Informatics, Volume 83*, Issue 2, Pages 89–98, ISSN 1386-5056, https://doi.org/10.1016/j.ijmedinf.2013.11.001

3 Nurses delivering care in a digitised environment

Jen Bichel-Findlay, Kathleen Dixon
and Nathaniel Alexander

Chapter objectives

This chapter will offer the reader:

- Insight into the definitional evolution of nursing informatics.
- A description of the transformation of data within the healthcare landscape.
- An outline of the key informatics innovations and issues facing nurses in the primary health setting.
- An outline of the key informatics innovations and issues facing nurses in the acute care setting.
- An overview of future trends in health informatics that will impact on nurses delivering care.

Introduction

The digitisation of the healthcare environment impacts all sectors and services across Australia and has the potential of reducing errors at the point of care, improving service efficiency, reducing healthcare costs, and identifying health problems early. Nurses will be able to make decisions based on the aggregation of real-time data rather than waiting for data to be collated and become available. Nursing practice can be enhanced through to predicting which patients are at risk of problems and issues and being able to implement strategies so that these do not eventuate or are managed with minimal impact on the patient's quality of life. The discipline of nursing informatics is now firmly embedded in healthcare, requiring all nurses to be digitally proficient, data enabled and innovation aware. The current landscape is an exciting one for nurses, who will not only become more discriminate users of patient information but will also create and advance new ways of using technology to sustain quality nursing practice.

The term digitally proficient refers to staff being both comfortable and skilled in the use of technology. The term data enabled refers to staff reviewing the data that has been collected and making choices that enhance the effectiveness of the organisation's goals, particularly patient's health outcomes.

Nursing informatics defined

Nursing informatics was initially described as a combination of computer, information and nursing science, designed to assist in the management and processing of nursing data, information and knowledge to support the practice of nursing and the delivery of nursing care (Graves & Corcoran, 1989). Thirty years later it is a recognised field of nursing that focuses on how nurses, essentially knowledge workers, interact with data and information to produce more granular and meaningful information, knowledge or wisdom so that better decisions are made that benefit patients and improve healthcare outcomes. As nurses are the largest frontline health workforce, and any change in nursing workflow has impacts on the overall delivery of healthcare, it is essential that nurses have input into digital transformation projects. Each state and territory in Australia is aiming towards having a Chief Nursing & Midwifery Information Officer, who will be responsible for supporting and guiding nurses and midwives on issues related to information and communication technology, and act as a conduit between nursing and midwifery services and the information management and technology staff.

> The term knowledge worker was first used by Peter Drucker in 1959 and refers to a person who applies theoretical and analytical knowledge in their daily work activities to solve complex problems. In other words, they are paid to think rather than to perform manual tasks.

Transformation of data to wisdom

The Data-Information-Knowledge-Wisdom (DIKW) framework, initially referred to as the Nelson Continuum (Snipes, 2019), describes the relationship between data, information, knowledge and wisdom.

- **Data** is the collection of numbers, characters or facts that are assembled according to a foreseen need for analysis and are generally numeric or alphabetic code (Hebda & Czar, 2018). An example is the number *500*. Data is focussed on naming, collecting and organising (McHugh, 2011).
- **Information** is the compilation of interpreted data, often examined for patterns and structure (Hebda & Czar, 2018). An example is *a urine output of 500 millilitres*. The central point of information is organising and interpreting (McHugh, 2011).
- **Knowledge** is a synthesis of information derived from several sources to produce a validated single concept or idea that can be used again (Hebda & Czar, 2018; McHugh, 2011). An example is *the daily urine output in a healthy individual is >500 millilitres per day*.
- **Wisdom** emerges when knowledge is used accordingly to manage and resolve problems (Hebda & Czar, 2018). An example is *advice for a renally compromised individual is to avoid oliguria by maintaining a daily urine output >500 millilitres*.

For most of the last three decades, data in health has been structured, or in other words, data that fits neatly within fields and columns in either paper records or a database. Structured datum is generally stored in a relational database (that is, able to recognise relations between stored items) and is easily searchable. Examples include post codes, mobile phone numbers, and people's last names. Unstructured datum, on the other hand, is datum that has internal structure but is not structured via predefined data models or schema. Unstructured data can be stored within a non-relational database, are not easily searchable, and includes formats such as audio, video, social media postings, digital photographs, websites, and text messages. Currently there is much more unstructured data than structured data in existence, and tools to analyse unstructured data are limited and expensive but are developing. While this type of data is perceived as messy and difficult to store and search at the present time, it has a much greater potential to help clinicians understand relationships and to predict outcomes. Another type of datum that represents less than 10% of total data is semi-structured, of which email is a common example. This type of data maintains internal tags and markings that recognise separate data elements, which facilitates information grouping and hierarchies.

The Internet of Things (IoT) is gradually encroaching on every facet of life, and health is no exception. The IoT describes any device that communicates with the Internet and has become a large network of 'smart' connected things that have embedded software and sensors that allow them to interoperate without involving human interaction. A smartphone is an example of a commonly used IoT device, and sensors installed into an elderly person's home to detect falls is an example of an IoT device used in healthcare. Most IoT devices have basic learning capabilities, which permit them to learn and adapt to their input data and adjust their output behaviour accordingly. They can be programmed to respond to indicators, both external and internal, and therefore their value in remotely monitoring patients in real-time has significantly enhanced care delivery and improved disease management. IoT devices permit nurses to be more engaged in care delivery while simultaneously decreasing the amount of time and energy needed to care for each patient. The IoT will also mean that nurses will no longer be reliant on often incomplete or inaccurate patient self-reporting. Nurses will play a central role in teaching patients how various IoT devices work and why the increased technology is beneficial, however will need to be aware of how effective their communication is in realising patient goals without the patient feeling less cared for in a digitally dominated landscape.

Primary health setting

The Australian primary health sector provides a wide range of services and is often the first point of contact people have with the health system. General Practitioner (GP) attendances have been steadily increasing over the last seven years, with Australians now visiting a GP 6.1 times a year (Australian Institute of Health and Welfare, 2018). The Care Track Australia study (Runciman et. al., 2012) highlighted that appropriate care (that is, care based on evidence or consensus guidelines) is only provided to just over half of the patient population and in some patients only a third receive the recommended care. In addition, care delivery is often uncoordinated, due to a lack of communication between care providers, and this leads to services being duplicated. One approach to improve care coordination is to use a longitudinal electronic record that captures episodic patient-focused summary information from clinical systems traversing primary health, community, hospital and specialist care.

Electronic health record

Australia commenced their electronic health record (EHR) journey in 1999, with the deployment of the Personally Controlled EHR in 2009 and later renamed My Health Record (MHR) in 2012. The MHR stores an individual's health information such as allergies, medicines, discharge summaries, event summaries from emergency departments, radiology and pathology reports, and other relevant information. It enables secure sharing of health information between an individual's healthcare providers, whilst enabling the individual to control who can access their information. It was originally anticipated that the MHR would lead to faster, safer and more streamlined treatment (Australian Digital Health Agency, 2019), and studies are currently being undertaken to identify if these benefits are being realised. Emergency department nurses, for example, will be able to access the patient's health history provided the individual has consented to this. A patient's MHR can be identified so that nurses know to undertake a risk assessment, monitor a particular attribute, or just be aware of a potential vulnerability. It will also improve communication as it can be used to share information between acute, community and primary healthcare providers, public and private healthcare professionals, state and territory healthcare providers and different healthcare professionals.

The national deployment of the MHR in Australia, coordinated by the Australian Digital Health Agency, has not been without issue. Traditionally, all health information has been under the control of clinicians and the shift to patient control of their health records has led to debate over why the record is patient controlled rather than clinician controlled, how secure the system is, and what legislative changes are required. Placing the patient in control of their health record is a significant change, as MHR enables patients to control what information is shared with particular clinicians and what information is withheld. This would seem to contradict some of the objectives of MHR which is to enable a complete and accurate record of a patient's medical history, to provide a holistic care by clinicians caring for the patient.

Furthermore, concerns have been raised as to health literacy levels of patients who access their information from MHR without necessarily consulting their primary healthcare provider. This is of particular concern for patients with low levels of health literacy who may access information in MHR without guidance from their primary healthcare provider, potentially resulting in confusion and ill-informed decisions about their health. The traditional model of health education places the clinician as the key controller of access to health information and the interpretation of that information. With the patient now in control of health information, their ability to make a decision as to what to do with that information creates potential risk and challenges the clinician-controlled health information model.

The MHR also presents challenges in relation to issues of privacy and health law. In Australia, the My Health Records Act, 2012 governs the use of the EHR. Its primary purpose is to ensure that patients' healthcare records are non-fragmented and offer clinicians with point of care information to guide clinician decision making. The system, however, is not without risk and security of digital data is one of the most pressing concerns. Breaches through unauthorised access have cost implications including financial, reputational and personal. Although patient confidentiality, privacy and security are well documented areas of concern, nurses have identified there is a need for attention to issues such as system bypasses, false entries and workarounds (Ayatollahi, Mirani & Haghani, 2014; McBride, Tietze, Hanley & Thomas, 2017).

System bypass refers to a flaw in the system that allows hackers to go around the system to access data. False entries result from incorrect or missing information due to either intentional or unintentional actions. Workarounds are informal temporary practices that are not part of normal workflow. For instance workarounds arise when there is a mismatch between the work intentions of a nurse and the workflow dictated by the EHR.

In 2016, the Australian Red Cross experienced a significant data breach resulting from the accidental publication of 55,000 blood donors' personal data on a public website (Daly, 2018). A more recent example of a data breach at the Australian National University Canberra illustrates the risks associated with digital data storage. According to a statement from the Vice Chancellor, personal staff, student and visitor data extending back 19 years was accessed and included information such as academic records of students, names, addresses, dates of birth, phone numbers, personal email addresses, emergency contact details, tax file numbers, payroll information, bank account details and passport details (Australian National University, 2019). Of all reported data breaches across all sectors in 2018/2019, healthcare has reported the most with 203 breaches in total (Office of the Australian Information Commissioner [OAIC], 2019). Notifiable Data Breaches Statistics Reports from the OAIC identify the leading cause of healthcare data breaches is phishing (fraudulent attempt to acquire sensitive information such as passwords and credit card details by masquerading as a trustworthy entity in an electronic communication), however more than a third of all notifiable data breaches are directly due to human error (OAIC, 2019). These findings highlight the importance of healthcare providers ensuring they deploy robust security practices to protect sensitive personal data.

Acute care setting

The digitisation of the acute care sector has been a challenge, due in part to the complex and complicated nature of the environment and the often-inordinate costs. Australian hospitals, both public and private, are currently implementing a range of digital solutions that will improve communication and remove the reliance on paper documentation, including patient administration systems, electronic medical records, clinical decision support systems, computerised provider order entry and electronic medication management to name a few. While some healthcare organisations are nearly all digital, others have just commenced the journey and are in a hybrid state of electronic and paper-based documentation.

Electronic medical record

Rather than being a summary of information accessed by multiple healthcare providers across multiple healthcare organisations like the MHR, an electronic medical record (EMR) is a dynamic record that contains comprehensive information that is created and resides within a single healthcare organisation such as a health service to which a patient has been registered or admitted. This digital version of a patient's chart, the EMR contains the patient's medical history, diagnoses, treatments, referrals, progress notes, assessments, observations, nursing activities, advanced care planning and so on. The information is collected once but used many times and can be viewed by multiple healthcare providers from multiple locations, such as a nurse in a specific unit, a physiotherapist in his/her office and a medical officer in a medical centre all accessing a patient's EMR at the same time. Information about the patient, including previous admissions, can be easily obtained by healthcare providers, even at remote locations, without the need to instigate a 'hunt' for the medical chart that is common in a paper-based hospital.

All EMRs require a Patient Administration System (PAS), which holds the master patient index or database that maintains consistent and accurate information about each patient registered by a healthcare organisation. The PAS tracks the patient/client/consumer across care settings, and holds details such as name, date of birth, unique healthcare identifier, gender, ethnicity, address and so on. Most EMRs offer computerised provider order entry (CPOE), allowing healthcare professionals to electronically order laboratory, radiology, referral, procedure and medication orders. Order sets can then be developed locally relevant to casemix (mix of types of patients treated by a healthcare facility) and current nationally endorsed guidelines. An example is the response to chest pain in patients presenting to the emergency department. A chest pain order would entail, in one mouse click, the ordering of a chest X-ray, electrocardiogram and biochemistry. A nursing example is a triage nurse in the emergency department having an order set for simple and obvious wrist and arm fractures, allowing the nurse to order radiology for the affected site and some basic blood tests and pain relief. Order sets reduce the time the patient is waiting for assessment and treatment, decrease underservicing and over servicing, and promote the correct items to be included in each service.

Electronic medication management

Most acute healthcare facilities are implementing electronic medication management (EMM), comprising systems that support the prescribing, ordering, checking, reconciling, dispensing and recording the administration of medication. EMM increases the legibility on medication orders, reduces medication errors and associated adverse events, and minimises variance in prescribing patterns, particularly if combined with bar coding and radio-frequency identification technology (Australian Commission on Safety and Quality in Health Care, 2019; Pearce & Whyte, 2018). A number of healthcare facilities are implementing automated patient dispensing from pharmacy to the inpatient setting, allowing the nurse to administer medication that is specifically barcoded for a particular patient. This has resulted in changes to nursing workflows, as the traditional role of a second checker of medication is made redundant. In addition to CPOE and EMRs, EMMs may also have clinical decision support (CDS) – a system that analyses entered data and assists the healthcare professional to make safer decisions. CDS can provide alerts and reminders about upcoming activities. It is particularly valuable in medication administration, as it can identify near misses such as medication allergies, drug-to-drug interactions, drug-to-disease interaction and so on. These systems reduce the risk of nurses administering the wrong drug, the wrong dose of a drug, selecting the wrong route, the wrong time for a drug to be administered and a drug being administered to the wrong patient.

The benefits of electronic clinical information systems are improved documentation and a reduction in the time that nurses devote to documentation. The information captured in these systems ensure consistency and completeness of structured data and facilitates efficiency in nursing activities such as worklist prompts, clinical pathways, nursing care plans, medication administration and information and discharge information. Increased uptake of electronic clinical information systems is not without challenges, and is currently creating huge data reservoirs, that will require nurses to have high level data management skills and be well versed in the legal and ethical implications of data management (Risling, 2017). As well, there are unintended consequences, which can result and include issues with usability, implications for patient safety, disrupted nurse-patient relationships and provider moral distress. (McBride, Tietze, Robichauz, Stokes & Weber, 2018). For example, usability challenges arise when a nurse is unfamiliar with the operational requirements of the system, which can lead to unintended consequences such as a delay in the delivery of patient care, potentially compromising patient safety and causing the nurse moral distress. The potential for patient safety implications may also be due to overreliance on clinician decision support, and can be addressed through integrated clinical education and training that realises the full benefits of both a clinician decision support electronic system and clinician autonomy in decision making. Furthermore, disrupted nurse-patient relationships may be remedied through optimisation of clinical workflow processes that account for the use of technology in the delivery of healthcare. These solutions may reduce provider moral distress.

The term data reservoir refers to a place that allows data to be accumulated and provides self-service access to data scientists and business users for business purposes such as integration and analysis.

The Registered Nurses Standards for Practice issued by the Nursing & Midwifery Board of Australia (NMBA) and underpinned by the Health Practitioner Regulation National Law requires nurses to critically think and analyse nursing practice and deliver care that is supported by comprehensive assessments. The CDS system overrides aspects of this critical thinking by the practitioner as it mandates certain actions by the clinician as defined in the organisation's policies and procedures. Overreliance on the CDS system has the potential to result in inadequate or inappropriate care being delivered. Although the organisation bears the legal and corporate risk associated with these decisions, a nurse's professional accountability to the Board based on the Standards of Practice may be compromised if the standards are not reflective of contemporary practice.

Social media

Social media is now being used in healthcare, particularly in educating patients and promoting healthy behaviours, to engage with the public, to share information and to debate policy and practice issues. Social media is a form of electronic communication through which users share information, ideas, personal messages and other content with online communities (Sipes, 2019). Microblogging platforms such as Twitter, Tumblr and Instagram are ideal for nurses to develop short messages for patients to consume. Facebook, YouTube, blogs and Wikis can also be used by nurses to educate patients and caregivers such as family on acute and chronic disease management. Several social networks have been providing self-help groups, or peer-to-peer healthcare, where people seek others with similar health concerns to obtain information and how to overcome challenges. Examples include MedHelp, Cure Together, Vitals, Daily Strength, PatientsLikeMe, Inspire and Face2Face Health. This peer-to-peer healthcare is expanding, as it exposes people to information and also to others who are confronting the same challenges (Fox, 2011).

Although the use of social media is beneficial to the nursing profession, the lack of theoretical and evaluation models for the use of social media by nurses adds to the concerns about privacy, confidentiality and anonymity (Sipes, 2019; Skiba, Knafel & Lee, 2015). Nurses and students need to understand the implications, including their professional ethical responsibilities in their use of social media (Casella, Mills & Usher, 2014). The ethical principles, autonomy, non-maleficence, beneficence and justice provide a contemporary framework for ethical decision making (Johnstone, 2016). Nurses should refer to these principles, along with their professional codes and guidelines to help guide their use of social media and other digital technology. It is important that nurses and students are aware that boundary violations in the use of social media can cause harm to patients, family members, the nurse's employers and fellow staff members and that even with privacy settings in place, information on social media sites is public information (Westrick, 2016). Inappropriate use of social media by nurses, whether on or off duty, is subject to professional sanction and may result in disciplinary action.

A recent decision in the Civil and Administrative Tribunal of New South Wales (NCAT) highlights the serious consequences for nurses who commit boundary violations in the use of social media. A number of complaints were made by the Health Care Complaints Commission against a nurse, including that the nurse inappropriately accessed a patient's clinical records for nonclinical purposes, which breached *Health Privacy Principle 10* of the *Health records and Information Privacy Act 2002*. In addition, the nurse inappropriately engaged in an online friendship with the patient through social media and inappropriately used information obtained in the course of his clinical duties to maintain an online friendship. The findings of the Tribunal were that the nurse was guilty of Unsatisfactory Professional Conduct and Professional Misconduct and as a result the nurse was deregistered for a period of four years (Health Care Complaints Commission v Mackie – NSW CaseLaw).

Most employers mandate adherence to organisational values when regulating the use of social media. The NMBA stipulates in their social media policy (NMBA, 2014) what is required of nurses when utilising social media. Where social media is used to deliver health information from a personal account, the nurse is professionally held to account on the information provided. If social media posts are in contradiction to accepted health values and evidence, the nurse may be in breach of their Code of Conduct. Lachman (2013) found that many nurses are unaware of the privacy settings of their social media accounts, and do not know or appreciate the pervasive nature of posts on social media (Hao & Gao, 2017). Healthcare facilities can be the subject of harmful commentary based on a single nurse posting inappropriate humour. Having been identified as working for a particular facility, the nurse may find themselves excluded from their current employment and future employment opportunities as employers view the ability of their staff to provide professional unbiased and nonjudgemental nursing care to the community is paramount (Edge, 2017). This is an emerging area of ethics and regulation and will continue to evolve in the years ahead.

Future trends

Precision healthcare

As technology is always evolving and innovating, nurses need to acknowledge that future initiatives may impact on nurses and how they care for patients. Precision healthcare is one such emerging area that will require more involvement of nurses, and a number of Australian states and territories are currently developing nursing workforce capabilities. Precision healthcare aspires to deliver optimised treatments for disease based on more comprehensive and granular information about the patient and their condition, often through capturing the patient's genome sequence (person's total genetic information). This vast dataset can be interrogated to diagnose or determine carrier status and predisposition of practically every known condition, as well as response to disease and treatment. This personalised medicine proposes better outcomes for patients and reduced costs of care for healthcare providers by identifying targeted treatment, minimising unproductive procedures and avoiding adverse responses to therapy. The abundance of information poses the conundrum of how much information should be returned to the individual and when. Nurses should focus on expanding their knowledge of and comfort with this area, particularly in advocating for patients undergoing diagnostic testing and considering treatment regimes. There are always high expectations that new approaches will solve today's problems in isolation, however all components of the system need to function synchronously, and ethical questions need to be carefully considered by the nursing profession in regard to precision healthcare. Nurses have always experienced ethical challenges in their work, precision healthcare will present new and unique ethical tensions with which nurses will have to contend. Having a deeper understanding and knowledge of these challenges may assist nurses in responding to the tensions created by this future initiative.

Artificial intelligence

Artificial intelligence (AI) is the ability to enable machines to think and act like humans by teaching computers to acknowledge images and sounds, and then make decisions based on them. The benefits of AI are two-fold – it can automate mundane tasks and offer creative insight. AI employs sophisticated algorithms to discover clinically relevant information from a large volume of healthcare data in real-time and utilises the gained insights to assist nursing care delivery. It is also capable of learning and improving its accuracy based on feedback, referred to as machine learning. AI has the potential to revolutionise the way nurses deliver care, such as automatically generating alerts, detecting threats and problems related to patient safety, and predicting the length of stay of patients. Recent developments include bottles which automatically issue reminders to patients to drink or take medication, nappies that sound an alert when soiled and require changing, and sensor-equipped stoma pouches that let the patient know that the bag is almost full (Matheson, 2018). This will allow nurses to devote more time to focus on critical thinking and problem solving.

Healthcare facilities often encounter productivity issues, where nurses are unable to undertake patient activities due to performing mundane repetitive tasks. A number of organisations have developed 'virtual nurse technologies' to augment or support nurses in carrying out their activities. These virtual nurses are often computer-generated, on-screen nurses with whom the patient can interact, and are intended to be informative, social and empathetic to present patients with a more natural interaction that maintains the comfort they might feel when interacting with a nurse. AI also plays a fundamental role in robotics, of which the development and deployment of nursing care robots or nursebots are increasing in response to an ageing population and chronic nursing shortages. Nursebots can assist immobile patients with simple activities and are typically located in the patient's room in a hospital or at home. They can carry out laundry services, household chores, remind patients or care recipients when to eat, drink, take medication, and perform exercises (Grasso, 2018). A US patent exists for an autonomous, intelligent and interactive robot that performs the functions of an operating room scrub nurse (Frazier et al., 2019). Townsville Hospital in far north Queensland has been trialling 'Pepper', a humanoid social robot that acts as a concierge by answering simple questions from patients. Pepper tracks faces and turns toward voices, greeting and engaging patients by providing advice on where to park, where to eat and answering questions about smoking (Fernbach & Raffferty, 2018).

Conclusion

The health landscape is changing with the increasing digitisation of healthcare services. Expert software not only streamlines nursing documentation, but also will automate it through the use of technologies. Digitisation presents an opportunity to increase the capacity to predict, improving the quality of care and resulting in increased patient safety. Having instant access to patient data and information from electronic records can reduce errors and costs as well as improving service efficiency and effectiveness. Both the primary health and acute care settings have completed significant digitisation, and both environments are investigating the use of assistive approaches such as AI, machine learning and genomics. Nurses need to remain relevant in a technologically advanced future and encouraging more nurses to be involved in the development of technology would ensure that the human caring perspective is assured. Technology has the potential to perform routine tasks so that nurses can devote more time to patient interaction. It is important that undergraduate and postgraduate educational programs recognise the growing role of digitisation and promote options to increase awareness, develop skills and promote potential opportunities.

Online resources

1 Australasian Institute of Digital Health (AIDH) Nursing and Midwifery Community of Practice: https://digitalhealth.org.au/communities-of-practice/nursing-and-midwifery/
2 International Medical Informatics Association – Nursing Informatics Special Interest Group: https://imia-medinfo.org/wp/sig-ni-nursing-informatics/
3 Australian College of Nursing – Nursing Informatics Community of Interest: https://www.acn.edu.au/membership/coi/coi-leads#nurse-informatics
4 Health Information Management Systems Society: https://www.himss.org/

References

Australian Commission on Safety and Quality in Health Care (ACSQHC). (2019). *Electronic medication management systems: a guide to safe implementation*. (3rd ed). Sydney, Australia: ACSQHC.

Australian Digital Health Agency. (2019). How my health record benefits you. Retrieved from https://www.myhealthrecord.gov.au/for-you-your-family/my-health-record-benefits

Australian Government. (2012). My Health Records Act 2012. Canberra, Australia: Australian Government.

Australian Institute of Health and Welfare (AIHW). (2018). *Australia's health 2018*. Canberra, Australia: AIHW.

Australian National University. (2019). Message from the Vice Chancellor 4 June 2019. Retrieved from https://www.anu.edu.au/news/all-news/message-from-the-vice-chancellor

Ayatollahi, H., Mirani, N., & Haghani, H. (2014). Electronic health records: What are the most important barriers? *Perspectives in Health Information Management, 11*(Fall), 1–12.

Casella, E., Mills, J., & Usher, K. (2014). Social media and nursing practice: Changing the balance between the social and technical aspects of work. *Collegian, 21*(2), 121–126.

Daly, A. (2018). The introduction of data breach notification legislation in Australia: A comparative view. *Computer Law & Security Review, 34*, 477–495.

Edge, W. (2017). Nursing professionalism: Impact of social media use among nursing students. *Journal of Healthcare Communications, 2*(3), 28.

Fernbach, N., & Rafferty, S. (2018). *Townsville Hospital hosts humanoid robot in Australian first trial*. ABC News, 24 August 2018. Retrieved from https://www.abc.net.au/news/2018-08-24/townsville-hospital-trials-robot-helper/10157200

Fox, S. (2011). Peer-to-peer health care. Pew Research Center. Retrieved from http://www.pewinternet.org/2011/02/28/peer-to-peer-health-care-2/

Frazier, R. M., Carter-Templeton, H., Wyatt, T. H., & Wu, L. (2019). Current trends in robotics in nursing patents – a glimpse into emerging innovations. *CIN: Computers, Informatics, Nursing, 37*(6), 290–297.

Grasso, C. (2018). Challenges and advantages of robotic nursing care: a social and ethical analysis. The corporate social responsibility and business ethics blog. Retrieved from https://corporatesocialresponsibilityblog.com/2018/06/26/robotic-nursing-care/

Graves, J. R., & Corcoran, S. (1989). The study of nursing informatics. *Journal of Nursing Scholarship, 21*(4), 227–231.

Hao, J., & Gao, B. (2017). Advantages and disadvantages for nurses of using social media. *Journal of Primary Health Care and General Practice, 1*(1), 1–3.

Health Care Complaints Commission v Mackie – NSW Caselaw. (2018). NSWCATOD 174.

Hebda, T., & Czar, P. (2018). *Handbook of informatics for nurses and healthcare professionals*. (6th ed.). Boston, MA: Pearson.

Johnstone, M-J. (2016). *Bioethics: A nursing perspective*. Chatswood, Australia: Elsevier.

Lachman, V. D. (2013). Social media: Managing the ethical issues. *MEDSURG Nursing, 22*(5), 326–329

Matheson, R. (2018). Startups building integrated nursing ecosystems with AI. *Healthcare IT News*. Retrieved from https://www.healthcareitnews.com/news/startups-building-integrated-nursing-ecosystems-ai

McBride, S., Tietze, M., Hanley, M., & Thomas, L. (2017). Statewide study to assess nurses' experiences with meaningful use-based electronic health records. *CIN: Computers, Informatics, Nursing, 35*(1), 18–28.

McBride, S., Tietze, M., Robichaux, C., Stokes, L., & Weber, E. (2018). Identifying and addressing ethical issues with use of electronic health records. *Online Journal of Issues in Nursing, 23*(1), 1–12.

McHugh, M. H. (2011). Computer systems basics. In V. K. Saba &K. A. McCormick (Eds.), *Essentials of nursing informatics*. (5th ed.) (pp. 603–617). New York City, NY: McGraw-Hill.

Nursing & Midwifery Board of Australia (NMBA). (2014). *Social media policy*. Canberra: NMBA. Retrieved from https://www.nursingmidwiferyboard.gov.au/Codes-Guidelines-Statements/Policies/Social-media-policy.aspx

Office of the Australian Information Commissioner (OAIC). (2019). Notifiable data breaches statistics reports. Retrieved from https://www.oaic.gov.au/privacy/notifiable-data-breaches/notifiable-data-breaches-statistics/

Pearce, R., & Whyte, I. (2018). Electronic medication management: Is it a silver bullet? *Australian Prescriber, 41*(2), 32–33.

Risling, T. (2017). Educating the nurses of 2025: Technology trends of the next decade. *Nurse Education in Practice, 22*, 89–92.

Runciman, W. B., Hunt, T. D., Hannaford, N. A., Hibbert, P. D., Westbrook, J. I., Coiera, E. W., …Braithwaite, J. (2012). CareTrack: Assessing the appropriateness of health care delivery in Australia. *Medical Journal of Australia, 197*(2), 100–105.

Skiba, D. J., Knafel, S., & Lee, C. (2015). Social media in the connected age: Impact on healthcare education and practice. In V. K. Saba & K. A. McCormick (Eds.), *Essentials of nursing informatics*. (6th ed.) (pp. 631–642). New York City, NY: McGraw-Hill.

Snipes, C. (2019). *Application of nursing informatics: Competencies, skills, decision-making*. New York City, NY: Springer.

Westrick, S. J. (2016). Nursing students' use of electronic and social media: Law, ethics, and e-professionalism. *Nursing Education Perspectives, 37*(1), 16–22.

4 Career pathways for registered nurses

An expanding horizon

Mahnaz Fanaian, Christine Chisengantambu-Winters, Irene Mayo and Amanda Johnson

Chapter objectives

This chapter will offer the reader:

- An overview of roles post qualification
- Opportunities related to advanced practice
- An overview of future challenges in career pathways for registered nurses

Introduction

This chapter provides an overview of opportunities in nursing post qualification. In this chapter, career paths have been divided into 4 broad areas: Clinical, Management, Education and Research and Policy development. These broad areas are also the reflective of the registered nurse scope of practice (Nursing and Midwifery Board of Australia (NMBA), 2016a). Nursing career paths are not linear and often combine one or more of these paths. Throughout the chapter examples are provided to illustrate the diversity of career paths nurses can choose across their career and the list is not intended to be exhaustive. New careers and roles continue to emerge reflective of changing population and health service needs. Regardless of the career path chosen, the need to engage in lifelong learning and achieve further qualifications underpins many opportunities to grow and move into new areas of practice. Qualifications include those related to clinical specialisation through post graduate study, for example neonatal or palliative care and those with a focus on research, for example Master by Research, PhD and postdoctoral positions.

Section 1: Clinical pathway

Commonly, the clinical environment is where Registered Nurses (RNs) start their career. This is the environment in which RNs consolidate their undergraduate education by engaging in practice to further acquire competence and confidence in patient care.

This section will explore the role of nurses in primary healthcare settings specifically as a growing area for nursing before exploring senior roles that relate to both primary and tertiary healthcare settings, inclusive of specialisations.

Primary health care

Primary health care is considered the first level of contact that individuals have with the health care system (Skrobansk et al., 2019). RNs who work in primary health care settings can be based in medical centres or community hubs and their role includes health promotion, immunisation, health assessment and the management of chronic diseases. There are a range of settings within primary health care including: general practice, residential aged care, custodial or detention facilities, and educational settings such as schools (Australian Primary Health Care Nurses Association, 2012). There are around 11,000 practice nurses in Australia (Australian Medicare Local Alliance, 2012) and there is a growing demand for RNs to work in primary health care settings (Thomas et al., 2017).

Becoming a clinical nurse specialist (CNS) or a clinical nurse educator (CNE)

Following the consolidation of experience and practice, opportunities to move into specialised roles may be available for nurses working in all settings. RNs who have at least three years' experience within a relevant specialty area and have a post-graduate qualification within the specialty, can seek opportunities to work as a CNS. The role of the CNS involves a mixture of patient care and further responsibilities such as those that promote professional development of the self, others and their speciality.

A CNE is normally an RN who also has at least three years' experience working within a specific nursing speciality and has attained a post-graduate qualification specific to nursing or adult education. Like the CNS, the CNE role involves a mixture of patient care but specifically focusses on the education and development of nursing staff within their workplace. The CNE role also includes supporting new staff such as new graduate nurses, providing training sessions and conducting competency assessments with staff (Cofeey & White, 2019).

Box 4.1 - Clinical pathway scenario

Mandy is a registered nurse who qualified three years ago and began her career as an RN in a general medical ward in a large urban hospital. Mandy worked on the ward for three years and took up opportunities to work in Intensive Care Unit while completing in-house training courses. Mandy decided she wanted to move into the role of CNS in ICU and enrolled in a graduate certificate course in ICU. After finishing her 6 months course and working 2 more years in ICU, she applied for Master of Science in clinical nursing to give her the background and qualification she needed to progress whilst also continuing to develop her clinical experience. During her master's degree study, a position of CNS in ICU became available and she applied for it and successfully started her career as a CNS.

Reflective questions:
1   What further studies or qualifications would a clinical nurse specialist involve?
2   If you are thinking three years post qualifications to become a clinical nurse specialist, what support strategies would you put in place now?
3   What do you think would be the main responsibilities of a clinical nurse specialist that is different to a registered nurse?

Advanced practice: The clinical nurse consultant and nurse practitioner

A CNC is an advanced practice nurse in Australia and is a pathway for experienced RNs, usually with at least five years post registration experience and a postgraduate qualification in the speciality area, who want to maintain a clinical role in a defined specialty. CNCs are important members of the clinical team as they possess an advanced level of clinical judgement and are source of expertise. CNCs have a wide array of skills and participate in clinical care, leadership, teaching and research within their specialities.

Nurse practitioners (NP) are advanced practitioners and the title of NP is legislatively protected and individuals endorsed by the NMBA (2017). Their ability to prescribe some medications, order and interpret diagnostic investigations are some of the extended capabilities that differentiate this role from that of the CNC. The NPs can work in a variety of settings (Masso and Thompson, 2014). The NP role requires the completion of a relevant Master's degree and at least 3 years full-time advanced practice experience to meet the Nursing and Midwifery Board of Australia (NMBA) National Practice Standards for the NP, followed by endorsement by the NMBA (2016).

Section 2: Management pathway

Management roles embrace both managerial and leadership roles. This section explores the roles and responsibilities of the different types of nurse manager and the roles that range from bed side nursing to corporate executive.

Overview of managerial roles

Managers are involved in the implementation of organisational activities; from execution of daily activities to strategic policy development and innovation. Managers lead the organisation, driving them forward and increasing their business and core functions to achieve its desired goal (Australian College of Nursing, 2015; Daly et al., 2014 Thomas et al., 2016). Management involves the art of planning, organising, leading and directing, monitoring, delegating and motivating employees to facilitate the production of services (Dalton, 2010).

Arguably, the use of the term 'manager' can be used loosely to denote the oversight of the execution of activities and at the same time it denotes the different levels of 'power positions' within an organisation (Singh, 2000). Within the health profession, Nurse Managers are 'at the centre of establishing and delivering primary and patient care activities and they are the "go-to" people within the organisation'" (Chisengantambu et al., 2017, p.1).

From clinical practice to senior leadership

The position and roles of nurse managers vary according to their titles, functions, demand and responsibilities and Figure 4.1 is an example of career pathways in Royal Children Hospital (RCH). Some acronyms here are: AUM (Associate Unit Manager), RN Division 1 = work in settings such as hospitals, aged care, mental health and education. A Div 2 is an EN who may or may not be medication endorsed.

The RCH Nursing Career Pathway

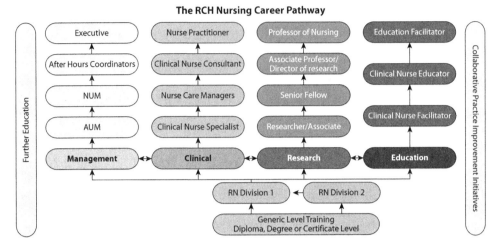

Figure 4.1 The royal children's hospital career pathway

Source: Royal Children's Hospital Melbourne

Nurse unit manager (NUM)

The NUM is a middle level management position that is responsible for managing small teams, configuring schedules, addressing staff issues, managing the ward/unit budget and addressing and minimising patient complaints and issues. Nurse unit managers operate as both clinicians and managers at the same time (Chisemgantambu et al., 2017) contributing to both care delivery and strategic decisions of the organisation. Overall, the NUM position is pivotal to the coordination of patient care, ward management and leadership for the professions of nursing and midwifery with the goals of delivering high-quality patient care and efficient use of resources (NSW Government, n.d).

After hours nurse manager (AHNM)

The After-Hours Nurse manager role was established to increase the level of clinical leadership and supervision across nursing afterhours (Fossum et al. 2019). The AHNM position is concerned with ensuring that wards/units are staffed, while at the same time ensuring patient and staff movement in order to apply and meet triage standards and early discharge protocols and policies, ultimately creating bed availability and providing staff that have the experience to meet care demands. The AHNM role requires clinical and managerial experience, and knowledge of the different operational policies concerned with admissions, discharges, transfers and ward protocols and staffing. This position also requires AHNMs to liaise and coordinate activities with other service providers both within and outside the hospital inclusive of other hospitals, care institutions e.g. aged care nursing homes, police, ambulance services and patient transport.

Director of nursing (DON) at hospital level/group of services

The Director of Nursing (or equivalent title) is a senior executive level in the health care setting. The DON plans, organizes, develops and directs the overall operations of the nursing service within the hospital setting. Nursing leaders such as the DONs work with other health service providers to maintain quality standards of care in accordance with Federal, State and facility standards, guidelines and regulations. DONs inform the strategic direction of Australia's health system and help drive change within organisations (Australian College of Nursing, 2017).

There are DONs for different services, for instance; Director of Clinical Services, Regional Director of Nursing, Director of Community Services and other speciality areas, e.g. aged care and mental health. This position holds oversight of the provision of quality patient care, provided in accordance with professional demands and standards (Greenwood, n. d). The DON position is a leadership position and DONs cultivate empowerment through their leadership practices and influence in the work environment (Rao & Evan, 2015). DONs provide leadership and engage clinical nurses as decision-making partners, while at the same time they are responsible for ensuring level of service and the quality of services is at the ultimate level to which the organisation can provide (Dyess et al., 2016).

Chief nurse (state and territory)

The chief nurse is the highest executive position at state/territory level within the Department of Health. This is highest position one can attain at country/national level. It also applies for a person working for global/international organisations like WHO and UNICEF and holds a position of a geographical regional director. The chief nurse position is a pivotal and critical role that mandates and oversees all nursing policies at the state level from strategic and directionally position. According to Queensland Department of Health (2013) The chief nurse create a compelling vision for the professional practice of nursing and midwifery through strategic thinking, nurses and midwifery workforce and organisational development, and business planning. More broadly and importantly they create and lead clinical practice; influencing the degree of innovation and excellence at every level of a health At this level, the concern is ensuring care delivery portfolio, growing, supporting and sustaining the workforce; and ensuring budget demands, and research and development and application of policies are carried in the areas that will provide the combined best benefit outcomes of service provision. The minimal qualification is often a Master's degree and other formal training such as certification in health management and or executive training can be of an advantage to this role.

Chief executive officers (CEO)

The role of the CEO is to lead the execution of strategies developed for the organization and to set the future direction of the organization/institution, (Keller, 2007 & Half, 2019). Managing large and complex organisations and institutions demand acumen of leadership and management skills. In today's complex business orientated work environment, organisations are expected to ensure the operation of the organisation are viable (Keller, 2007).

CEOs are the highest officers in an organisation. Nurses who become CEOs have positioned themselves by taking on different leadership operational roles that demonstrate leadership qualities.

Most CEOs have a degree and may also have Master's or PhD usually in management or business administration topped up with short courses e.g. executive management and other leadership short courses. Usually the additional credentials are attained even when one is already a CEO. Overall, literature reveals most CEOs need to have varied experience, to have worked in different areas of the health institutions, to have held various portfolios and have a good record of operational successes. The responsibilities of a CEO include overseeing, setting and establishing the business and management operations of the institution/organisation.

Section 3: Education pathway

It is important that nurses undertake learning to meet the challenges of a dynamic and ever-changing health care system (Qanbari Qalehsari et al., 2017). The nurses in education have many roles and include: hospital based clinical educator; hospital educator (or coordinator of professional development); lecturer in TAFE or other Registered Training Organisation (RTO), and academic within the university setting. Hospital based educator roles can take on many forms and are defined by the organisation. A clinical nurse educator is an RN with several years of nursing experience, but also has passion for teaching others. While some nurse educators have bachelor's degrees, it is more common for organisations to require clinical nurse educators to hold advanced degrees related to their field as well. Nurse educators in health care have a dynamic leadership role as clinical experts, role models, and mentors for junior nursing staff (Sayers et al., 2015)

Lecturers in nursing are mostly employed to prepare diploma level nurses (Enrolled Nurses) at a Technical and Further Education facility (TAFE) or RTO, or registered nurses through a degree program that leads to registration at a University. To work at a TAFE or RTO a 'Certificate IV in Training and Assessment' is required and to work as a lecturer in a University setting, a Master's degree or PhD are required.

Overview of academic roles

Teaching

Lecturers (University, TAFE or RTO) contribute to the teaching of the next generation of nurses at degree or diploma level and can include undergraduate and post-graduate studies. Some RNs change their career from clinical work to combine academic and clinical work or an academic role alone. A clear career structure is set out in academia with the opportunity to progress from the starting position of lecturer through to senior lecturer, associate professor, and professor of nursing, midwifery, or research.

Research pathway

Clinical research underpins evidence-based practice and improvement in nursing practice and health outcomes. The research career pathway provides nurses the opportunity to build a career that is intrinsically interlinked with practice and there are a number of roles in the research pathway outlined in Table 4.1.

Many hospitals and universities are affiliated with research centres and may offer secondments or research positions to build the research capacity of nurses. One example is the Nursing Research Institute (NRI), a collaboration between Australian Catholic University, St Vincent's Health Australia Sydney and St Vincent's Hospital Melbourne, see https://www.acu.edu.au/about-acu/institutes-academies-and-centres/nursing-research-institute for more information.

Table 4.1 Clinician researcher career pathway (Smith et al., 2018)

Role title	Min required qualification	AQF Level	Role expectation
Research Assistant	RN, Current good Clinical research practice (CRN) cert., Least 1-yr FTE post registration experience	5–7	Literature searches, data collection, conducting interview, data entry, and administrative functions
Predoctoral or doctoral clinical research fellow	Honours degree; Master of philosophy or Master of Research; Current CRN certificate, Least 3 years FTE post registration, with 2 years speciality experience	8–9	Initiates, conducts, and disseminates the findings of locally based research in their speciality. • Awarded internal or external research funding • Publishes >5 papers per year in peer reviewed journals, the majority as first author • Participates as a co-investigator with limited supervision on larger studies and contributes to dissemination of findings • Presents research at national conferences • Manages research projects • Responsible for the research funds and annual reporting expenditure
Postdoctoral clinical research fellow	PhD; Current good CRN certificate, Least 5 years FTE post registration, with 3 years speciality experience	10	• Conducts independent and/or team research • Builds a program of research in speciality practice • Publishes >7 papers per year in peer reviewed journals, the majority as first author. • Invited speaker at national conferences and/or chairs sessions at national and international conferences • Supervises honours and master's research students • Applies for external research project and fellowship funding • Volunteers for community presentations
Senior clinical research fellow	PhD; Current good CRN certificate, Least 7 years FTE post registration, with 5 years speciality experience	10	• Acts as a principal researcher in large scale research studies, that attract national research funding • Demonstrates leadership in research by developing research teams for local and small scale studies • Publishes >10 papers per year in peer reviewed journals, as first author for >30%. • Supervises PhD students and research support staff • Oversees the research group financial management, • Engages across organizations and with charitable bodies • Invited international speaker • Significant national and state involvement and leadership in professional activities

(Continued)

Table 4.1 Clinician researcher career pathway. (Smith et al., 2018) (*Continued*)

Role title	Min required qualification	AQF Level	Role expectation
Clinical associate professor	PhD; Current good Clinical research practice certificate	10	• Recognized as a research leader in their specialist field • Makes major contributions to the research activities • Awarded significant research funding • Conducts independent and team research and authors conference and seminar papers • Publishes as a senior author on publications • Supervises research support and administrative staff, • Takes a major role in all aspects of major research projects including management and/ or leadership of large research projects or teams • Prepares and supports others to prepare research funding submissions and provides oversight of financial management and reporting of monies received • Initiates and establishes, and promotes research links with national and or international bodies • Involvement and leadership in professional activities including invited speaker at national and international conferences and seminars in the field of expertise • Makes occasional contributions to teaching programs in affiliated universities • Substantial role in research capacity building and development of a research culture • Supervises higher degree research students involvement in the development of research policy, attendance at meetings associated with research or the work of the organizational unit.
Chair or clinical professor	PhD; Current good Clinical research practice certificate	10	• Same as Clinical associate professor, plus: • Demonstrates leadership and the pursuit of excellence in research in own area of research, in the organizational unit, within the affiliated university and within the scholarly and the wider community • involvement in the development of research policy, attendance at meetings associated with research or the work of the organizational unit to which committee work

Abbreviation: AQF, Australian qualifications framework

Research pathway scenario

Lara is a registered nurse who qualified four years ago with Bachelor of Nursing and began her career as an RN in Oncology ward in a large tertiary hospital. Lara was interested in research and applied for Master of clinical Nursing with specialisation in Oncology. After finishing her study, she worked two more years while getting involved in several research studies based in the ward. This experience increased her desire to be more involved in research. She applied to study a PhD in Nursing and worked as research assistant, collecting data, interviewing participants and analysing data, at the same university that she was studying.

Reflective questions

1 What do you think a PhD involves and what are the benefits of becoming a doctor in nursing?
2 If you are thinking of doing a PhD, what would be three steps to take to accomplish this?
3 What do you think would be the main responsibilities of a nurse researcher?
4 How do you see the role of a researcher in the disciplines of nursing or midwifery?

Section 4: Future challenges in career pathways for registered nurses

The future roles of registered nurses are influenced by many variables and include: population demographics; new technologies; funding; new treatments; and new infectious diseases. What is not always known is how this will look and predicting future career paths for the registered nurse is challenging.

However, we know that the health care system is dynamic and ever changing and therefore this necessitates a workforce which is adaptable and able to acquire new knowledge and skills and translate these to known and new care setting or models of practice. An example faced by the Australian health care system is an aging population and the high presence of multimorbidity (Johnson & Chang, 2021 in press). As Australia's ageing population continues to grow, demand for aged care workers will also grow (AIHW, 2000). This creates opportunities for people looking to pursue a career in aged care, but also creates challenges for the sector in attracting, training and retaining sufficient workforce. Indeed, these challenges are already being faced across the sector with providers reporting skills shortages and significant difficulties recruiting and retaining appropriately qualified staff. In order to meet future needs it will be crucial for the sector to adapt and adopt strategies that will ensure its ability to attract and retain a highly skilled and well-trained workforce. According to Ryan et al. (2018), nursing is one of the professions where there is recurrent shortage attributed to an ageing workforce, an ageing population and increased demands for health care.

Successfully managing your professional nursing career pathway requires careful consideration and planning. A deliberate and purposeful plan needs to be made to articulate the stages, the processes and preparation required to meet the desired goal. It is important to appraise your own personal performance and invite constructive feedback to encourage career development. It is also important to celebrate and document your success and achievements and to share these with others.

References

Australian College of Nursing (ACN). (2017). Nurse Leadership, ACN, Canberra. Retrieved from: https://www.acn.edu.au/wp-content/uploads/2017/10/acn_nurse_leadership_white_paper_reprint_2017_web.pdf

Australian College of Nursing. (2015). Nurse leadership white paper by ACN 2015. Retrieved from: https://www.acn.edu.au/wp-content/uploads/2017/10/acn_nurse_leadership_white_paper_reprint_2017_web.pdf

Alvernia University. (2019). The Herniary of Nursing, Retrieved from https://online.alvernia.edu/program-resources/hierarchy-of-nursing/

Australian Primary Health Care Nurses Association (APNA). (2019). Nursing in Primary Health Care Program Retrieved from: https://www.apna.asn.au/profession/niphc

Australian Primary Health Care Nurses Association. (2012). Definition of primary health care nursing. Retrieved from: https://www.apna.asn.au/files/DAM/2%20Careers/Primary%20health%20care%20nursing/DefinitionOfPrimaryHealthCareNursing.pdf

Australian Medicare Local Alliance. (2012). General practice nurse national survey report. Retrieved from: http://apna.asn.au

Australian Government Department of Health. (2016). Nurse and Midwives NHWDS. Retrieved from: https://hwd.health.gov.au/webapi/customer/documents/factsheets/2016/Nurses%20and%20Midwives%202016%20-%20NHWDS%20factsheet.pdf

Australian Nurses Midwifery Federation, (ANMF). (2018). Nurse and midwife unit manager new classification frequently asked questions. https://www.anmfvic.asn.au/~/media/cea05f54bdc249ee85fb97f6134aba40.pdf

AIHW (Australian Institute of Health and Welfare) (2000). Disability and ageing Australian population patterns and implications. Retrieved from: https://www.aihw.gov.au/reports/disability/disability-and-ageing-australian-population/contents/table-of-contents

Azad, N., Anderson, H.G., Brooks, A., Garza, O., O'Neil, C., Misty M. Stutz, M. M., & Sobotka, J. L (2017). Leadership and management are one and the same. *American Journal of Pharmaceutical Education*, *81*(6), 1–5. doi: 10.5688/ajpe816102

Baraz, S., Memarian, R., & Vanaki, Z. (2015). Learning challenges of nursing students in clinical environments: A qualitative study in Iran. *The Journal of Education and Health Promotion* 4(1), 52, 1–10,. DOI:10.4103/2277-9531.162345

Bettencourt, E. (2016). The Importance of Strong Nurse Management. Diversity Nursing Com. Retrieved from http://blog.diversitynursing.com/blog/the-importance-of-strong-nurse-management

Carter McNamara, C. (2019). Roles and Responsibilities of Chief Executive Officer of a Corporation. Retrieved from https://managementhelp.org/chiefexecutives/job-description.htm

Cashin, A., Stasa, H., Gullick, J., Conway, R., & Buckley, T. (2014). Clarifying clinical nurse consultant work in Australia: A phenomenological study. *Collegian*, *22*, 405–412. DOI: http://dx.doi.org/10.1016/j.colegn.2014.09.002

Chisengantambu, C., Robinson, G. M., & Evans, N. (2017). Nurse managers and the sandwich support model. *Journal of Nursing Management 26*(4), 192–199. https://doi.org/10.1111/jonm.12534

Coffey, J. S., & White, B. L. (2019). The clinical nurse educator role: A snapshot in time. *The Journal of Continuing Education in Nursing*, *50*(5), 228–232. DOI:10.3928/00220124-20190416-09

Creasey, T., (n.d). In Introduction to Change Management. Prosci, retrieved from https://cdn2.hubspot.net/hubfs/367443/2.downloads/ebooks/An-Introduction-Guide-to-Change-Management-guide.pdf?__hstc=59013810.8c77143d5bcc9cd394824b376d4b5541.1573514485456.1573514485456.1573514485456.1&__hssc=59013810.1.1573514485456&__hsfp=888501586

Croteau, J. D., & Wolk, H. G. (2010). Defining advancement career paths and succession plans: Critical human capital retention strategies for high-performing advancement divisions. International Journal of Educational Advancement, *10*(2), pp. 2, 59–70. Retrieved from file:///H:/Book%20Manuscript/Croteau-Wolk2010_Article_DefiningAdvancementCareerPaths.pdf

Daly, J., Jackson, D., Mannix, J., Davidson, P. M., & Hutchinson, M. (2014). The importance of clinical leadership in the hospital setting. *Journal of Healthcare Leadership*, *2014*(6), pp. 75–83.

Dalton, K. (2010). *Leadership and Management Development: Developing Tomorrow's Managers* (First Ed). Pearson Education: Canada.

DeLaune, S. C., Ladner, P. K., McTier, L., Tollefson, J., & Lawrence, J. (2020). *Fundamentals of nursing* (2nd ed). South Melbourne, VIC: Cengage.

Dixit, S. K., & Sambasivan, M. (2018). A review of the Australian healthcare system: A policy perspective. *SAGE Open Med.*, 6: 1–14, doi: 10.1177/2050312118769211. Retrieved from https://www.ncbi.nlm.nih.gov/pmc/articles/PMC5900819/

Duggal, N. (2019). What's the Difference Between Leadership and Management? Retrieved from https://www.simplilearn.com/leadership-vs-management-difference-article?source=frs_author_page

Dyess, S., Sherman, R., Pratt, B., & Chiang-Hanisko, L. (2016). "Growing Nurse Leaders: Their Perspectives on Nursing Leadership and Today's Practice Environment". *OJIN: The Online Journal of Issues in Nursing, 21*(1), DOI: 10.3912/OJIN.Vol21No01PPT04

Englebright, J. (2008). *The chief nurse executive role in large healthcare systems, 32*(3), 188–194. doi: 10.1097/01.NAQ.0000325175.30923.ff

Fossum, M., Hewitt, N., Weir-Phylandb, J., Keoghb, M., Stuart, J., Fallonb, K., & Bucknall, T. (2019). Providing timely quality care after-hours: Perceptions of a hospital model of care. *Collegian, 26*, pp. 16–21.

Glick, M. B. (2011). The Role of Chief Executive Officer. *Advances in Developing Human Resources (ADHR), 13*(2), pp. 171–207.

Greenwood, B. (n.d) The qualities of a nurse manager. *Work - Chron.com*, Retived from qualities-nurse-manager-6812.html. http://work.chron.com/Accessed 26 August 2019.

Halcomb, E., & Ashley, C. (2016). Australian primary health care nurses most and least satisfying aspects of work. *Journal of Clinical Nursing, 26*, 535–545. DOI 10.1111/jocn.13479.

Half, R. (2019). How to become a CEO: What makes a great chief executive? Retrieved from https://www.roberthalf.com.au/blog/jobseekers/how-become-ceo-what-makes-great-chief-xecutive

Health Education and Training Institute (HETI). (2019). Retrieved from https://www.heti.nsw.gov.au/about-heti

Jerome, N. (2013). Application of the Maslow's hierarchy of need theory; impacts and implications on organizational culture, human resource and employee's performance. *International Journal of Business and Management Invention, 2*(3), 39–45. Retrieved from https://pdfs.semanticscholar.org/b0bc/c8ca45193eaf700350a8ac2ddfc09a093be8.pdf

Joseph, M. L., & Huber, D. L. (2015). Clinical leadership development and education for nurses: Prospects and opportunities. *Journal of Healthcare Leadership, 7*, pp. 55–64. Doi: 10.2147/JHL.S68071

Keller, S. P. (2007). The CEO's role in leading transformation. McKinsey & Company Retrieved from https://www.mckinsey.com/business-functions/organization/our-insights/the-ceos-role-in-leading-transformation

Masso, M., & Thompson, C. (2014). Nurse practitioners in NSW 'gaining momentum': rapid review of the nurse practitioner literature. Retrieved from: https://www.health.nsw.gov.au/nursing/practice/Publications/nurse-practitioner-review.pdf

McGagh, J., Marsh, H., Western, M., Thomas, P., Hastings, A., Mihailova, M., & Wenham, M. (2016). Review of Australia's research training system: Report for the Australian Council of Learned Academies. Retrieved from: www.acola.org.au

New South Wales Health (n.d). Nursing and Midwifery. Heading in the right direction for a career in Nursing/Midwifery Management. Retrieved from https://mnclhd.health.nsw.gov.au/wp-content/uploads/NurseMidwiferyManager.pdf

Nursing and Midwifery Board of Australia. (2016). Registration standard: Endorsement as a nurse practitioner. Retrieved from: https://www.nursingmidwiferyboard.gov.au/Registration-Standards/Endorsement-as-a-nurse-practitioner.aspx

Nursing and Midwifery Board of Australia. (2016a). Registered nurse standards for practice: Retrieved from: https://www.nursingmidwiferyboard.gov.au/Codes-Guidelines-Statements/Professional-standards/registered-nurse-standards-for-practice.aspx

Nursing and Midwifery Board of Australia. (2017). Nurse practitioner standards for practice – effective from 1 January 2014. Retrieved from: https://www.nursingmidwiferyboard.gov.au/Codes-Guidelines-Statements/Professional-standards/nurse-practitioner-standards-of-practice.aspx

Nursing Research Institute (NRI). Retrieved from: https://www.acu.edu.au/about-acu/institutes-academies-and-centres/nursing-research-institute

NSW Government (n.d.). Nursing and Midwifery: Heading in the right direction for a career in Nursing/Midwifery Management. Retrieved from: https://mnclhd.health.nsw.gov.au/wp-c

Peters, K., McInnes, S., and Halcomb, E. (2015). Nursing students' experiences of clinical placement in community settings: A qualitative study. *Collegian, 22,* 175–181. Retrieved from: https://www.collegianjournal.com/article/S1322-7696(15)00016-5/pdf

Qanbari Qalehsari, M., Khaghanizadeh, M., & Ebadi, A. (2017). Lifelong learning strategies in nursing: A systematic review. *Electronic Physician Excellence in Constructive Peer Review,* 9(10), doi: 10.19082/5541, pp. 5541–5550.

Queensland Department of Health. (2013). The nurse executive role in quality and high performing health services: a position paper. Retrieved from: https://www.health.qld.gov.au/data/assets/pdf_file/0023/147353/nurrseexecpos.pdf

Rao, D., & Evans, L. K. (2015). The Role of Directors of Nursing in Cultivating Nurse Empowerment. *Annals of Long-Term Care: Clinical Care and Aging,* 23(4), pp. 27–32.

Royal Children's Hospital Melbourne Retrieved from: https://www.rch.org.au/nursing/nursing_opportunities/Nursing_Career_Pathway/

Ryan, C., Bergin, M., White, M., & Well, J.S.G. (2018). Ageing in the nursing workforce – a global challenge in an Irish context. *International Nursing Review,* 66(2), 157–164. https://doi.org/10.1111/inr.12482

Sayers, J., Lopez, V., Howard, P. B., Escott, P., & Cleary, M. (2015). The leadership role of nurse educators in mental health nursing. *Issues in mental health nursing,* 36(9), 718–724.

Singh, S. (2000). Relationship between managers' authority power and perception of their subordinates' behaviour. *Indian Journal of Industrial Relations,* 35(3), 275–300. Retrieved from: https://www.jstor.org/stable/27767664

Skrobanski, H., Ream, E., Poole, K., & Whitaker, K. L. (2019). Understanding primary care nurses' contribution to cancer early diagnosis: A systematic review. *European Journal of Oncology Nursing,* 41, 149–164. DOI: https://doi.org/10.1016/j.ejon.2019.06.007

Smith, S., Gullick, J., Ballard, J., & Perry, L. (2018). Clinician researcher career pathway for registered nurses and midwives: A proposal. *International Journal of Nursing Practice,* 24(3), 1–10. https://doi.org/10.111/ijn.12640.

Smolowitz, J., Speakman, E., Wojnar, D., Ellen-Marie Whelan, E. M., Ulrich, S., Hayes, C., & Wood, L. (2014). Role of the registered nurse in primary health care: Meeting health care needs in the 21st century. *Nursing Outlook,* 63(2), pp. 130–136.

Thomas, T. W., Seifert, P. C., & Joyner, J. C. (2016). Registered nurses leading innovative changes. *The Online Journal of Issues in Nursing,* 21(3), 1–15. DOI:10.3912/OJIN.Vol21No03Man03

Thomas, T. H. T., Bloomfield, J. G., Gordon, C. J., & Aggar, C. (2017). Australia's first transition to professional practice in primary care program: Qualitative findings from a mix-method evaluation. *Collegian,* 25, 201–208. DOI: http://doi.org/10.1016/j.colegn.2017.03.009.

World Health Organization. (2014). Primary health care. Retrieved from http://www.euro.who.int/en/health-topics/Health-systems/primary-health-care

5 Mental well-being and resilience of nurses

Lynette Cusack and Janie Brown

Chapter objectives

This chapter will offer the reader:

- An understanding of what is well-being
- An understanding of why well-being is part of nursing students and registered nurses ongoing professional responsibilities
- An understanding of why a well workforce provides good quality and safe care
- An outline of the factors associated with poor well-being
- A description of resilience and some strategies for building and sustaining resilience

Introduction

As nursing students move through their undergraduate program, they will take on more professional responsibility, particularly while on clinical placement. Towards the end of the final year they will prepare for transition to registration and plan for future employment as new graduates. Throughout their years of training, nursing students will have had moments of high anxiety, which may have been very stressful, as well as moments of great satisfaction. Frequent changes of clinical placements in different health service environments, the introduction to shift work as well as the everyday challenges of maintaining commitments to study, family and friends and casual or part time work are difficult activities to juggle. Students and new graduates encounter stressors everyday within the education and practice environment. If nursing students or new graduates are not mindful of factors in the environment that cause them stress and the cumulative effect of these, they may become unwell, resulting in compassion fatigue and burnout (Rees et al 2016). Preparing for stressful situations and applying effective coping strategies (Alshahrani, Cusack, Rasmussen 2018) for these high stress times are important skills for nurses to learn as students and to take with them as new graduates in their registered nurse (RN) role. This chapter offers nursing students and new graduates insights into why their wellness and resilience matters for themselves and for the patients in their care. The chapter describes some strategies to help students and new graduates to recognise when they need to take extra care of themselves and how to build their resilience.

Definition of well-being

Well-being is a state of health (World Health Organisation, 1948). The World Health Organization's (WHO) 1948 definition of health as a 'state of complete physical, mental and social wellbeing and not merely the absence of disease or disability' is still relevant today. Health is a dynamic condition resulting from the body's constant adjustment and adaptation in response to stresses and changes in the environment. This response maintains an inner equilibrium called homeostasis. Proceedings from the 'First International Conference on Health Promotion', in 1986 in Ottawa recognised that to reach a state of complete physical, mental and social wellbeing, an individual or group must be able to identify and to realize aspirations, to satisfy needs, and to change or cope with the environment (World Health Organisation, 2009). Health promotion and building resilience strategies assist to achieve and maintain well-being.

Importance for health professionals to maintain their well-being

In Australia, nursing and midwifery are regulated professions under the Health Practitioner Regulation National Law 2009 (the National Law), in force in each state and territory. The Nursing and Midwifery Board of Australia (NMBA) has specific roles under the National Law. One of the NMBA's main roles is to protect the public. It does this by developing standards, codes and guidelines that together establish a professional practice framework that sets out the expectations for professional and safe practice of nurses and midwives (Please refer to Chapter 1). One of the important documents within the professional practice framework is the Code of Conduct (Nursing and Midwifery Board of Australia, 2018). Within the Code of Conduct, Principle 7: Health and Well-being states that there is an expectation that nurses, midwives and students 'promote health and well-being for people and their families, colleagues, the broader community and themselves ...' (p14).

The National Law states that students undertaking clinical training placements in a health profession must be registered in the interests of protecting the public's safety in much the same way that health practitioners must be registered. Nursing students are registered by their education provider with the Australian Health Practitioner Regulation Agency (AHPRA) for the NMBA. There are no fees for student registration. Students must be aware that the National Boards can act on student impairment matters or when there is a legal conviction of a serious nature that may impact on public safety (Health Practitioner Regulation National Law (South Australia) Act 2009). Therefore, it is important that students learn to look after their own mental and physical well-being early on in their education program as well as when they register and practice in their profession.

It is well reported in the literature that nurse burnout can potentially impact clinical performance, patient safety, and increase the turnover of nurses (Foureur, Besley, Burton, Yu, & Crisp, 2013; Hall, Johnson, Watt, Tsipa, & O'Connor, 2016). If a student or RN is not feeling well either physically or mentally, then concentrating and making critical decisions can be difficult. This has the potential to lead to mistakes that can have serious consequences for patients for example, not checking medications correctly before they are administered to a patient. Also the ability to empathise, have patience and effectively communicate may be affected, which could lead to the nurse being rude and/or aggressive to patients, their families/carers and colleagues resulting in a complaint about their behaviour. No matter in what context you practice nursing, whether it is in the emergency department, paediatrics, medical wards or aged care there are different stressors in the environment that affect people differently. Being mindful and aware about how one is feeling emotionally and physically is an important attribute that will be discussed later in this chapter.

Factors associated with poor well-being

At times throughout our personal and working lives we all experience periods of sadness, worry, emotional fragility and unusual physical symptoms. We can often isolate a reason for our feelings. Perhaps there may be strained relationships within the family or there is an impending event such as an exam. Usually the symptoms are short lived and over a period of time our feelings tend to return to where they were before the event. We may experience many similar episodes of momentary anxiety or distress throughout our lives, but we can usually continue with our daily activities and the levels of anxiety or stress subside.

However, sometimes we experience situations or events that provoke feelings that are not as transient and from which we may not recover as easily or as quickly. This is especially the case for people who work in high stress, high stakes, chaotic and traumatic environments and roles. Many student nurses and new graduates are exposed to these types of environments in clinical practice. The events experienced while on clinical placement or in a transition to practice program can be unpredictable and may expose students and new graduates to a range of occupational stressors. This can include exposure to a violent patient, lack of resources, failed resuscitation of a deteriorating patient, and family grief due to a dying patient.

It is likely that students and new graduates will be exposed to situations where patients and their families are experiencing traumatic and life changing events. Repeated exposure to these types of experiences may cause vicarious or secondary trauma for the student or new graduate.

> Nurses are continually exposed to stressful events in their day-to-day work and are at risk for the negative effects of stress. A potential consequence of such caring work has a negative and profound effect on nurses, and it is sometimes referred to as compassion fatigue or secondary traumatic stress (Sabo, 2006 quoted by Yang & Kim 2012)

Where coping strategies are ineffective, students can feel a heightened sense of concern and vulnerability as they are not able to disconnect from the situations. This inability to disconnect may be experienced through a continued feeling of sadness about a patient's situation. Another example is when an incident at work continues to be replayed in their mind over and over again, which leads to a feeling of anxiety and affects the ability to sleep. The first signs that a student or new graduate might be having difficulty coping with their situation are prolonged emotional reactions that manifest as more than sadness and concern. Students may start to experience anxiety, depression and changes in their ability to think and reason clearly and react appropriately.

Anxiety is a treatable mental health disorder. The experience of anxiety is a normal part of the human condition. Everyone experiences anxiety in varying degrees. Anxiety disorders range from feelings of uneasiness to immobilizing bouts of terror. It is characterised by feelings of extreme nervousness about an upcoming event, dread or even a sense of impending doom. Physical symptoms may include shortness of breath, palpitations, dry mouth, sweating, diarrhoea and elevated blood pressure (Muir-Cochrane, O'Kane, & Harrison, 2017). If people experience ongoing anxiety they may adopt poor coping strategies that involve the use of alcohol and other drugs or avoidance of situations that make them anxious. Depression can be experienced both short term and long term if the feelings of depression and distress persist or keep on reoccurring. Depression can be caused through particular traumatic events in a person's life or are emotional problems associated with neurological and brain diseases (Beech, 2017).

Secondary traumatic stress comes about as a result of continual exposure to traumatic events that occur to people we know or care for. Students and new graduates are at risk of secondary traumatic stress because of the types of situations that arise in the clinical environment. They will also be witness to the struggles of classmates and peers when they are studying and working together (Figley, 1995; Hegney, Rees, Eley, Osseiran-Morrison, & Francis, 2015).

When constantly exposed to stressors in the absence of effective coping strategies, there is a potential for students, new graduates and experienced registered nurses to develop burnout and compassion fatigue. Burnout comprises a number of feelings and symptoms including emotional exhaustion that often comes with a loss of energy, a decreased enthusiasm for work and personal life, and feelings of self-doubt and lack of control.

Due to the nature of caring work it is also possible that nursing students and nurses develop compassion fatigue, which is a type of occupational burnout (Pines & Maslach, 1978; Rees, Breen, Cusack, & Hegney, 2015). This occurs because the constant need to provide compassion and empathy can simply become overwhelming.

Ideally students and new graduates should derive satisfaction with their work and with their achievements. This is called compassion satisfaction when applied to work undertaken by caring for people and is characterised by the positive feelings that come from helping someone else during a traumatic experience (Craigie et al., 2016; Stamm, 2010). When students and new graduates notice that there are more negative feelings such as stress, anxiety and depression than positive feelings such as compassion satisfaction, they are becoming vulnerable to burnout and compassion fatigue. Taking stock of the situation early can provide the opportunity to intervene.

Box 5.1 - Case study (Jenny)

Jenny, a final year nursing student, had been assigned to a paediatric ward while on clinical placement where she looked after a number of children who were terminally ill. Jenny felt the intense grief of the children's parents, grandparents and siblings. On graduation, Jenny started work as a RN on an adult palliative care ward where once again she experienced the death of patients and the grief of their family. Jenny started to have the same intense feeling of sadness that she had previously expereinced on the peadiatric ward and became so overwhelmed with sadness that all she wanted to do was sleep. She became withdrawn and stopped going out with her friends. She also felt that she was failing as a new graduate and started to avoid going to work. This change in behaviour was noted by the nurses on the ward who, concerned for Jenny, contacted the Nurse Unit Manager (NUM). The NUM made time to meet with Jenny to discuss the observations of the changes in behaviour and Jenny's increased use of sick leave. The NUM offered extra support, provided helpline/counselling information as well as encouragement for Jenny to contact her general practitioner.

Maintaining resilience and staying well

Not everyone finds the same situations to be stressful. Two nursing students can be exposed to the same situation and have completely different reactions. One may be able to continue with daily life largely unaffected, while the other experiences some or all of the emotional and physical symptoms described earlier for a prolonged period of time. The ability to cope in stressful situations on an ongoing basis is known as resilience.

> There are a number or definitions for resilience however psychological resilience has been defined as the ability of a person to recover, rebound, bounce-back, adjust or even thrive following misfortune, change or adversity (Garcia-Dia et al., 2013)

Many people describe resilience as being able to bounce back after a traumatic event rather than snapping under pressure, a bit like a tree bending but not snapping in a strong gust of wind and returning to its upright position after the storm. While many students and new graduates are naturally resilient people, there are periods in life when we are all more susceptible to negative consequences as a result of the stressors we face. It is important, therefore, to build resilience and sustain it throughout our careers. It is also important to ensure that nursing students and new graduates are able to cope in the workplace, because patient safety depends on it and nurses are more likely to leave the profession if they are experiencing negative psychological consequences such as anxiety, depression, stress and burnout (Mealer et al., 2012; Perry et al., 2017). Being resilient has been found to increase the likelihood that an individual will persist with work and/or study while experiencing difficulties. Being resilient also enables some people to grow personally from these difficult experiences (Cope, Jones, & Hendricks, 2016).

There are a number of things that students and new graduates can do to remain emotionally well despite the stressors that they encounter. They can engage in reflective practices such as writing down the events that have caused emotional feelings that won't go away and identifying strategies to deal with them. Little changes can make a big difference. For instance, if leaving the house on time in the mornings is stressful, consider preparing everything the evening before and setting the alarm for 15 minutes earlier. However, strategies to help address stressors are not always as straightforward as being more prepared and resetting the alarm clock. We can't always change things, so we need to develop strategies to cope with stress from the situations we do experience but cannot control. Some effective strategies include developing and maintaining a good balance between study or work and other enjoyable activities. The Headington Institute Self Care and Lifestyle Balance Inventory (link is provided at the end of the chapter) provides an indicator of your own work life balance and in doing so highlights a number of ways to get the balance right. Using these approaches has been shown to be effective in lowering rates of burnout and improving coping in nursing students (Rees et al., 2016). It is important to note that sometimes we can make individual change, but on its own this may not be enough to make us feel better. The environment we are in when learning or working as health professionals may also need to change, to promote resilience in individuals (Cusack et al., 2016; Rees et al., 2019).

Box 5.2 - Case study (Annabelle)

Annabelle, a new graduate who has been working in a health service for 7 months, finds that her father has been diagnosed with lung cancer. She is finding it difficult to cope with the demands of her work in intensive care, and with her parents and siblings anxiety and grief. She has also recently bought a house with a large mortgage repayment. The concerns about making the mortgage repayments weigh heavily on her mind. Annabelle starts to find that she is unable to concentrate at work. She receives constant anxious phone calls from her mother and siblings while she is at work. Her colleagues start to become less supportive as time goes on due to Annabelle's increasing unreliability while at work. One of her colleagues asked at a tea break if she was okay. Annabelle discloses that she is not sleeping, feels anxious all the time and struggles to get to work. Her colleague gives her the number of the EAP, assuring her that interactions with the EAP are confidential. Annabelle contacts the program where counsellors are able to assist her to access other resources, to develop a plan to move forward and to adopt positive coping strategies.

Summary

In this chapter we have discussed why it is important to become and remain well. Nursing students and new graduates are an important part of a regulated profession because they are the future nursing workforce. This means that there are responsibilities that individuals working within the profession must consistently meet. These are responsibilities for safe care to patients, maintaining community trust in the profession and to look after your own well-being. It is therefore necessary that all students and new graduates take the time to consider their own feelings of well-being, to put in place coping strategies for the challenges ahead, and to sustain the ability to bounce back and grow. Most important of all is to know when to get help.

Resources

- Nurse Midwife Support: 24-hour free confidential telephone counselling service for nurses, midwives and nursing and midwifery students.
- Every University has a student counselling service. Find out what they offer and keep the contact details with you. (You may have to pass it onto a friend.)
- Health Service Employers also have an Employee Assistance Programs (EAP) that you can access once you are registered and working. Take the time to find out the name of the EAP and contact details.
- There are also some Mindfulness Training Apps that can be downloaded onto your phone for regular access.
- Learn to relax. Explore meditation, a sporting or any other activity that positively helps you to relax.

Online resources

1 Proqol: https://www.proqol.org/
2 The Headington Institute Self Care and Lifestyle Balance Inventory: https://www.headington-institute.org/files/test_self-care-and-lifestyle-inventory_best_76305.pdf

References

Alshahrani, Y., Cusack, L., & Rasmussen, P. (2018). Undergraduate nursing students' strategies for coping with their first clinical placement: Descriptive survey study. *Nurse Education Today*, Oct; *69*, 104–110.

Beech, I. (2017). The person who experiences depression. In M. Chambers (Ed.), *Psychiatric and mental health nursing: The craft of caring* (3rd ed.). New York: Routledge.

Cope, V., Jones, B., & Hendricks, J. (2016). Why nurses chose to remain in the workforce: Portraits of resilience. *Collegian, 23*(1), 87–95.

Craigie, M., Osseiran-Moisson, R., Hemsworth, D., Aoun, S., Francis, K., Brown, J., … Rees, C. (2016). The influence of trait-negative affect and compassion satisfaction on compassion fatigue in Australian nurses. *Psychological Trauma: Theory, Research, Practice and Policy, 8*(1), 88–97.

Cusack, L., Smith, M., Hegney, D., Rees, C. S., Breen, L. J., Witt, R. R., … Cheung, K. (2016). Exploring environmental factors in nursing workplaces that promote psychological resilience: Constructing a unified theoretical model. *Front. Psychol.*, 13 May 2016, *7*(600), 1–8. doi: 10.3389/fpsyg.2016.00600

Figley, C. R. (1995). *Compassion fatigue: Coping with secondary traumatic stress disorder in those who treat the traumatized.* New York: Brunner/Mazel.

Foureur, M., Besley, K., Burton, G., Yu, N., & Crisp, J. (2013). Enhancing the resilience of nurses and midwives: Pilot of a mindfulness based program for increased health, sense of coherence and decreased depression, anxiety and stress. *Contemporary Nurse, 45*(1), 114–125.

Garcia-Dia, M.J., DiNapoli, J.M., Garcia-Ona, L., Jakubowski, R., & O'Flaherty, D. (2013). Concept analysis: Resilience. *Arch.Psychiatr.Nurs., 27*, 264–270. doi: 10.1016/j.apnu.2013.07.003

Hall, L. H., Johnson, J., Watt, I., Tsipa, A., & O'Connor, D. B. (2016). Healthcare staff well-being, burnout, and patient safety: A systematic review. *PloS One, 11*(7), e0159015–e0159015.

Health Practitioner Regulation National Law Act 2009 (Queensland)

Hegney, D., Rees, C. S., Eley, R., Osseiran-Morrison, R., & Francis, K. (2015). The contribution of individual psychological resilience in determining the professional quality of life of Australian nurses. *Front. Psychol.*, 21 October 2015. https://doi.org/10.3389/fpsyg.2015.01613

International Council of Nurses. (2012). *The ICN code of ethics for nurses.* Geneva.

Mealer, M., Jones, J., Newman, J., McFann, K. K., Rothbaum, B., & Moss, M. (2012). The presence of resilience is associated with a healthier psychological profile in intensive care unit (ICU) nurses: Results of a national survey. *International Journal of Nursing Studies, 49*(3), 292–299.

Muir-Cochrane, E., O'Kane, D., & Harrison, K. (2017). The person who expereinces anxiety. In M. Chambers (Ed.), *Psychiatric and mental health nursing: The craft of caring.* New York: Routledge.

Nursing and Midwifery Board of Australia. (2007). A national framework for the development of decision-making tools for nursing and midwifery practice.

Nursing and Midwifery Board of Australia. (2016a). *Guidelines for continuing professional development.* Melbourne: NMBA.

Nursing and Midwifery Board of Australia. (2016b). *Registered nurse standards for practice.*

Nursing and Midwifery Board of Australia. (2018). *Code of conduct for nurses* Retrieved from https://www.nursingmidwiferyboard.gov.au/Codes-Guidelines-Statements/Professional-standards.aspx

Perry, L., Xu, X., Duffield, C., Gallagher, R., Nicholls, R., & Sibbritt, D. (2017). Health, workforce characteristics, quality of life and intention to leave: The 'Fit for the Future' survey of Australian nurses and midwives. *Journal of Advanced Nursing, 73*(11), 2745–2756.

Pines, A., & Maslach, C. (1978). Characteristics of staff burnout in mental health settings. *Psychiatric Services, 29*(4), 233–237.

Rees, C. S., Breen, L. J., Cusack, L., & Hegney, D. G. (2015). Understanding individual resilience in the workplace: The international collaboration of workforce resilience model. *Front. Psycol.* 6:73. doi: 10.3389/fpsyg.2015.00073

Rees, C. S., Eley, R., Osseiran-Moisson, R., Francis, K., Cusack, L., Heritage, B., & Hegney, D. G. (2019). Individual and environmental determinants of burnout among nurses. *Journal of Health Services Research & Policy*, *24*(3), 191–200.

Rees, C. S., Heritage, B., Osseiran-Moisson, R., Chamberlain, D., Cusack, L., Anderson, D., ... Hegney, D. G. (2016). Can we predict burnout among student nurses? An exploration of the ICWR-1 model of individual psychological resilience. *Front. Psychol.*, 19 July 2016. https://doi.org/10.3389/fpsyg.2016.01072.

Rozo, J, A., Olson, D. M., & Thu H. (2017). Situational factors associated with burnout among emergency department nurses. *Workplace Health & Safety*, *65*(6): 262–265.

Stamm, B. (2010). *The Concise ProQOL Manual.*

World Health Organisation. (1948). Constituion. https://www.who.int/about/who-we-are/constitution.

World Health Organisation. (2009). *Milestones in health promotion: Statements from global conferences*, Geneva, Switzerland.

Yang, Y. H. & Kim, J. K., (2012). A literature review of compassion fatigue in nursing. *Korean Journal of Adult Nursing*, *24*(1), 38–51.

6 Aboriginal and Torres Strait Islander health

Faye McMillan, Linda Deravin and Glenda McDonald

Chapter objectives

This chapter will offer the reader:

- An understanding of the meanings of health from an Aboriginal and Torres Strait Islander perspective
- A brief overview of the impact of European colonisation on Aboriginal and Torres Strait Islander peoples in relation to health outcomes
- An overview of the Australian health care system including Australian Indigenous health services
- An understanding of culturally appropriate care when delivering health services to Aboriginal and Torres Strait Islander people.

Introduction

European colonisation of Australia has had a significant impact on the health and well-being of Aboriginal and Torres Strait Islander peoples (Aboriginal and Torres Strait Islander Social Justice Commissioner, 2005). It is well recognised that Aboriginal and Torres Strait Islander people have higher mortality and morbidity rates and that the gap in life expectancy is approximately 10 years less for both males and females compared to that of the Australian non-Indigenous population (Australian Bureau of Statistics, 2018). For a nation that prides itself on being advanced and a 'lucky' country for its people this is an unacceptable state of affairs. Since the Australian government's official 'Apology' to the Aboriginal and Torres Strait Islander people in 2008, especially to the members of the Stolen Generations and their descendants, substantial steps have been taken towards improving Aboriginal and Torres Strait Islander people's general health and well-being through the Closing the Gap initiative (Australian Indigenous HealthInfoNet (AIHW), 2015; Council of Australian Governments, 2008). Still more can be done before actual and sustained health improvements are felt by Aboriginal and Torres Strait Islander communities across the country.

This chapter will explain Aboriginal and Torres Strait Islander meanings of the term 'health'. It will also examine the impact of past treatment and historical government policies on the Aboriginal and Torres Strait Islander peoples of Australia and provide a critical commentary on the delivery of health services for this population. Finally the importance of providing culturally safe and appropriate nursing care will be explained and the contribution that nurses can make to influence health outcomes for Aboriginal and Torres Strait Islander people will be explored.

Meanings of health from Aboriginal and
Torres Strait Islander perspectives

Perspectives of health and health service delivery are universal topics of interest and concern, and they continue to evolve to meet market and sector demands worldwide. The experience of health for Indigenous peoples across the globe is specifically referenced in the United Nations Declarations on the Rights of Indigenous People (UN General Assembly, 2007), where health is positioned as a human right. The World Health Organization (WHO), in the Constitution of 1946, stated it was envisaged that '...the highest attainable standard of health [is] a fundamental right of every human being' (WHO, 2017, p1). However, the Australian health care landscape is fraught with institutional and interpersonal racism that affects organisations, individuals and communities (AIHW, 2018; Bourke, Marrie & Marrie, 2019).

If the premise of understanding health is the WHO definition and the Constitution of 1946, then health is determined through the perspectives of individuals and populations. The concept of health as experienced by Aboriginal and Torres Strait Islander peoples is complex and influenced by a number of factors. For Aboriginal and Torres Strait Islander people, culture is a considerable part of identity. Identifying which **mob** they may belong to, connections with **country** along with cultural history and ways of knowing, being and doing shape an individual's understanding of themselves, how they are within the world and how to interact with the world.

For Aboriginal and Torres Strait Islander peoples, the notion of health goes well beyond the physical health of the individual, to include the 'social, emotional and cultural well-being of the whole community' (Dudgeon, Wright, Paradies, Garvey, & Walker, 2014, p26). This perspective contributes to a holistic understanding of health. It speaks to the understanding that wellness is experienced outside of the 'Biomedical/ Medical Model' of health. It understands disease processes by considering how they impact on individual systems and the body as a whole (Chapman, 2018). Social, cultural, political and historical determinants all impact on health and well-being as parts of the holistic nature of health. Gee et al (2014, pp.57,63) illustrated the determinants of health (social and emotional well-being) for Aboriginal and Torres Strait Islander people and the influence of these determinants in the following diagrams (see figures 6.1 and 6.2).

The critical factor in understanding health from Aboriginal and Torres Strait Islander perspectives is acknowledging the dependent and interdependent relationships within and between these determinants and embedding this knowledge in the delivery of health services. The consultative process undertaken by the Australian Government upheld the centrality of culture when defining health for Aboriginal and Torres Strait Islander peoples and the right of individuals to experience a safe, healthy and empowered life (Department of Health and Ageing, 2013, p.9). This approach has also been expressed in the National Aboriginal and Torres Strait Islander Health Plan 2013–2023.

'Mob' refers to a group of people where traditional kinship ties exist. This collection of people includes immediate and extended family, a language group or people who identify as being part of a cohesive group with similar traditions, values and beliefs

'Country' is more than a geographical location for Indigenous people. It refers to a place where a community's traditions, law and culture are centred and includes the physical landscape, stories and special places that have particular meaning for that community

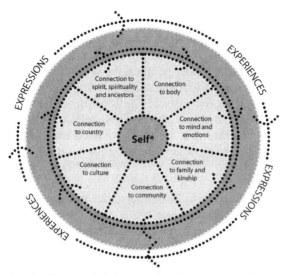

*This conception of self is grounded within a collectivist perspective that views the self as inseparable from, and embedded within, family and community.

©*Gee, Dudgeon, Schultz, Hart and Kelly,* 2013
Artist: Tristan Schultz, RelativeCreative.

Figure 6.1 The determinants of health for Aboriginal and Torres Strait Islander people (Part I)

Source: RelativeCreative

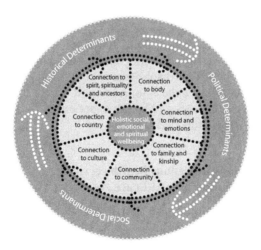

©*Gee, Dudgeon, Schultz, Hart and Kelly,* 2013
Artist: Tristan Schultz, RelativeCreative.

Figure 6.2 The determinants of health for Aboriginal and Torres Strait Islander people (Part II)

Source: RelativeCreative

Influence of history on Aboriginal and Torres Strait Islander health

The impact of colonisation on the health and well-being of Aboriginal and Torres Strait Islander peoples has been profound. However, the influence of history on Aboriginal and Torres Strait Islander peoples, the oldest living cultures on the planet as told from their histories, is truly remarkable. Aboriginal and Torres Strait Islander people's health was based on their direct relationship to the land and water within and external to the Nation (Behrendt, 2012). These relationships established and fostered positive health outcomes that were experienced individually but also collectively. This knowledge has been largely unrecognised within a colonised discourse, as Behrendt (2012) stated:

> Because Indigenous peoples built neither cities nor monuments, European cultures have tended to describe their societies as 'primitive'. This view assesses Indigenous cultures only from a comparison with technology in other parts of the world and fails to appreciate that, although many modern cultures are thousands of years old, Aboriginal cultures have been around for more than 60,000 years and, over that period of time, were able to manage all of the major issues that face a society — social cohesion, environmental destruction and degradation, sustainable population growth and renewable resources. On this assessment, some would argue that Aboriginal cultures are 'advanced' and some other modern cultures are "developing".

The process of colonisation within Australia and the impact of colonial practices upon Aboriginal and Torres Strait Islander peoples began a cycle of poor health outcomes for individuals and communities (Behrendt, 2012). Prior to colonisation the health status of Aboriginal and Torres Strait Islander peoples in Australia was significantly better than that experienced today. With colonisation came the introduction of diseases that had never been experienced on this continent and an interruption of sustainable living practices (Behrendt, 2012). Since colonisation, although the health outcomes of Australians have improved in general, they have not for Aboriginal and Torres Strait Islander peoples. This disparity is the continuing legacy of the processes, policies and laws introduced since the colonial establishment of Australia in 1788 that have directly impacted on the lives and health experienced by Aboriginal and Torres Strait Islander peoples (Behrendt, 2012).

Contemporary Australian Indigenous health services, organisations and distribution of healthcare resources

There are a variety of factors that have contributed to poor health outcomes within the Aboriginal and Torres Strait Islander population of Australia. Apart from the history of human rights and social injustices that have been inflicted upon Aboriginal and Torres Strait Islander peoples, the lack of access to the social determinants of health has further compounded poor health outcomes including; high unemployment rates, barriers to accessing health services, poor diet and nutrition, lack of housing or poor living conditions (Marmot, 2011). Reports from multiple agencies, including the Federal Government, have identified that health outcomes continue to be a major concern for the health and well-being of Aboriginal and Torres Strait Islander peoples

(Commonwealth of Australia, 2017; Deravin, Anderson, & Francis, 2018; Wright & Lewis, 2017). The Federal Government has tasked public health services with reducing this gap in health equity by making Aboriginal health a priority in the delivery of programs and services. However, public health services in Australia use the **Western medical model** of health care delivery, which itself is part of the problem as these services have historically not provided culturally safe or respectful health care (Molloy, 2017; Nielsen, Stuart, & Gorman, 2015). Hence, the establishment of health services led by a primary health care model and provided by Aboriginal Community Controlled Health Services has been crucial for improving the health and well-being of Aboriginal and Torres Strait Islander communities (Adams, 2009; Panaretto, Wenitong, Button, & Ring, 2014).

The Western medical model is a biomedical model of care that focuses on biological factors of health and does not consider psychological, environmental, spiritual and social influences that also have an impact on the health of individuals

---

To understand the need for the development of Aboriginal Community Controlled Health Services, it is relevant to review the health system. In Australia, nurses work within a complex and multifaceted system; incorporating both public and private organisations that provide health care to Australian citizens and residents who reside within its geographical boundaries. This system has been in place since the 1950's (Miles & Francis, 2019). The Commonwealth Government funds some nurses and midwives and other allied health professionals, such as Aboriginal Health Workers, to provide primary care services through the Medicare levy (Miles & Francis, 2019). The distribution of health care resources is based on population size within geographical areas and the national health priorities. The focus is on illness and treatments, whereas Aboriginal and Torres Strait Islander understandings of health extend beyond this. Until recently, mainstream health services did not accommodate for cultural differences. This is now changing through affirmative action from groups such as the Congress of Aboriginal and Torres Strait Islander Nurses and Midwives (CATSINaM) raising awareness regarding the lack of cultural safety and the need for health staff and systems to modify their approaches (McMurray & Clendon, 2015; Nagle, 2018). Chapter 2 has further information about the structure of the Australian health system.

An Aboriginal community controlled health service is a primary health care service which is managed by an elected Board of local Aboriginal community members. These services exist to deliver holistic and culturally appropriate health care to the community.

For over 30 years Aboriginal Community Controlled Health Services have demonstrated their ability to meet the needs of Aboriginal and Torres Strait Islander peoples through the provision of holistic and culturally safe care (Adams, 2009; Coombs, 2018). These services are also funded by the Commonwealth. The national peak body for Aboriginal health care, representing every community-controlled health service throughout Australia, is the National Aboriginal Community Controlled Health Organisation (NACCHO).

Primary Health Networks, which are independent companies funded by government, have historically provided financial support for Aboriginal Community Controlled Health Services. As Primary Health Networks are based on the Western model of health care delivery, have had limited engagement with ACCHSs and lack their understanding of Aboriginal health issues, the self-determination of Aboriginal Community Controlled Health Services is now at risk (Coombs, 2018). This situation appears contradictory to supporting Aboriginal and Torres Strait Islander peoples to access culturally appropriate health care and undermines their choice in determining where they wish to access health services (Coombs, 2018). In order to provide culturally safe and appropriate care to Aboriginal and Torres Strait Islander peoples a range of supportive health care strategies are needed (Campbell et al., 2018).

Cultural safety and culturally appropriate care

As discussed previously, the health system experiences of Aboriginal and Torres Strait Islander people have not always been positive. Encounters with Western medicine, inappropriate care and discriminatory treatment by health staff and systems have resulted in their reluctance to engage with mainstream health services. Nurses can help to bridge this gap in engagement by working alongside Aboriginal and Torres Strait Islander partners to affect changes within the health system and improve health outcomes (Deravin, Anderson, & Francis, 2017). The first step in this process is to gain an understanding of other cultures and to develop **cultural humility and capability** oneself (Department of Aboriginal and Torres Strait Islander Partnerships, 2016; Nagle, 2018).

Cultural humility – Recognising the difference between other cultures and your own with the intent of interacting in a non-discriminatory or unbiased way.

Cultural capability – the skills required to deliver services in a culturally respectful way

---

The provision of culturally safe environments within health services will require considerable effort from both organisations and individuals. In 2018 **cultural safety** became a professional requirement of registered nurses and midwives in Australia (Nursing and Midwifery Board of Australia (NMBA), 2018). This approach refocuses the evaluation of health care from the providers to the 'receivers'. The emphasis is on co-creation of health care environments and encounters that Aboriginal and Torres Strait Islander peoples determine are safe for them to engage in.

Measures to support a change in the health system environment started with raising awareness of cultural differences through staff education and training in the 1990's. This was extended to incorporate system-wide factors and the term **cultural respect** was adopted by governments as a way of strengthening relationships between Aboriginal and Torres Strait Islander peoples and the health care system (Bainbridge, McCalman, Clifford, & Tsey, 2015). Since the early 2000's the term **cultural competence** has evolved, with tertiary education organisations and health systems supporting staff to attain 'competence' in relation to Aboriginal and Torres Strait Islander peoples and cultures. However, cultural competence depends on the willingness of individuals who work in the health system to examine their preconceived ideas and beliefs about Aboriginal and Torres Strait Islander people. Only then is there any possibility of achieving the goal of cultural humility and capability, which is a combination of knowing, being and doing (see figure 6.3).

> The cultural safety of health professionals and services is determined by Aboriginal and Torres Strait Islander peoples and organisations themselves.

> Cultural competence: to gain an understanding of another person's culture through the development of an individual's knowledge and skill which allows that individual to work ethically in a range of personal and professional intercultural settings.

Education is a powerful tool in changing cultural attitudes within health services; however education needs to be supported by governments and policy (Commonwealth of Australia, 2017; Workforce Planning and Development, 2016). There are several ways this is being done in Australia. The Aboriginal and Torres Strait Islander Health Curriculum Framework (Commonwealth of Australia, 2016), provides guiding principles to tertiary educational institutions on how to incorporate Indigenous knowledge and understanding in courses for the health professions. The framework states that health professionals should undertake a discrete Indigenous health subject within approved and accredited health education programs. The Australian Nursing and Midwifery Accreditation Council (ANMAC) require all under-graduate nursing courses to include content specific to Aboriginal and Torres Strait Islander peoples. Laying the

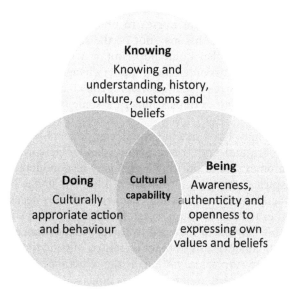

Figure 6.3 Adapted from the cultural capability framework

Source: Department of Aboriginal and Torres Strait Islander Partnerships, 2016

foundational work for future practitioners to adopt culturally safe practices is a good beginning. The existing health workforce also requires this education (McMurray & Clendon, 2015; Stuart & Nielsen, 2011).

The Nursing Standards for Practice in Australia direct that all nurses are to conduct themselves in a way that is respectful of Aboriginal and Torres Strait Islander cultures and experience (Australian Nursing and Midwifery Accreditation Council, 2017; Nursing and Midwifery Board of Australia, 2016, 2018). Failure to adhere to these standards may result in professional **censure**.

Censure – expression of disapproval and possibly disciplinary procedures.

Public health services in most states have mandated that all health staff should undertake cultural awareness training, such as Respecting the Difference in New South Wales (Health Education and Training Institute, 2019), or the South Australian Aboriginal Cultural Learning Framework (Department for Health and Ageing, 2017). Private health organisations and the aged care sector do not currently have these requirements but are strongly encouraged to show evidence of culturally safe practices when undertaking facility **accreditation**.

Accreditation – A system of independent external review that measures quality of services provided.

Cultural differences

Rituals, traditions, behaviours and beliefs differ between various Aboriginal nations across Australia. It is important for nurses to understand the local traditions, yet it should be acknowledged that this may not be the same for every Aboriginal and Torres Strait Islander person they come into contact with. Gaining an understanding of cultural differences may contribute to better engagement and communication between Aboriginal and Torres Strait Islander peoples and the staff who operate health services. The following examples illustrate some cultural differences for the nurse to consider.

Funerary practices may have specific ritual components, which are immensely important for an Aboriginal and Torres Strait Islander person and their community. Smoking ceremonies (use of burning herbs) may be conducted to encourage the deceased person's spirit to go away (McGrath & Phillips, 2008). This is a challenge within acute care facilities. 'Sorry' business occurs when it is necessary for communities to come together to mourn a family or community member's passing. For some Aboriginal people this may mean the need to travel great distances to participate in days of mourning and concurrently contact is limited outside the community group. Another custom in some Aboriginal nations is the reluctance to speak the deceased person's name for a period of 12 months. This is done so that the deceased person is not called back from the afterlife (McGrath & Phillips, 2008).

A common misunderstanding regarding communication in health services is the avoidance of eye contact when an Aboriginal person presents for care. For an

Aboriginal person, the avoidance of looking someone directly in the eye is a measure of respect whereas commonly within 'white' culture, avoiding eye contact is considered rude or could be perceived as the person not paying attention to what is being said.

Hierarchical and extended family responsibilities are different for Aboriginal and Torres Strait Islander people than for the mainstream Australian community. For example, the next of kin for an Aboriginal person, meaning the person who has the authority to consent (or not) to medical treatment, may not necessarily be the next direct blood relative. It may be a community Elder who holds this responsibility.

Conclusion

Nurses can make a significant difference in the health and well-being of Aboriginal and Torres Strait Islander peoples by supporting and providing culturally safe places wherever health services are delivered (Deravin et al., 2018). Through understanding the culture and history of Aboriginal and Torres Strait Islander peoples and acting as advocates for equality, understanding and respect, nurses can be the agents of change for improving health systems. The way Aboriginal and Torres Strait Islander peoples experience health services can be significantly improved. Recognising that an Aboriginal person has the right to self-determination in how they wish to engage with health services and respond to their own health needs, including using traditional healing methods as part of their treatment regime, should be supported and respected.

Resources

Australian Health Ministers' Advisory Council. (2017). *Aboriginal and Torres Strait Islander health performance framework- 2017 report.* Retrieved from https://www.pmc.gov.au/sites/default/files/publications/2017-health-performance-framework-report_1.pdf

Australian Human Rights Commission. (2009). Track the history timeline: The stolen generations. Retrieved from https://www.humanrights.gov.au/track-history-timeline-stolen-generations

Australian Indigenous HealthInfoNet. (2015). What is the history of Closing the Gap? Retrieved from http://www.healthinfonet.ecu.edu.au/closing-the-gap/key-facts/what-is-the-history-of-closing-the-gap

Australian Institute Health and Welfare. (2018). Aboriginal and Torres Strait Islander health performance framework (HPF) report 2017. Retrieved from https://www.aihw.gov.au/reports/indigenous-health-welfare/health-performance-framework/contents/tier-3-effective-appropriate-efficient/3-03-health-promotion

Gulanga Program. (2016). Preferences in terminology when referring to Aboriginal and/or Torres Strait Islander peoples. Retrieved from https://www.actcoss.org.au/sites/default/files/public/publications/gulanga-good-practice-guide-preferences-terminology-referring-to-aboriginal-torres-strait-islander-peoples.pdf

National Congress of Australia's First Peoples. (2016). Redfern Statement. Retrieved from https://nationalcongress.com.au/redfern-statement/

References

Aboriginal and Torres Strait Islander Social Justice Commissioner. (2005). Social justice report 2005 (Research Report No. 3/2005). Retrieved from https://www.humanrights.gov.au/sites/default/files/content/social_justice/sj_report/sjreport05/pdf/SocialJustice2005.pdf

Adams, M. (2009). Close the Gap: Aboriginal community controlled health services. *Medical Journal of Australia, 190*(10), 593–593. doi:10.5694/j.1326-5377.2009.tb02574.x

Australian Bureau of Statistics. (2018). Estimates of Aboriginal and Torres Strait Islander Australians, June 2016. Retrieved from http://www.abs.gov.au/ausstats/abs@.nsf/mf/3238.0.55.001

Australian Indigenous HealthInfoNet. (2015). What is the history of Closing the Gap? Retrieved from http://www.healthinfonet.ecu.edu.au/closing-the-gap/key-facts/what-is-the-history-of-closing-the-gap

Australian Institute of Health and Welfare. (2018). *Closing the gap targets: 2017 Analysis of progress and key drivers of change*. Canberra: AIHW.

Australian Nursing and Midwifery Accreditation Council. (2017). *Enrolled nurse accreditation standards 2017*. Retrieved from https://www.anmac.org.au/standards-and-review/enrolled-nurse

Bainbridge, R., McCalman, J., Clifford, A., & Tsey, K. (2015). *Cultural competency in the delivery of health services for Indigenous people*. Retrieved from https://apo.org.au/sites/default/files/resource-files/2015/07/apo-nid56408-1188591.pdf

Behrendt, L. (2012). *Indigenous Australia for dummies* (1st ed.). Milton, Qld: Wiley & Sons.

Bourke, C., Marrie, H., & Marrie, A. (2019). Transforming institutional racism at an Australian hospital. *Australian Health Review, 43*(6), 611–618. doi.org/10.1071/AH18062

Campbell, M., Hunt, J., Scrimgeour, D, Davey, M., & Jones, V. (2018). Contribution of Aboriginal community-Controlled Health Services to improving Aboriginal health: an evidence review. *Australian Health Review, 42*(2), 218–226. doi:10.1071/AH16149

Chapman, D. (2018). Understanding the biomedical model. Retrieved from https://www.nursespost.com/understanding-the-biomedical-model/

Commonwealth of Australia. (2016). *Aboriginal and Torres Strait Islander Health Curriculum Framework*. Retrieved from http://www.health.gov.au/internet/main/publishing.nsf/Content/72C7E23E1BD5E9CFCA257F640082CD48/$File/Health%20Curriculum%20Framework.pdf

Commonwealth of Australia. (2017). *Closing the gap: Prime Minister's report 2017*. Retrieved from https://www.pmc.gov.au/resource-centre/indigenous-affairs/closing-gap-prime-ministers-report-2017

Coombs, D. (2018). Primary Health Networks' impact on Aboriginal Community Controlled Health Services. *Australian Journal of Public Administration, 77*(S1), S37–S46.

Council of Australian Governments. (2008). *National partnership agreement on closing the gap in Indigenous health outcomes*. Retrieved from http://www.federalfinancialrelations.gov.au/content/npa/health_indigenous/ctg-health-outcomes/national_partnership.pdf

Department for Health and Ageing. (2017). *SA Health: Aboriginal Cultural Learning Framework*.

Department of Aboriginal and Torres Strait Islander Partnerships. (2016). Cultural Capability Matters: Queensland Government Aboriginal and Torres Strait Islander Cultural Capability Training Strategy. Retrieved from https://www.datsip.qld.gov.au/resources/datsima/involved/cultural-capability-training-strategy.pdf

Department of Health and Ageing. (2013). National Aboriginal and Torres Strait Islander Health Plan 2013–2023 Retrieved from https://www1.health.gov.au/internet/main/publishing.nsf/content/B92E980680486C3BCA257BF0001BAF01/$File/health-plan.pdf

Deravin, L., Anderson, J., & Francis, K. (2017). Choosing a nursing career: Building an Indigenous nursing workforce. *Journal of Hospital Administration, 6*(5), 27–30. doi:10.5430/jha.v6n5p27

Deravin, L., Anderson, J., & Francis, K. (2018). Closing the gap in Indigenous health inequity: Is it making a difference? *International Nursing Review, 65*(4), 477–483. doi:10.1111/inr.12436

Dudgeon, W., Wright, M., Paradies, Y., Garvey, D., & Walker, I. (2014). *Working together: Aboriginal and Torres Strait Islander mental health and wellbeing principles and practice* (pp. 3–24). Commonwealth Department of Health.

Gee, G., Dudgeon, P., Schultz, C., Hart, A., & Kelly, K. (2014). Aboriginal and Torres Strait Islander social and emotional wellbeing. *Working together: Aboriginal and Torres Strait Islander mental health and wellbeing principles and practice, 2*, 55–68.

Health Education and Training Institute. (2019). Aboriginal culture: Respecting the difference. Retrieved from https://www.heti.nsw.gov.au/education-and-training/courses-and-programs/aboriginal-culture-respecting-the-difference

Marmot, M. (2011). Global action on social determinants of health. *Bulletin of the World Health Organization, 89*(10), 702–702. doi:10.2471/BLT.11.094862

McGrath, P., & Phillips, E. (2008). Insights on end-of-life ceremonial practices of Australian Aboriginal peoples. *Collegian, 15*(4), 125–133.

McMurray, A., & Clendon, J. (2015). *Cultural inclusiveness: Safe cultures, healthy Indigenous people Community health and wellness: primary health care in practice* (5th ed.). Chatswood: Churchill Livingstone Elsevier.

Miles, M., & Francis, K. (2019). The Australian and New Zealand health care systems. In L. Deravin &J. Anderson (Eds.), *Chronic care nursing: A framework for practice* (2nd ed.). London: Cambridge University Press.

Molloy, L. (2017). Nursing care and Indigenous Australians: An autoethnography. *Collegian, 24*(5), 487–490. doi:10.1016/j.colegn.2016.10.011

Nagle, C. (2018). *Person first and business second: Towards cultural competence in nursing and midwifery* (Vol. 26, pp. 44–44). Australian Nursing & Midwifery Federation.

Nielsen, A. M., Stuart, L. A., & Gorman, D. (2015). Confronting the cultural challenge of the whiteness of nursing: Aboriginal registered nurses' perspectives. *Contemporary Nurse, 48*(2), 190–196. doi:10.1080/10376178.2014.11081940

Nursing and Midwifery Board of Australia. (2016). *Registered nurse standards for practice.* Retrieved from http://www.nursingmidwiferyboard.gov.au/Codes-Guidelines-Statements/Professional-standards.aspx

Nursing and Midwifery Board of Australia. (2018). *Midwife standards for practice.* Retrieved from https://www.nursingmidwiferyboard.gov.au/Codes-Guidelines-Statements/Professional-standards.aspx

Panaretto, K. S., Wenitong, M., Button, S., & Ring, I. T. (2014). Aboriginal community controlled health services: Leading the way in primary care. *Medical Journal of Australia, 200*(11), 649–652.

Stuart, L., & Nielsen, A-M. (2011). Two Aboriginal registered nurses show us why black nurses caring for black patients is good medicine. *Contemporary Nurse, 37*(1), 96–101. doi: 10.5172/conu.2011.37.1.096

UN General Assembly. (2007). United Nations declaration on the rights of Indigenous peoples. *UN Wash, 12*, 1–18.

Workforce Planning and Development. (2016). *Good Health - Great Jobs: Aboriginal Workforce Strategic Framework 2016–2020.* Retrieved from https://www1.health.nsw.gov.au/pds/ActivePDSDocuments/PD2016_053.pdf

World Health Organization. (2017). Human rights and health. Retrieved from https://www.who.int/news-room/fact-sheets/detail/human-rights-and-health

Wright, P., & Lewis, P. (2017). *Progress and priorities report 2017: Close the Gap Campaign Steering Committee.* Retrieved from https://www.humanrights.gov.au/sites/default/files/document/publication/Close%20the%20Gap%20report%202017.pdf

Part II

Nursing practice in Australia

Contemporary issues

Part II: Section I: Nursing in acute care contexts

7 Perioperative nursing

Christine Minty-Walker, Paul L Donohoe,
Suzanne E Hadlow and Nathan J. Wilson

Chapter objectives

This chapter will offer the reader:

- Insight into the perioperative nursing environment; history and the present.
- An outline of the three core areas of perioperative nursing.
- A description of contemporary contexts and the challenges faced by perioperative nurses.
- An overview of future challenges to nursing in the perioperative context.

Introduction

Perioperative nursing refers to patient care supporting transition through the preoperative, intraoperative and post-operative stages. Sometimes referred to as Operating Room, Operating Theatre or Operating Suite nursing, which relate mainly to the intraoperative stage, perioperative nursing encompasses far more than this. Unique to perioperative nursing is the responsibility of the nurse to be an advocate for the patient during every transitional stage of the perioperative journey where patient anxiety and fear are common. Perioperative nurses require expert knowledge and skills related to surgical procedures, methods of anaesthesia, technological equipment, effective communication skills, and to be constantly alert to the potential for rapid change in patient status. This chapter will unpack these issues to give both undergraduate and newly graduated nurses a rich insight into the complexities, challenges and rewards of perioperative nursing.

History of perioperative nursing

Until the development of modern anaesthetics, undergoing a surgical procedure was likely a painful and unpleasant experience. The first archaeological evidence of brain surgery was recorded by Hippocrates (460–355 BC) when cranial trepanation was performed; known today as a burr hole. This drilling into the skull relieved pressure on the brain or was used on mentally ill patients to release evil spirits (Arani, Fakharian & Sarbandi, 2012). Surgery, as it is known today, likely started around the 1800s. At this time, the operating theatre, where surgical procedures took place, were literally tiered theatres, where the public or students could observe, from above, the surgeons performing surgery. An example of this was the early 19th century gallery style operating theatre of St Thomas's Hospital in London. This was totally a unsterile environment, and during at that time the surgeons wore their everyday street clothes, used unsterilised instruments, and operated with their bare hands. Further, some procedures, such as limb amputations, took place while the patients were given alcohol or opium to numb the pain; the use of effective anaesthetics took some time to develop.

In the 1800s, the agent diethyl ether, or in 1847 Chloroform, was used to provide pain relief and induce loss of consciousness. These were effective, however were imperfect, especially Chloroform due to its delayed poisoning of patients (Thorpe & Spence, 1997). From 1956 a safer, non-toxic and non-combustible inhalation agent called halothane was introduced (Jones, 1990). Infection control practices also advanced and surgical instruments were boiled for sterilisation. Today heat is still used as a form of sterilisation for surgical instruments (Atkinson, 1992). The importance of aseptic technique emerged in the late 1800s with Joseph Lister's antiseptic principles of surgery that were built upon Louis Pasteur's germ theory (Callahan, Seifi & Holt, 2016). This meant that the wearing of caps, boots and gowns started to be required; these items of clothing are now known as theatre scrubs.

The existence of microscopic organisms – germs, can lead to disease (*Ouyang*, 2015)

The term perioperative nursing was adopted from the 1970s, where previously the term operating theatre nursing was applied (Hamlin, Richardson-Tench & Davies, 2009). Operating theatre nursing was a very prestigious profession from the 1800s onwards and was even embedded into the nursing curriculum in 1880. However, in the 1960s, the role of the perioperative nurse was increasingly seen as highly technical, and the perioperative nurse was seen more as the surgeon's handmaiden and hence the nursing specialty area started to lose its historical prestige (Wade, 2012).

Operating room technicians were employed in Canada in the 1980s partly in relation to a shortage of nurses (Wade, 2012). Today in places such as New Zealand, there are still anaesthetic technicians, in the United Kingdom there are non-nursing roles, and in the United States scrub technologists are employed (Hamlin, Davies, Richardson-Tench & Sutherland-Fraser, 2016). Within Australia, the Australian College of Perioperative Nurses (ACORN) advocates for the roles of scrub, scout, anaesthetic and recovery room to be performed by a nurse, and strongly resists these roles being replaced by ancillary workers (ACORN, 2012). ACORN have introduced professional practice standards for perioperative nursing, to set a public standard for what patients can expect from perioperative nurses. Additionally, ACORN provides educational events and activities to support the continuing professional development of perioperative nurses.

The present context of perioperative nursing

Perioperative settings are located in both public and private hospitals where surgical procedures are either elective/emergency or trauma. Major trauma facilities are located within larger public hospitals where trauma classification systems indicate the priority of treatment (Warren, Morrey, Oppy, Pirpiris & Balogh, 2019).

Surgical specialties include neurosurgery, ear, nose and throat, head and neck, dental, cardiothoracic, vascular, general, colorectal, gastroenterology, endoscopy, bariatric, orthopaedics, plastic and reconstructive, faciomaxillary, obstetrics and gynaecology, ophthalmology, paediatrics, and urology. Peripheral, or feeder facilities, tend to perform only certain categories and acuity of surgery, whilst larger metropolitan facilities cater for major trauma, burns and high acuity procedures such as organ transplant, robotic and laser surgery. Intensive care, high dependency and close observation units are also sized and funded to support the relevant operating facilities.

Many student nurses are first exposed to the operating suite during clinical placements where they learn that this area of nursing offers a trifecta of opportunity: anaesthetic, clinical (scrub and scout) and recovery room roles. Although different roles, critical to optimum patient outcomes are teamwork and collaborative practice between all members of the health care team. Perioperative nursing involves a patient journey as they transition through the various stages, where multiple handovers occur between the different nursing roles. An important role of perioperative nurses is patient advocacy, especially when the patient is anaesthetised or sedated. This role ensures that the patient's safety is protected, and the nurse will speak up on behalf of the patient if there is potential for harm (Hamlin, Davies, Richardson-Tench & Sutherland-Fraser, 2016). Being an advocate for the patient is aligned with the Code of Conduct for Nurses in Australia; taking a person-centred approach and being an advocate when necessary (Nursing and Midwifery Board of Australia, 2018).

Most operating suites around Australia will also have a day surgery unit adjacent to, or in close proximity to the operating suite. Over several decades, there has been an increased and improved flow of patients having day surgery procedures via day surgery admission. This gradual change has primarily been the result of major technological advances, shorter acting anaesthetics, and effective analgesia (Barnett, 2016). For example, a laparoscopic tubal ligation previously required open surgery, now performed using Minimally Invasive Surgery (MIS) techniques. MIS techniques can include a single-incision laparoscopic surgery (SILS) or natural-orifice transluminal endoscopic surgery (NOTES) (Hamlin, Davies, Richardson-Tench & Sutherland-Fraser, 2016). A secondary benefit to the increase in day surgery procedures has been the increased availability of hospital beds, as the patient admission and discharge occurs on the day of surgery.

Minimally Invasive Surgery (MIS) is undertaken with a small incision or no incision at all, using a cannula with laparoscope or an endoscope. (*Hamlin, Davies, Richardson-Tench & Sutherland-Fraser* 2016, p.387).

Preadmission clinics

With the ageing population and improvements in surgical techniques and equipment, together with advancement in anaesthesia, patients with many co-morbidities are now presenting for surgery. To enable timely and cost-effective admission of these patients, pre-admission clinics have been developed. A pre-operative patient may attend a pre-admission clinic up to a week before their surgery. This is an opportunity for surgical 'workup' or preparation to be attended and a review by the anaesthetist to determine baseline data and develop a plan for anaesthesia during surgery. This may include arranging for blood tests, electrocardiogram (ECG), cross matching of blood for the possibility of a blood transfusion, completion of health history, and appropriate referrals prior to the patient arriving for their surgery. Examples of nurse-initiated referrals might include to an occupational therapist where a patient is having major orthopaedic surgery and will likely require some home modifications to be in place after surgery and discharge.

This time is also a valuable opportunity for the nurse to discuss with the patient, the expectations and adjuncts such as patient controlled analgesia, sequential compression devices, oxygen and intravenous therapy. Strategies that a nurse may use to provide education include demonstrations with the actual device or going over education leaflets specific to a procedure. The clinics are effective in early preparation for patients with co-morbidities and have the potential to reduce the number of issues that can arise on admission to the ward environment on the day of surgery and the risk of cancellation of surgery.

> *A* sequential compression device is a sleeve-like device used on patients undergoing surgery to minimise the chance of a deep vein thrombosis in their legs (*Obi et al.*, 2015)

Anaesthetics nurse

Advances in surgery have been in conjunction with advances in anaesthetics science and pharmaceuticals. General anaesthesia is administered by anaesthetists, doctors who have undergone 12 years of training and are medical consultants in their own right (Wise, 2019). There are many different types of anaesthesia: general, local, sedation, or regional (i.e., spinal or epidural). General anaesthesia is administered either as a volatile gas with oxygen or as total intravenous anaesthesia. The anaesthetic nurse's responsibility is to assist the anaesthetist during all phases of the anaesthetic – preparation, induction, maintenance and emergence (ACORN, 2012). A thorough understanding of anaesthetic medications and equipment is paramount in the role of an anaesthetic nurse as is skills in dealing with emergency situations such as anaphylactic shock, airway complications or the rare hereditary muscle disorder malignant hyperthermia.

The anaesthetic nurse will prepare for the required type of anaesthesia according to the individual patient and their anatomical structures. The checking and functioning of all equipment is critical prior to surgery. A protocol must be followed for the checking of the anaesthetic delivery system or anaesthetic machine confirming correct assembly, appropriate pressures and alarm functions (Australian and New Zealand College of Anaesthetists, 2014). There are ranges of monitoring from basics such as pulse oximetry, non-invasive blood pressure and ECG, to more advanced monitoring such as arterial blood pressures and entropy monitoring.

> Entropy monitoring is a method of assessing the effect of anaesthetics on the brains EEG, such that an accurate assessment of depth of anaesthesia is administered (Chhabra, Subramaniam, Srivastava, Prabhakar, Kalaivani & Paranjape, 2016).

The anaesthetic nurse will sign the patient into the operating theatre after receiving a handover from the ward nurse. The preoperative checklist will be completed along with the first section of the surgical safety checklist. Patient comfort will be ensured, particularly warmth as the theatre is a very cold environment. The temperature can range between 18–24°C as a means to reduce bacterial growth (Australian College of Operating Room Nurses, 2016). To counter these cold temperatures and ensure the patient remains normothermic, forced air-warming devices and warm fluids are required, especially for paediatric patients or for long surgical procedures.

The basic responsibilities of the anaesthetic nurse are:

1 Anticipate and provide equipment.
2 Monitoring and assessment of the patient.
3 Documentation on the fluid balance chart.
4 Accessing S8 medications.
5 Transfer and positing of the patient (Hamlin, Davies, Richardson-Tench & Sutherland-Fraser, 2016; ACORN, 2012).

Circulating and instrument nurses

The circulating nurse is typically referred to as the scout nurse. The scout nurse is the link between the sterile and unsterile field. Prior to the patient arrival the scout nurse will be preparing the operating theatre according to the surgeons' preference. This will include the positioning of the table, lighting, diathermy machine, suction cannisters and sequential compression device. Depending on the procedure, specialised equipment such as laser, argon-beam coagulator or laparoscopic towers will be required.

The scout nurse will then greet the patient in the anaesthetic bay and using tools such as the preoperative checklist, will confirm the admission process, including but not limited to, patient identification, a valid consent, fasting status, and the marking of the surgical site (ACORN, 2012). A therapeutic relationship with the patient is established ensuring the patient feels comfortable prior to entering to the operating room.

Whilst the instrument nurse is scrubbing, the scout nurse has the responsibility of opening all sterile supplies, checking sterility indicators, expiration dates and integrity as well as commencing the documentation prior to the surgical count. To summarise the basic responsibilities of the scout nurse are:

1 Opening of all instruments using aseptic techniques whilst ensuring the integrity and sterility of all supplies.
2 Ensuring the safe transfer and positioning of the patient.
3 Performing the surgical count and documenting accordingly.
4 Checking and connecting all equipment such as the diathermy and suctioning.
5 Anticipate the needs of the scrub nurse and surgical team.
6 Observe for breaches in aseptic technique (Hamlin, Davies, Richardson-Tench & Sutherland-Fraser, 2016; ACORN, 2012).

The instrument nurse is typically referred to as the scrub nurse. The scrub nurse ensures all instruments, trays, sutures and equipment are available, functional and ready prior to surgery as per the surgeon's preference list. Preparation is vital, as unavailable equipment can delay the surgical start time. Expert knowledge of the surgical procedure and anatomy is required. The scrub nurse also greets the patient confirming the patient identity, procedure and allergy status. Once the scout and scrub nurse agree that the operating theatre is ready for surgery, the scrub nurse performs a surgical scrub and dons a sterile gown and gloves. The scrub nurse will set up the sterile field as the scout uses aseptic technique to pass equipment. Simultaneously, the scout and scrub nurse will perform a surgical count of all accountable items and check the items on each tray against the tray list. Once the surgeon is scrubbed, the patient can be draped and prepped. The scrub nurse must continually anticipate the needs of the surgeon, passing the necessary instruments at the correct time. The scrub nurse also relies on the scout to provide sponges or sutures at the correct time. The surgical team works in a synchronised flow to ensure safe patient outcomes and the continued flow of the procedure. To summarise, the basic responsibilities of the scrub nurse are:

1 Obtaining all equipment on the surgeon's preference card.
2 Expert knowledge of the surgical procedure and equipment.
3 Performing the surgical counts with the scout nurse.
4 Working closely with the surgeon to pass the instruments and items required.
5 Anticipate the needs of the surgical team.
6 Maintain and adhere to the principles of aseptic technique (Hamlin, Davies, Richardson-Tench & Sutherland-Fraser, 2016; ACORN, 2012).

Together the scrub and scout nurse work in conjunction to advocate for the patient, provide a safe environment, best patient outcomes, and participate in risk management processes. Reducing postoperative complications such as pressure injuries and deep vein thrombosis is vital, as well as applying aseptic techniques and a surgical conscience to prevent or reduce the possibility of wound infections. Cleaning and infection control procedures between patients are essential, as well as monitoring traffic flow of sterile and contaminated supplies.

Overall the scrub nurse is responsible for the surgical count ensuring no items are left unaccounted for (Staunton & Chiarella, 2013), including items left inside the patient's body which are classified as an adverse event. Both the scrub and scout nurse will ensure the correct labelling of specimens and handling of a prosthesis. To help ensure safe surgery, all members of the surgical team are involved in the team time-out before skin incision. This involves using the World Health Organisations Surgical Safety Checklist to confirm the correct patient, site, and procedure to name a few items. The majority of adverse events in the operating theatre are linked to time-out issues, hence the implementation of this mandatory procedure (Papadakis, Meiwandi & Grzybowski, 2019). The role of the scrub and scout is interchangeable on each shift and depends on the skill mix relating to different surgical procedures. Some surgery lasts for many hours and can be highly complicated and stressful, so the scrub must be prepared to stand for the procedure, which can cause both mental and physical fatigue.

Recovery room nursing

Recovery room nursing is typically either referred to as the Post Anaesthetic Care Unit (PACU) or the Recovery Room. The role of the PACU nurse is to optimise positive

---

Box 7.1 - Case study (Annabelle)

Annabelle, a 10-year old female, arrived to the operating theatre for an Open Reduction Internal Fixation of her left distal radius fracture after falling off her bike. Her mother accompanied her to reduce any anxiety. Annabelle is wheeled into the operating room and the anaesthetic induction commences. The anaesthetic nurse now takes Annabelle's mother to the waiting room. The scout nurse commences the 'time out' in the absence of the surgeon who is running late.

Reflective questions:

1 Should the scout nurse commence the 'time out' without all team members present?
2 Annabelle's X-rays have been left in the day only ward. Are these required for a 'time out'?
3 Explain why the surgical safety checklist is important.

---

outcomes as patients make the transition from their surgery and being anaesthetised. The basic responsibilities of PACU staff are:

1 Airway management and oxygenation of patients who have had general anaesthesia,
2 Monitoring vital signs and, depending on the complexity of the surgery and patient co-morbidities, more invasive monitoring such as arterial pressures,
3 Assessment and treating post-operative pain with opiates through to simple analgesia as required. This can include setting up and monitoring Patient Controlled Analgesia (PCA) pumps, epidurals, or monitoring of spinal or regional anaesthesia,
4 Treat post-operative nausea and vomiting, and
5 Monitor the surgical site for bleeding, swelling and haematoma, and wound assessment including neurovascular observation downstream from the surgical site.

Major risks to the patient

The transition from surgery and general anaesthesia is a time where the patient is at increased risk of adverse events. These include laryngospasm, respiratory arrest, cardiac arrhythmia, and cardiovascular instability. Another key issue that requires specific nursing intervention/s is known as emergence delirium (Luckowski, 2019).

Emergence delirium either presents as agitation or excessive drowsiness that occurs during the postop period after emergence from general anaesthesia.

In addition, managing and prioritising the other needs of the patient maximises positive outcomes and a safe transition to the ward or other department. With these risks in mind, the initial transfer from operating room to the PACU requires the handover of accurate clinical information not only from the surgical team, but most importantly from the anaesthetist such as the drugs used, pain relief administered and vital signs. The handover from the scrub nurse must include, but is not limited to, factors such as the type of operation/procedure the patient had, the presence of any drains/catheters, and whether the patient has any known allergies.

A structured communication between all health professionals working in the perioperative context promotes clear and accurate communication. A commonly used and evidence-based framework for handovers is the Identification, Situation, Background, Assessment, and Recommendation (ISBAR) (Kitney, Tam, Bennett, Buttigieg, Bramley & Wang, 2016). Likewise, the ISBAR can also be used by the PACU nurse when discharging a patient and transferring them to a ward or other department. Other evidence-based handover tools have been tested however, such as the Post☐Anaesthetic Care Tool, and should always be considered for practice (Street, Phillips, Haesler & Kent, 2018). Most critically, however are the uses of PACU discharge criteria where a patient must meet a certain summary score for their vital signs, pain, consciousness, circulation, and physical activity.

Issues for PACU nurses

The PACU is an environment where nurses work in close quarters with anaesthetists and surgeons and there is potential to develop great professional and personal relationships. This can have both positive and negative consequences as familiarity may lead to decreased attention and distraction. Nevertheless, the PACU unit can be incredibly stressful when dealing with untoward events and challenging situations, and a good team dynamic will make these situations easier to manage. For instance, watching a child turning blue as you desperately attempt to maintain oxygenation during laryngospasm is not uncommon. Likewise, the PACU nurse is often the first contact with patients after potentially traumatic surgery, such as a female patient who has just had a mastectomy. These are opportunities where the nurse's empathic care and communication skills can greatly affect the patient on gaining consciousness.

As with most nursing contexts, there are often budget constraints, staffing and rostering shortages, and skill mix challenges. Nurse understaffing is associated with significantly higher incidence and severity of hypoxaemia and hypotension (Kiekkas et al. 2019). Care quality and patient safety are benchmarks that need to be met with a matching patient acuity and sufficient and appropriately skilled nursing staff. There are often peaks and troughs with admissions to PACU from theatre. Predictive models maybe encouraged to identify appropriate nurse to patient ratios and to minimise shortages. Ultimately however, regardless of PACU staffing levels, the anaesthetist should not leave until the PACU nurse is able to take handover and be at the bedside for 1:1 nursing while the patient is unconscious and or has an artificial airway in situ (Kiekkas et al, 2019). Most importantly, good planning and flexibility are pivotal in managing both the needs of the unit and the patients being cared for in the PACU. Situations and patient condition can change dramatically in an instant; the PACU is a very rewarding context to work but can also be highly stressful and is not without its tragic moments that can be emotionally draining.

Current challenges and tensions facing perioperative nurses

The acuity of surgery in each specialty area is demanding the segregation of nurses into modules of surgeries. Historically theatre nurses were multi-skilled, however, with the variety of specialties, nurses are being specialised for one area, for example cardiac surgery only. Each surgical specialty has continued to advance with revolutionary technical advancements in medical equipment and consumables, leading to the requirement that perioperative nurses are adept with audio-visual, computerised, and technically elaborate equipment. This can be quite challenging and confronting and may influence an individual nurse's decision towards perioperative nursing as technology continues to advance at a rapid pace.

The average Body Mass Index (BMI) is increasing among the population which means that people presenting as overweight or obese is also increasing, and these patients present unique perioperative challenges. To abide by Work Health and Safety polices, appropriate equipment must be utilised to ensure patient safety and reduce injury to the health care team. Their transfer and positioning require thoughtful and planned approaches by a team of staff, sometimes using lifting equipment e.g. HoverMatt® or bariatric ceiling hoists. All patient movements are governed by the anaesthetist in the theatre setting where they have the control and responsibility of the patient's airway. The increased neck circumference of people classified as overweight or obese can cause issues while performing airway management. It is imperative the patient is correctly and safely positioned for optimal access during the surgery, as well as addressing the patients increased risk for pressure injury and venous thromboembolism due to a high BMI (Van Wicklin, 2018). The scrub nurse must also ensure the instrumentation is of an adequate length to suit the anatomical structure of the patient. Operating tables are designed to be narrow, to prevent back strain in the surgical team, and hence require additional pieces to increase their width to accommodate bariatric patients. This creates potential postural issues for the surgical team, which may be alleviated by operating from an increased height by standing on a footstool.

Future challenges facing the field of perioperative nursing

The projected shortfall of registered nurses in Australia will affect all specialties of nursing, however the perioperative environment will be increasingly affected. Undergraduate nursing students' decreased exposure to the perioperative environment, coupled with the absence of content about perioperative nursing within the nursing curriculum, will result in less students opting to work in this specialty post-graduation (Doyle, 2018; ACORN, 2012). An increase in clinical placements, or short visits following patients through their perioperative experience, could assist to counter this problem (Hamlin, Davies, Richardson-Tench & Sutherland-Fraser, 2016).

The scope of practice of perioperative nurses has, and will continue to evolve into the future as technology and practice evolves. For instance, the scope of practice has already evolved beyond the traditional roles to include the Perioperative Nurse Surgeon's Assistant. This advanced role requires the nurse to work in the pre-, intra- and post-operative areas of patient care, either employed by the surgeon or being self-employed (ACORN, 2012). The perioperative nurse practitioner is another advanced role that will become more important over time, as are the evolution of highly specialised roles such as the nurse endoscopist and nurse sedationist (Hamlin, Davies, Richardson-Tench & Sutherland-Fraser, 2016).

Technology is rapidly advancing, and perioperative nurses must remain abreast of these changes. Advances such as 'surgical robots, navigation systems, hybrid theatres, 3D organ printing and 4D augmented reality including holographic and virtual keyboards' will be available in the future (Smith & Palesy, 2018, p.25). These changes will require other roles such as robotic coordinators or nursing informatics experts to help decrease the occupational stress created when adapting to such rapid and complex change (Saletnik, L. 2018).

Online resources

1 Australian College of Perioperative Nurses (ACORN): www.acorn.org.au
2 Australian Commission on Safety and Quality in Health Care. Surgical Safety Checklist: www.safetyandquality.gov.au/our-work/communicating-safety/patient-identification/patient-procedure-matching-protocols/surgical-safety-checklist
3 Australian and New Zealand College of Anaesthetist: www.anzca.edu.au

References

Arani, M.G., Fakharian, E., & Sarbandi, F. (2012). Ancient legacy of cranial surgery. *Archives of Trauma Research*, *1*(2), 72–74. doi: 10.5812/atr.6556

Atkinson, L.J. (1992). *Berry & Kohn's operating room technique* (7th ed.). St Louis, Missouri: Mosby-Year Book

Australian and New Zealand College of Anaesthetists. (2014). ANZCA Guidelines on checking anaesthesia delivery systems. Retrieved from http://www.anzca.edu.au/documents/ps31-2014-guidelines-on-checking-anaesthesia-deliv.pdf

Australian College of Operating Room Nurses. (2016). *ACORN standards for perioperative nursing 2016–2017*. Adelaide: Australian College of Operating Room Nurses.

Australian College of Operating Room Nurses. (2012). *ACORN standards for perioperative nursing: Including nursing roles, guidelines, position statements and competency standards 2012–2013*. Adelaide: Australian College of Operating Room Nurses.

Barnett, G. (2016). Developing an effective day surgery service. *Update in Anaesthesia*, *31*, 9–13.

Callahan, B.C., Seifi, A., & Holt, G.R. (2016). The scrub revolution: From hospital uniform to public attire. *Southern Medical Journal*, *109*(5), 326–329. doi: 10.14423/SMJ.0000000000000455

Chhabra A., Subramaniam R., Srivastava A., Prabhakar H., Kalaivani M., & Paranjape S. (2016). Spectral entropy monitoring for adults and children undergoing general anaesthesia. *Cochrane Database of Systematic Reviews*, *3*, 1–57. doi: 10.1002/14651858.CD010135.pub2.

Doyle, D. J. (2018). Succession planning and the future of perioperative nursing leadership. *Association of periOperative Registered Nurses (AORN)*, *108*(2), 191–194. doi 10.1002/aorn.12308

Hamlin, Richardson-Tench, & Davies. (2009). *Perioperative nursing an introductory text*. Chatswood, Australia: Elsevier Australia.

Hamlin, Davies, Richardson-Tench, & Sutherland-Fraser. (2016). *Perioperative nursing: An introduction* (2nd ed.). Chatswood, NSW: Elsevier Australia.

Jones, R.M. (1990). Desflurane and sevoflurane: Inhalation anaesthetics for this decade? *British Journal of Anaesthesia*, *65*, 527–536.

Kiekkas, P., Tsekoura, V., Aretha, D., Samios, A., Konstantinou, E., Igoumenidis, M., Fligou, F. (2019). Nurse understaffing is associated with adverse events in post anaesthesia care unit patients. *Journal of Clinical Nursing*, *28*(11-12), 2245–2252. doi: 10.1111/jocn.14819

Kitney, P., Tam, R., Bennett, P., Buttigieg, D., Bramley, D., & Wang, W. (2016). Handover between anaesthetists and post-anaesthetic care unit nursing staff using ISBAR principles: A quality improvement study. *ACORN: The Journal of Perioperative Nursing in Australia*, *29*(1), 30–35.doi.org/10.26550/2209-1092.1001

Luckowski, A. (2019). Safety priorities in the PACU. *Nursing 2019*, *49*(4), 62–65. doi: 10.1097/01.NURSE.0000554246.74635.e0

Nursing and Midwifery Board of Australia. (2018). Code of conduct for nurses. Retrieved from https://www.nursingmidwiferyboard.gov.au/Codes-Guidelines-Statements/Professional-standards.aspx

Obi, A. T., Alvarez, R., Reames, M., Moote, M.J., Thompson, M.A., Wakefield, T.W., & Henke, P.K. (2015). A prospective evaluation of standard versus battery-powered sequential compression devices in postsurgical patients. *The American Journal of Surgery, 209(4)*, 675–681. doi: 10.1016/j.amjsurg.2014.06.017

Ouyang, B. (2015). The resistance to antisepsis in the 19th century: A briefing on two European antisepsis proponents, *University of Toronto Medical Journal, 92*(3), 92–94.

Papadakis, M., Meiwandi, A., & Grzybowski, A. (2019). The WHO safer surgery checklist time out procedure revisited: Strategies to optimise compliance and safety. *International Journal of Surgery, 69*, 19–22. doi: 10.1016/j.ijsu.2019.07.006

Saletnik, L. (2018). Technology in the perioperative environment. *Association of periOperative Registered Nurses (AORN), 108*(5), 488–490. doi: 10.1002/aorn.12414

Smith, J., & Palesy, D. (2018). Technology stress in perioperative nursing: An ongoing concern. *Journal of Perioperative Nursing, 31*(2), 25–28. doi: org/10.26550/2209-1092.1028

Street, M., Phillips, N.M., Haesler, E., & Kent, B. (2018). Refining nursing assessment and management with a new post anaesthetic care discharge tool to minimize surgical patient risk. *Journal of Advanced Nursing, 74(11)*, 2566–2576. doi: 10.1111/jan.13779

Staunton, P., & Chiarella, M. (2013). *Law for nurses and midwives* (7th ed.). Sydney: Churchill Livingstone Elsevier.

Thorpe, C.M., & Spence, A.A. (1997). Clinical evidence for delayed chloroform poisoning. *British Journal of Anaesthesia, 79*(3), 402–409. doi: org/10.1093/bja/79.3.402

Van Wicklin, S.A. (2018). Challenges in the operating room with obese and extremely obese surgical patients. *International Journal Safe Patient Handling & Mobility (SPHM), 8*(3), 120–131.

Wade, P. (2012). Historical trends influencing the future of perioperative nursing. *Operating Room Nurses Association of Canada (ORNAC). Journal, 30*(2), 22–35.

Warren, K.J., Morrey, C. Oppy, A. Pirpiris, M., & Balogh, Z.J. (2019). The overview of the Australian trauma system. *Orthopaedic Trauma Association International, 2*(1). doi: 10.1097/OI9.0000000000000018

Wise, J. (2019). How to become an anaesthetist. *The British Medical Journal (BMJ), 366*:l4665, 1–2. doi: 10.1136/bmj.l4665

8 Nursing adults in general medical or surgical contexts

*Gladis Kabil, Sheeba Thomas, Peter Lewis,
Kathryn Steirn and Amanda Johnson*

Chapter objectives

This chapter will offer the reader:

- An outline of the current medical and surgical setting in Australia
- A description of contemporary key practice challenges that medical and surgical nurses face
- A description of pathways to practice in medical and surgical nursing
- An overview of future challenges to nursing and nurses who practice in this area.

Introduction

Despite the attraction of high profile, specialist areas of nursing practice such as oncology and critical care, more than a quarter of nurses are registered in Australia for practice in the fields of acute, general medical and surgical nursing. Medical and surgical nursing can be highly complex in practice for a number of reasons, including the complicated nature of patient presentation. The most recent edition of the *Clinical Companion to Medical Surgical Nursing* lists about 200 different conditions from acute abdominal pain to varicose veins, from headache to hernia, and it lists a range of interventions from amputation to oxygen therapy (Hagler et.al. 2020). Furthermore, the Australian Institute of Health and Welfare (AIHW, 2018) has calculated that 50% of people admitted to general medical or surgical wards will have a chronic condition; 45% will have a mental illness; 63% will be overweight or obese; and 18% will possess some form of disability. Any combination of these conditions might constitute a presenting problem for hospitalised patients, but their presence adds a layer of complexity to the care of any patient who presents to hospital with a medical diagnosis or who is in need of surgery. Therefore, nurses working within acute, general medical and surgical contexts require a broad range of well- developed clinical skills in order to deliver high quality care to people with a range of illnesses and health conditions.

Key practice issues

Key practice issues that pose significant challenges in the delivery of care in medical and surgical wards are presented here in two categories. The first relates to organisational factors to do with the organisation of nursing work. The second relates to patient-related factors of an ageing population, multimorbidity and polypharmacy.

Organisation of nursing work

In the Australian medical surgical setting, the two most common ways of organizing nursing work are patient allocation and team nursing. Primary nursing and task-based allocations are not usually practiced in medical and surgical wards because a significant proportion of the workforce now comprises inexperienced, newly graduated registered nurses (Duffield, Roche, Diers, Catling-Paull, & Blay, 2010). Inexperienced nurses working alone in primary and task-based nursing models can compromise patient safety and erode the confidence of a newly registered nurse. Both patient allocation and team nursing models require higher ratio of qualified, experienced registered nurses than either or the other two approaches (Duffield et al., 2010).

> Primary nursing means that a specific nurse is assigned to one patient on admission and is responsible for the coordination, if not the direct delivery, of care for that patient throughout their admission. Patient allocation means that one nurse, usually a registered nurse, is allocated to undertake total care for one or a number of patients throughout a nursing shift. Task allocation means that nursing work is divided into tasks to be shared between registered nurses and ancillary staff. Each nursing staff member is then responsible for the completion of their tasks in the care of all patients on the ward. Team nursing means that a group of two or more nurses provide all the care to a group of patients.

Box 8.1 - Case study – work organisation

When registered nurse Karen arrives on her 20 bed general surgical ward one Saturday morning, she is informed by night staff that two of the nurses rostered on for the shift have rung and informed sick, and only one has been replaced by a nurse from the hospital's casual pool. This leaves the ward short-staffed.

When Karen reviews the condition of patients on the ward she realises that the ward's usual method of patient allocation will not work for the current shift and, in fact, is likely to be dangerous for patients and nurses. She decides, instead, to use a system of team nursing. She will care for 10 patients with the less experienced but regular ward staff member, Julie. Karen's friend of many years, Stephanie, will care for the other 10 patients with the pool nurse, Grace.

Each pair of nurses works out their priorities for patient care before systematically working through those priorities from patient to patient. They even factor in time for a short break in during which one nurse from each pair will retreat to the nurses' tea room to sit down for a quick cuppa.

By the end of the shift, all four nurses are exhausted and aware of the small, caring actions that they would normally like to provide that they have been unable to give. But they are also pleased with what they have achieved as a team – the delivery of safe, essential care for all patients.

Reflective question:

1   Imagine you were in Karen's situation. Is there anything that you would have done differently?

The availability of skilled registered nurses in acute medical and surgical settings is reportedly inadequate and has proven to be detrimental to the provision of quality care (Chapman, Rahman, Courtney, & Chalmers, 2017). For example, in one study conducted in medical and surgical wards, 74% of nurses reported care left undone in their last shift. The stated reasons were inadequate staff-patient ratios, limited nurse skill mix, and the time of day when the shift took place. Care was most often incomplete during shifts that took place after hours (Ball et al., 2016). The increasing complexity of patient presentations in medical and surgical wards and associated treatment mandate the need for increased nursing staff to patient ratios (Duffield et al., 2010). Furthermore, it has been demonstrated that improving nursing skill mix and decreasing staffing shortages can significantly lower patient mortality rates, and improve quality care and patient outcomes (Aiken et al., 2017).

Patient turnover

Reduced length of stay and increasing numbers of patient admissions has resulted in a high rate of patient turnover in some medical and surgical contexts. With advances in science, technology and medical practices, patients are no longer staying in hospital for extended periods of time. The average number of annual hospital admissions has been increasing 3.8% every year in Australia with a 2.7% increase in same-day acute care admissions. This means out of the 11 million patients admitted to hospital each year, an average of 6.3 million are admitted to same-day acute care services (AIHW, 2019).

In response to this, Australian hospitals are changing their care delivery infrastructure to incorporate more frequent short stay procedures and day surgeries for the resolution of acute episodes. High patient turnover has adverse consequences for the delivery of nursing care such as limited time to assess patient needs, prioritise and implement care, develop therapeutic relationships with patients and their families, and a decrease in continuity of care (Chapman et al., 2017).

However, medical and surgical nurses also care for patients with chronic illnesses and complex surgeries that require prolonged admissions that can last for months in some cases. Prolonged length of stay can result in complications for patients such as hospital acquired infections. Extended hospital stays have a significant impact on the economic cost of health care delivery (Damiani et al., 2011). However, lengthy hospital stays can provide the unique opportunity for establishing meaningful therapeutic relationships with patients. Medical and surgical nurses are able to liaise with the multidisciplinary team and act as care coordinators organizing post hospital care for patients whose length of stay is extended. This gives an opportunity for expansion of their scope of practice and an added dimension of interest in patient care.

Quality, safety culture and monitoring

Current nursing shortages and patient turnover have resulted in an increasing need for monitoring the quality of nursing care delivered in acute medical-surgical settings (Hegney et al., 2019). The landmark report by the Institute of Medicine 'To Err is Human' has highlighted the need to reduce medical errors and prevent serious events in healthcare (Sherwood & Barnsteiner, 2017). In response to this, the Australian Commission on Safety and Quality in Health Care (ACSQHC) standards and framework has been developed and is now being applied in many Australian hospitals. This framework enables hospitals to monitor and benchmark patient outcomes and effectiveness of clinical practice in order to ensure patient safety and the delivery of quality care (Wilcox & McNeil, 2016).

Patient outcomes depend on nurses' competency level in recognising, assessing and managing the deteriorating patient in medical and surgical units. Several organisation-wide systems of escalation of care have been implemented. These are commonly referred to as Medical Emergency Teams (MET), Rapid Response System (RRS) or Clinical Emergency Response System (CERS) across Australia (Clinical Excellence Commission, 2019). These systems have been shown to reduce patient mortality and facilitate timely identification of deteriorating patients. However, human factors such as communication failures and organisational and personal work practices can inhibit activation of RRS in medical-surgical settings (Mitchell, Williamson, & Molesworth, 2015). In light of this, face to face and online training, delivered on an annual basis, to achieve high levels of competence among the nursing workforce is considered to be highly beneficial for recognising and responding to deteriorating patients as well as being considered critical for the delivery of safe, high quality patient care.

The following case study highlights where the quality and safety of patients is compromised due to the challenges that our current healthcare system is facing.

Box 8.2 - Case study – quality and safety

Mr James is a 58-year-old man with a medical history of seizure disorder, hypertension, Atrial Fibrillation and Chronic Obstructive Pulmonary Disorder (COPD). Mr James presented to the hospital with wheezing and difficulty in breathing. The medical officer diagnosed Mr James as having acute exacerbation of his COPD.

Mr James was admitted to the medical ward and treated with oral steroids and an inhaled bronchodilator, which resulted in a gradual improvement in his respiratory function. He was also commenced on intravenous fluids for hydration and oral antibiotics.

Mr James gradually improved and was expected to be discharged from the hospital within the week. But on the third day of admission, Mr James voiced complaints of acute pain in his right leg to the nursing staff. The team ordered an ultrasound of the lower extremities and confirmed a blood clot in the leg (Deep Vein Thrombosis [DVT]). On admission, Mr James was not commenced on prophylactic anticoagulant therapy nor given any preventative education.

Reflective questions:

1 The **patient** did not receive standard treatment to prevent the formation of DVT. What are some possible reasons why this error occurred?
2 Can you suggest system process improvements that might reduce the likelihood of similar errors in the future?

Patient-related factors

The following section reviews patient-related factors that impact on the delivery of care in either a medical or surgical setting. The areas of ageing population, chronic disease, disability and multimorbidity and polypharmacy add a significantly complex and educationally demanding dimension to acute medical and surgical nursing.

Ageing population

The exponential rise of the Australian older population places an unprecedented demand on health services (AIHW, 2018). In 2017, 1 in 7 members of the Australian population were aged 65 years or older representing 15% of the total population. This means there are currently approximately 3.8 million Australians aged older than 65 years. This number is projected to grow steadily in coming decades (AIIIW, 2018). The majority of clientele in medical or surgical settings will be older people and the care required is multifactorial (Johnson & Chang, 2017).

It is important to understand the implications of ageing on exacerbation of chronic and acute conditions that patients in medical surgical units present with. For instance, wound healing post-surgery might be delayed in older adults. Older adults are more prone to developing pressure ulcers and they are at greater risk of sustaining falls, which are ever present risks in medical surgical units. Over 79% of falls in medical and surgical units occur in patients older than 70 years of age (Stephenson et al., 2015). Maintaining the health of older people in Australia will require a robust nursing work-force with adequate training in aged care. This further expands the scope of practice of the medical and surgical nurses.

Chronic disease, disability and multimorbidity

According to the AIHW, (2018) report, chronic diseases was a contributory factor to 37% of all hospital admissions in 2016 and 87% of all deaths. Further, 1 in 2 Australians report having at least one chronic condition and 1 in 4 having at least two or more (multimorbidity) (AIHW, 2018). Additionally, people experience disability such as poor eye sight or impaired hearing either separate to a chronic disease, as part of their disease process, or as a side effect to treatment, for example, in the case of chemotherapy for cancer and the resultant peripheral neuropathy (Johnson & Chang, 2018). More than a quarter of people with chronic conditions or disabilities who are admitted in the medical surgical wards require assistance for the activities of daily living such as bathing and dressing (Salmond & Echevarria, 2017). A recent study shows a 7% increase in the time taken to deliver nursing care in recent years due to the increased level of dependency of patients with chronic illnesses or disability in medical and surgical wards (Vallés, Valdavida, Menéndez, & Natal, 2018). This places additional burden on the already short-staffed medical and surgical wards.

Polypharmacy

Polypharmacy is defined as the prescription of 5 or more unique medications for an individual patient (Masnoon, Shakib, Kalisch-Ellett, & Caughey, 2017). Older Australians are at higher risk of polypharmacy than younger Australians. Approximately 1

Box 8.3 - Reflective questions

1 What impacts would polypharmacy have on an elderly patient admitted in a medical surgical unit?
2 How could you as the nurse rectify or work towards alleviating such issues prior to patient discharge?

---

million older Australians fit the criteria for polypharmacy in 2017, a 52% increase over a period of 10 years (Page, Falster, Litchfield, Pearson, & Etherton-Beer, 2019). More than one-fifth of older Australians admitted to medical wards take more than 10 medications (Hubbard et al., 2015). The Australian and New Zealand Society for Geriatric Medicine Position Statement Abstract: Prescribing in older people, (2018) affirm that the issue of polypharmacy presents a significantly increased risk of adverse drug reactions.

In addition, polypharmacy results in increased demand for care. A time in motion study in medical surgical settings found that polypharmacy increased the total cost of care by 72% as these patients often developed adverse reactions leading to prolonged hospital stay (van Oostveen, Gouma, Bakker, & Ubbink, 2015). Patients admitted to medical and surgical wards often receive concurrent treatment from several health care teams for their pre-existing co-morbidities. For instance, a patient admitted for orthopaedic surgery might also receive care from cardiology or nephrology teams during their admission. These multimodalities of treatment increase the risk of adverse drug reactions and weaken the immune system of the patient, which is already compromised by the surgery. Medical surgical nurses therefore need a thorough knowledge of drug interactions to provide individualised patient-centred care. In order to minimise patient harm, vigilance related to prescribing, dispensing, administration and monitoring high-risk medications is vital.

Future challenges

The final section of the chapter presents an outline of the future challenges to nursing practice in medical or surgical wards. Two challenges are presented: the need for ongoing education and ageing nursing workforce.

Education and training

The need for ongoing nursing education and training with the rapid advances in medical sciences and new models of nursing care poses a significant challenge for the newly graduated nurse in medical surgical settings. That challenge is: keeping abreast of new care options and the acquisition of new knowledge and skills to deliver optimal care. Importantly, while a nurse may have completed their pre-registration education, their commitment to remain engaged in life-long learning is paramount in an area of nursing that requires a broad knowledge base and a broad set of skills. Additional support that is provided to assist in the transition from nursing student to new graduate nurse include supernumerary days, in-service education and instruction, appointment of a preceptor, and specialty short courses or postgraduate courses conducted by Australian College of Nursing (Adams & Gillman, 2016).

Medical and surgical nurses make a significant contribution to advanced physical assessment, aiming for the best outcome for the patient (Zambas, Smythe, & Koziol-Mclain, 2016). This has led to increasing emphasis on performing holistic assessment in patients with complex issues and initiating escalation protocols in the hospitals. The nurse's role is pivotal in participating in the various quality and safety programs that serve to enhance and promote quality care, especially in a field of nursing in which quality care can have multiple meanings. This will integrate with quality and safety education in nursing, consequently, enhancing the future health needs of the healthcare system and developing a stronger workforce (Sherwood & Barnsteiner, 2017).

Ageing nursing workforce

Nationally, the Australian healthcare workforce faces significant challenges in managing such factors as an ageing population and increasing demands on the resources of the health care system (Buchan, Twigg, Dussault, Duffield, & Stone, 2015). The nature of healthcare in Australia is changing due to increasing incidence of chronic disease, emerging health technologies, and changing models of care. The ageing of the Australian nursing workforce will present challenges for the deployment of a balanced workforce and will likely contribute to a shortage in the nursing workforce of approximately 110,000 nurses by 2025 (Health Workforce Australia, 2014). A significant increase in nursing workload is likely to result which could lead to increasing incidence of burnout among nurses as well as reduced job satisfaction and stress (Ross, Rogers, & King, 2019). With more than 23% of total Australian nursing workforce working either in a medical or surgical ward, it is projected that there will be a deficit of 6000 medical surgical nurses by the year 2030 due to the ageing of the workforce (Health Workforce Australia, 2014). This workforce shortfall will have a significant and dangerous impact on the availability of nurses. On the other hand, it offers increased job opportunities for newly graduate nurses in medical surgical wards.

Scope of practice

In today's ever-changing healthcare system, the nursing profession has constantly evolved and grown rapidly in the medical and surgical context. Unlike critical care areas and emergency departments, nurses are not required to complete specialised training programs prior to working in medical and surgical wards. This makes jobs in medical surgical wards more accessible to newly graduate nurses.

Patients in the medical and surgical areas present with a wide array of problems such as cancers, chronic pain, palliation, cardiac conditions etc. Nurses in the medical and surgical wards therefore require a comprehensive body of knowledge derived from multiple sub-specialities (Lyneham, 2013). This provides opportunities for newly graduate nurses to acquire a wide range of experience and the possibility to specialise in any of the specialty areas in future based on their preference.

Nurses are part of the multidisciplinary team and contribute towards decision making in the clinical setting to achieve positive patient outcomes. They are also working as change agents to build a future healthcare system by involving in health policy making and rendering high-quality care through evidence-based practice (Crabtree et al., 2016). Hence, clinical leadership is one of the areas for nurses to excel in their career in the management of care delivery through problem-solving and hospital management (Scully, 2015). Accordingly, depending on the interest, registered nurses can advance their career through specialisations to become Clinical Nurse Consultant, Clinical Nurse Specialist, Clinical Nurse Educator, Advanced Nurse Practitioners, Nurse Unit Managers, or research project lead manager. For patients with chronic illness and disabilities with associated complex care needs, there is a need for specialised roles such as care coordinator. Medical and surgical nurses with their unique skill set, caring philosophy and management knowledge will be the most appropriate to assume such care coordination roles (Salmond & Echevarria, 2017).

Conclusion

Creating an efficient and robust workforce in the acute, general medical and surgical setting is particularly important where responsive solutions are required to increasing demands of patient care. Both the current model of healthcare in Australia and the changing patient demographics pose challenges. This chapter has provided an overview of these key challenges faced by medical and surgical nurses. It is important to ensure that the demographic change is seen as a transition rather than a crisis with challenges as well as opportunities. These opportunities bring a wider scope of practice for future nurses. This chapter provides a summary of these opportunities available to the newly emerging nursing workforce. Resources to assist with nursing skills development is provided at the end of this chapter.

Online resources

1 Australian College of Children and Young People's Nurses: https://www.accypn.org.au/
2 Australian College of Nursing: https://www.acn.edu.au/education/postgraduate-courses
3 Australian Day Surgery Nurses Association: http://adsna.info/
4 NSW Operating Theatre Association (OTA): https://www.ota.org.au/
5 Respiratory Nurses Interest Group of NSW: http://www.rnig.org.au/

References

Adams, J. E., & Gillman, L. (2016). Developing an evidence-based transition program for graduate nurses. *Contemporary nurse, 52*(5), 511–521.

Aiken, L. H., Sloane, D., Griffiths, P., Rafferty, A. M., Bruyneel, L., McHugh, M., … Ausserhofer, D. (2017). Nursing skill mix in European hospitals: Cross-sectional study of the association with mortality, patient ratings, and quality of care. *BMJ Quality & Safety, 26*(7), 559–568.

Australian and New Zealand Society for Geriatric Medicine Position Statement Abstract: Prescribing in older people (2018). *Australasian Journal on Ageing, 37*(4), 313–313. doi:10.1111/ajag.12577

Australian Institute of Health and Welfare. (2018). *Australia's Health 2018*. Canberra, Australia https://www.aihw.gov.au/reports/australias-health/australias-health-2018/contents/table-of-contents

Australian Institute of Health and Welfare. (2019). *Admitted patient care 2017–18: Australian hospital statistics*. Canberra: AIHW. https://www.aihw.gov.au/reports/hospitals/admitted-patient-care-2017-18/formats

Ball, J. E., Griffiths, P., Rafferty, A. M., Lindqvist, R., Murrells, T., & Tishelman, C. (2016). A cross-sectional study of 'care left undone' on nursing shifts in hospitals. *Journal of Advanced Nursing, 72*, 2086–2097.

Buchan, J., Twigg, D., Dussault, G., Duffield, C., & Stone, P. W. (2015). Policies to sustain the nursing workforce: An international perspective. *International Nursing Review, 62*(2), 162–170. doi:10.1111/inr.12169

Chapman, R., Rahman, A., Courtney, M., & Chalmers, C. (2017). Impact of teamwork on missed care in four Australian hospitals. *Journal of Clinical Nursing, 26*(1-2), 170–181. doi:10.1111/jocn.13433

Clinical Excellence Commission 2019 Policy Directive: *Recognition and management of patients who are deteriorating*. Retrieved from http://cec.health.nsw.gov.au/keep-patients-safe/Deteriorating-patients

Crabtree, E., Brennan, E., Davis, A., & Coyle, A. (2016). Improving patient care through nursing engagement in evidence-based practice. *Worldviews on Evidence-Based Nursing, 13*(2), 172–175.

Damiani, G., Pinnarelli, L., Sommella, L., Vena, V., Magrini, P., & Ricciardi, W. (2011). The Short Stay Unit as a new option for hospitals: a review of the scientific literature. *Medical science monitor: International medical journal of experimental and clinical research, 17*(6), SR15–SR19. https://doi.org/10.12659/msm.881791

Duffield, C., Roche, M., Diers, D., Catling-Paull, C., & Blay, N. (2010). Staffing, skill mix and the model of care. *Journal of Clinical Nursing, 19*(15-16), 2242–2251. doi:10.1111/j.1365-2702.2010.03225.x

Hagler, D., Harding, M., Kwong, J., Roberts, D., & Reinissch, C. (2020). *Clinical Companion to Lewis's Medical-Surgical Nursing: Assessment and management of clinical problems* (11th Ed.). Elsevier: St Louis

Health Workforce Australia. (2014). *Health Workforce 2025 – Doctors, Nurses and Midwives* (Volume 1) Retrieved from https://www1.health.gov.au/internet/main/publishing.nsf/Content/34AA7E6FDB8C16AACA257D9500112F25/$File/AFHW%20-%20Nurses%20overview%20report.pdf

Hegney, D. G., Rees, C. S., Osseiran-Moisson, R., Breen, L., Eley, R., Windsor, C., & Harvey, C. (2019). Perceptions of nursing workloads and contributing factors, and their impact on implicit care rationing: A Queensland, Australia study. *Journal of Nursing Management, 27*(2), 371–380.

Hubbard, R. E., Peel, N. M., Scott, I. A., Martin, J. H., Smith, A., Pillans, P. I., … Gray, L. C. (2015). Polypharmacy among inpatients aged 70 years or older in Australia. *Medical Journal of Australia, 202*(7), 373–377. doi:10.5694/mja13.00172

Johnson, A. & Chang, E. (2017). *Caring for older people. Principles for Practise* (2ⁿᵈ edn.). John Wiley & Sons, Australia

Johnson, A. & Chang, E. (2018). Chronic illness and disability: An overview. In: *Living with chronic illness and disability. Principles for nursing practice* (3rd edn.). Elsevier: Chatswood

Lyneham. J. (2013). A Conceptual Model for medical-Surgical Nursing: Moving Toward an International Clinical Specialty. *MedSurg Nursing*, Vol 22 no. 4 pp 215–220

Masnoon, N., Shakib, S., Kalisch-Ellett, L., & Caughey, G. E. (2017). What is polypharmacy? A systematic review of definitions. *BMC Geriatrics, 17*(1), 230. doi:10.1186/s12877-017-0621-2

Mitchell, R. J., Williamson, A., & Molesworth, B. (2015). Use of a human factors classification framework to identify causal factors for medication and medical device-related adverse clinical incidents. *Safety science, 79*, 163–174.

Page, A. T., Falster, M. O., Litchfield, M., Pearson, S-A., & Etherton-Beer, C. (2019). Polypharmacy among older Australians, 2006–2017: A population-based study. *Medical Journal of Australia, 211*(2), 71–75. doi:10.5694/mja2.50244

Ross, C., Rogers, C., & King, C. (2019). Safety culture and an invisible nursing workload. *Collegian, 26*(1), 1–7. doi:https://doi.org/10.1016/j.colegn.2018.02.002

Salmond, S. W., & Echevarria, M. (2017). Healthcare transformation and changing roles for nursing. *Orthopedic Nursing, 36*(1), 12–25. doi:10.1097/NOR.0000000000000308

Scully, N. J. (2015). Leadership in nursing: The importance of recognising inherent values and attributes to secure a positive future for the profession. *Collegian, 22*(4), 439–444. doi:https://doi.org/10.1016/j.colegn.2014.09.004

Sherwood, G., & Barnsteiner, J. (2017). *Quality and Safety in Nursing: A Competency Approach to Improving Outcomes.* Hoboken, United States: John Wiley & Sons, Incorporated.

Stephenson, M., McArthur, A., Giles, K., Lockwood, C., Aromataris, E., & Pearson, A. (2015). Prevention of falls in acute hospital settings: a multi-site audit and best practice implementation project. *International Journal for Quality in Health Care, 28*(1), 92–98. doi:10.1093/intqhc/mzv113

Vallés, S., Valdavida, E., Menéndez, C., & Natal, C. (2018). Impacto de la cronicidad en las cargas de trabajo de la enfermería hospitalaria. *Journal of Healthcare Quality Research, 33*(1), 48–53. doi:https://doi.org/10.1016/j.cali.2017.10.005

van Oostveen, C. J., Gouma, D. J., Bakker, P. J., & Ubbink, D. T. (2015). Quantifying the demand for hospital care services: A time and motion study. *BMC Health Services Research, 15*(1), 15. doi:10.1186/s12913-014-0674-2

Wilcox, N., & McNeil, J. J. (2016). Clinical quality registries have the potential to drive improvements in the appropriateness of care. *Medical Journal of Australia, 205*(S10), S21–S26. doi:10.5694/mja15.00921

Zambas, S. I., Smythe, E. A., & Koziol-Mclain, J. (2016). The consequences of using advanced physical assessment skills in medical and surgical nursing: A hermeneutic pragmatic study. *International Journal of Qualitative Studies on Health and Well-being, 11*(1), 32090. https://www.who.int/hrh/nursing_midwifery/global-strategic-midwifery2016-2020.pdf?ua=

9 Critical care nursing

Leanne Hunt and Sharon-Ann Shunker

Chapter objectives

This chapter will offer the reader:

- Insight into the role of the critical care nurse in providing patient and family centred care
- Understanding of the requirements and professional framework for a critical care nurse
- Insight into factors that impact patient flow from admission to discharge and transfer in and out of the critical care areas
- Opportunity to build a knowledge base and develop nursing skills specific to participating as an effective member of the multidisciplinary critical care team
- An understanding of the role of the critical care nurse in end of life care of the patient and process involved in organ and tissue donation

Introduction

Patients who require critical care are often physiologically unstable and are at an increased risk of dying and thus require intensive monitoring and treatment in order to improve outcomes and survival. Physiological instability may involve altered vital signs such as high or low heart rate, blood pressure, respiratory rate, temperature and oxygen saturation. Increased staff to patient ratios in critical care areas allow for close observation and continuous monitoring of the critically ill patient. In the critical care context, advanced technology and equipment provide supportive therapies such as ventilation, advanced hemodynamic monitoring, pacing, intra-aortic balloon pumps, renal replacement therapy and extracorporeal membrane oxygenators.

Florence Nightingale was one of the first nurses to advocate for the placement of patient's requiring 'intensive' nursing care close to the nurse's desk. This concept of gathering the sickest patients in a concentrated area to be cared for by specialised nurses was further developed from 1953 onwards where critical care has since progressed into sub-specialities with large financial investments in people, space and technology (Fairman & Lynaugh, 1998). This development was driven by a combination of patient needs, increased medical knowledge, greater government funding, professional interest and public expectations of care. In the current system, critical care comprises four sub-specialties: the Emergency Department (ED), Intensive Care Unit (ICU), Coronary Care Unit (CCU), and Perioperative Nursing, (discussed in Chapter 2.1.1). Each critical care area is a separate and self-contained unit with their own specialised staff and is dedicated to the management of acutely ill and complex patients. They provide clinical expertise and facilitate the support of vital organ functions of critical care patients (Agency for Clinical Innovation, 2015; Fairman & Lynaugh, 1998). Critical care units are usually classified via levels that provide a framework to describe the delineation of minimum support services, workforce and other requirements for clinical services to be delivered safely. Critical care units across Australia will vary based on unit size, the number, type and severity of illness of the patients admitted, staffing expertise, facilities and support services. (Agency for Clinical Innovation, 2018; College of Intensive Care Medicine of Australia and New Zealand, 2011; NSW Ministry of Health, 2019; Department of Health Queensland Government, n.d).

The emergency department

The emergency department (ED) provides access to emergency care, triaging, assessment, and management of patients. Delivering timely emergency care is an integral part of the health system and the quality of emergency care has a key role in determining health outcomes for patients. ED visits are often unscheduled and patients need a thorough primary assessment, with rapid decisions made, and rapid treatment actions delivered.

Patients are admitted to the ED as emergency presentations, trauma transfers by air or road ambulance, emergency admissions brought in by ambulance or GP referrals. They present with a variety of health-related issues such as; accidents, allergic reactions, and for urgent medical and surgical care. ED nurses need to be experts in primary assessment in order to quickly and accurately assess the needs of each patient, to prioritise care, intervene to stabilise the patient, treat the problem, discharge the patient after the emergency is over, or make arrangements for transfer to a different area of the hospital, or another hospital.

All patients that present to ED are triaged and assigned a category according to the Australian Triage Scale (ATS) (Australian College of Emergency Medicine, 2019). The triage process is a relatively quick and classifies patients on a scale of risk as a means to best identify those who require urgent medical assessment and intervention. The triage nurse must be trained in the area of triage and have well developed clinical skills. This is most often a more senior Registered Nurse (RN) as the triage role requires immediate and accurate patient assessment often on the basis of incomplete or ambiguous data.

> The Australian Triage Scale is a clinical tool used to establish the maximum waiting time for medical assessment and treatment of a patient (Australian College of Emergency Medicine, 2019).

Critical challenges facing ED nurses are varied, but include ambulance pressure, waiting times, the need to undertake primary assessment, and treat and transfer patients within reasonable timeframes to the most appropriate areas for ongoing management. Demands on the ED department and ED nurses have increased significantly in recent years and this trend is likely to continue. A significant proportion of elderly, complex, chronic health problems, acute mental health patients and other problems not traditionally seen as the domain of emergency care are now presenting to the ED (Victorian Government, 2007).

The intensive care unit

An intensive care unit (ICU) is dedicated to the management of patients with life-threatening illnesses and injuries, and monitoring of potentially life-threatening conditions. ICU provides specialist expertise and facilities for the support of vital functions and uses the skills of medical, nursing and other personnel experienced in the management of these problems (College of Intensive Care Medicine of Australia and New Zealand, 2011). Working as a nurse in ICU could also extend to the provision of services outside of the ICU such as being part of the Rapid Response or Medical Emergency Team (MET) and outreach services. Outreach services involve the senior critical care nurses following up patients post discharge from ICU and helping to prevent readmission (Garry, Rohan, O'Conner, Patton & Moore, 2018). Patients are admitted to ICU via ED, inter-hospital transfer (e.g. transfer for specialist care via road or air transport), or intra-hospital transfer (e.g. post MET call, OT, cardiac catheter lab). Admission of patients to ICU should extend to those with a reversible medical condition and reasonable expectation of survival or substantial recovery. Potential outcome of treatment should be taken into consideration, particularly when the benefit of treatment is unclear. Patients with low risk conditions and those with end-stage chronic diseases are least likely to benefit from Intensive Care. The status of patients admitted to ICU should be continuously reviewed to identify patients who may no longer need intensive monitoring, observation or treatment and are ready for discharge.

The level of intensive care available is often determined by the hospital and the facilities (such as having 24-hour pathology and radiology) and support services that can be offered, for instance the ability to care for complex trauma patients, cardiothoracic, or neurosurgery patients (NSW Health, 2019). As a nurse working in an ICU you will be expected to have a demonstrated commitment to being involved in research and attending education workshops that allow you to develop the knowledge and skills required to care for patients.

A Level III ICU is a tertiary referral unit for intensive care patients and should be capable of providing comprehensive critical care including complex multi-system life support for an indefinite period. As a nurse working in a Level III unit you will be expected to develop knowledge and skills to manage ventilators, renal replacement therapy, cardiac pacing, managing patients on intra-aortic balloon pumps, monitoring and treating patients with raised intra-cranial pressure and caring for patient on extracorporeal membrane oxygenation therapy (College of Intensive Care Medicine of Australia and New Zealand, 2013).

A Level II ICU provides care to less complex patients but should be capable of providing mechanical ventilation, renal replacement therapy and invasive cardiovascular monitoring for an indefinite period providing appropriate specialty support is available within the hospital. Where appropriate specialty support (e.g. neurosurgery, cardiothoracic surgery) is not available within the hospital, there should be an arrangement with a designated tertiary hospital so that patients referred can be accepted for specialty management. Some training and experience in managing critically ill children preferably with advanced paediatric life support provider status or equivalent, is desirable for medical and nursing staff in rural ICUs (College of Intensive Care Medicine of Australia and New Zealand, 2013).

A Level I ICU is one that is providing immediate resuscitation and short-term cardio-respiratory support for critically ill patients. Working as a nurse in this level unit you will be expected to understand basic concepts of ventilation and provide short-term support to the mechanically ventilated patient with simple invasive cardiovascular monitoring for a period of at least several hours, whilst awaiting transfer to a Level II or III unit. The patients most likely to benefit from Level I care include patients with uncomplicated myocardial ischemia, post-surgical patients requiring special observations and care, unstable medical patients requiring special observations and care beyond the scope of a conventional ward, and patients requiring short-term mechanical ventilation (College of Intensive Care Medicine of Australia and New Zealand, 2013).

The coronary care unit

CCUs are a component of Cardiac Care services. Cardiac Care nurses are involved in the continuum of patient care that involves the diagnosis, management and treatment of patients with cardiac disease. The network of Cardiac Care services involves specialised areas such as cardiothoracic surgery, interventional radiology, echocardiogram and rehabilitation services (South Australian Government, 2016). Admissions to the CCU can occur via ED, intra-hospital transfers (e.g. ICU or general wards) or inter-hospital transfers (e.g. another health facility).

CCUs provides intensive care for emergency and acute cardiac illness. The CCU nurse will be required to offer a high level of expert care and advanced monitoring of patients with acute and chronic cardiac problems. This will include monitoring and interpreting cardiac rhythms, performing 12 lead ECGs, monitoring cardiac enzymes and also providing supportive care with devices such as intra-aortic balloon pumps. The care CCUs provide has developed significantly from the treatment of acute myocardial infarction and arrythmia management to now becoming part of a supported network of cardiac care. Cardiac nursing also focuses on provision of patient education and rehabilitation (Australasian Health Infrastructure Alliance, 2018).

Contemporary issues in critical care

Professional development framework for a critical care nurse

Each critical care area requires an increasingly skilled nursing workforce underpinned by workforce growth, quality education, clinical practice guidelines and competencies (Williams, Kleinpell & Alberto, 2018).

> A skilled workforce is one that has specialised skills, training, knowledge and acquired ability related to their work. (OECD, 2011).

To begin working in critical care there are no additional educational, skill or years of practice requirements beyond a Division 1 Registered Nurse. Commencing work in critical care can be daunting due to the complexity of patients, technology and knowledge expectations. RNs new to critical care are supported by educators in transition to practice programs to develop their knowledge, skills and competence within the area. This model of practice development has been in place for many years and has been shown to provide an effective model of support for new practitioners to develop both skills and knowledge in caring for critically ill patients within the critical care environment. In addition to this support it is expected and recommended by a number of governing bodies (e.g., ACCCN, ACORN), that the majority of RNs gain a post-graduate qualification in their chosen critical care area.

Professional frameworks are being developed and used to guide practice development along the continuum of novice to expert practitioner. These frameworks include knowledge, skills and practice development guide. Each level from novice to expert has various competency assessments that are specific to the critical care area and are in addition to hospital competency requirements.

Competency assessments assess proficiency in knowledge, skills and competence. They are attached to learning packages and guidelines and are best assessed in a simulation or clinical practice environment.

Another aspect of education is the multidisciplinary focus to training and education of staff. Because no part of the health care team in critical care works individually there is an increasing trend to use multidisciplinary simulation training exercises in the workplace that mimic 'real life' scenarios and promote safe learning environments. This requires resources that include simulation environments, equipment, protected education time and the opportunity for debriefing and reflection. Simulation training is effective in helping to train and prepare staff for competency assessments (e.g. Advanced Life Support Assessments) where multidisciplinary input is required.

RNs working within critical care can develop advanced practice skills and be accredited to perform these as an independent operator. Advanced practice skills could be skills traditionally undertaken by medical officers but are now being performed by RNs (e.g. insertion of arterial line or central venous access devices). These advanced skills become particularly important in regional and rural settings where medical support may be off site or not immediately available, in these instances the RN can perform the intervention on the patient under the provision of an advanced practitioner.

Advanced practice nursing is a level of nursing practice that uses comprehensive skills, experience and knowledge in nursing care.

Patient flow

Smooth patient flow is the timely movement of patients in and out of ED, ICU and, CCU to ensure patients have access to the right care at the right time in the right place with minimum waiting times (Agency for Clinical Innovation, 2019). Critical care nurses play a pivotal role in facilitating the timely admission and discharge or transfer of patients into and out of units. The process involves all critical care area at different times in operational, tactical and, strategic ways (Cummings, Ellis, Georgiou, Keen, Showell & Turner, 2012).

Patient flow within critical care units is managed by a designated patient flow co-ordinator who is most often a RN or could be the team leader, clinical coordinator or medical officer. This coordinator liaises with the medical team to decide which patients are cleared for discharge to the ward. This is a fluid process and can occur multiple times per day. The overall hospital appointed patient flow manager allocates appropriate ward beds depending on availability. This flow of patients relies on patients in other areas of the hospital being cleared for discharge or transfer elsewhere for a bed to become available. If the bed is not available, then the patient remains in the critical care area and essentially 'blocks' the bed and admissions cannot be received into the unit.

Exit block occurs when patients requiring discharge or transfer out of critical care areas cannot gain access to appropriate beds within a reasonable time frame.

With the increasing complexity of patients and increasing technological capability the demand for critical care beds often outweighs the supply. The issue of patient flow is a critical issue throughout all hospitals within all areas of the hospital. Overall hospital bed occupancy rates have a significant impact on patient flow and the timely admission and discharge of patients to and from critical care areas (Agency for Clinical Innovation, 2019).

Multidisciplinary patient care

Each member of the team offers a unique background of information, training and technical skill, which can improve patient care and outcomes. The consolidation of all team members for multidisciplinary rounds that occur at a set time on a regular schedule is considered best practice. Rounds should emphasise a systematic approach to patient data presentation, the formation, documentation and communication of treatment plans, the order of team member input, and a summary of overall goals of care for the day.

Multidisciplinary care allows for discussion among various disciplines of the health-care team. This team may include critical care medical staff and specialist teams, nursing staff, allied health staff such as physiotherapists, dieticians, speech pathologists, pharmacists, social workers, patients and their families. Multidisciplinary meetings allow disciplines to discuss clinical information and address their goals, issues and concerns and give specialised input to the daily care plan. Consequently, this reduces the negative impact of delays or misunderstandings in communication. Communication failure among health care providers is one of the most frequently cited causes of preventable harm to patients (Sandeep, 2019). The critical care nurse brings a specialised level of knowledge, skill and caring to enhance delivery of a holistic, patient centred approach to care and is the essential link of communication between the various health professionals that are involved in the patients care, including social workers, physiotherapy, trauma teams, surgical teams, gastroenterology as well as providing their own clinical information about the patient (Williams, Kleinpell & Alberto, 2018). This link occurs because nurses are at the patient's bedside 24/7 and are best positioned to have a global understanding of what is happening with the patient.

Box 9.1 - Case study (50-year old patient)

You are the RN working in the ED of a Metropolitan Hospital. A 50-year old person presents with a history of 2 hours of chest pain associated with shortness of breath. An ECG shows ST elevation in the anteroseptal leads. Bloods have identified an elevated troponin.

The patient is transferred to the Cardiac Catheter Lab for emergency Percutaneous Coronary Intervention. During the procedure the patient becomes unstable and has a cardiac arrest. The patient is successfully resuscitated however requires intubation and advanced supportive therapy with inotropes and vasopressors.

This therapy will require the patient to be transferred to ICU and require a multidisciplinary approach to care.

- There are currently no available beds in ICU.

  - What are the principles of patient flow?
  - How may ICU exit block impact admissions into the unit?
  - How might ICU exit block affect the patient and their family?

- Who are the members of the multi-disciplinary team involved in care of this patient in ICU?
- What are some of the perceived benefits of a multidisciplinary approach to care?

In critical care the use of a multidisciplinary team approach with medical, nursing, allied health professionals working closely together is associated with a reduced patient length of stay (Sharma, Hashmi & Friede, 2019). Total days of mechanical ventilation, and prevention of complications such as stress ulcers, deep vein thrombosis, falls, skin breakdown, infection and readmissions also show significant improvement with the multidisciplinary approach. Staff satisfaction is also significantly improved with multidisciplinary rounds. Furthermore, participants in inter-disciplinary rounds have a greater understanding of patient care, more effective communication, and a better sense of teamwork than providers of traditional rounds (Sandeep, 2019).

Family member participation in care is a tremendous resource. Involving the family in daily rounds allows for information sharing with the team and with the family. The collaborative decision-making process can promote compliance with medical care as well as decrease associated anxiety and confusion about an illness and the recommended treatment.

End of life care

The goal of medical care is to preserve life and prevent suffering (South Western Sydney Local Health District, 2017). Despite all the available treatments there are times that people are too unwell to survive. When this occurs the RNs role is to provide comfort and dignity to the patient and support the patient and others through the process. RNs play a central role in planning end of life care. The planning of end of life care requires ongoing assessment, disclosure and consensus building with the patient and/or their family. At times families struggle to understand and come to terms with their relatives' condition. In this instance ongoing communication and discussion is necessary for family members' emotional wellbeing. It is imperative that consistent information is provided by all members of the team. End of Life Care Plans and Pathways improves the planning and delivery of end of life care.

Organ and tissue donation

The process of organ donation occurs exclusively within critical care areas. End of life care should include the opportunity to donate organs and tissue. The topic of organ and tissue donation is not accepted by all patients and families. Families should not be pressured to make decisions that they are not comfortable with. The critical care RN plays an important role in referring patients for organ and tissue donation to the hospital Donor Specialist Nurse (DSN). The DSN checks the Australian Organ Donor Registry, reviews the patient and determines their eligibility for donation. They will then plan the conversation with the family. Each state also has a state wide service that is available 24/7. Any conversation regarding donation is best conducted by staff that have undertaken the necessary training and are specialised in the field of organ & tissue donation.

Organ donation is governed by the Human Tissue Act 1993 and Ethical Practice Guidelines (https://www.legislation.nsw.gov.au/inforce/dae79cae-8043-47df-9c37-fe8d-1d7e38b3/1983-164.pdf). Organ donation can only be undertaken when there is confirmation of (a) Irreversible cessation of all function of the persons' brain (Brain Death) or (b) Irreversible cessations of circulation of blood in the person's body (Circulatory Death).

Patients and their families always remain the focus of care, whether or not organ donation is consented to. If the patient is for donation they require intensive nursing care to support and optimise organ function until retrieval. Priorities are to support and optimise the patients' hemodynamics and metabolic status, whilst liaising with the DSN about what interventions are to be undertaken prior to the donation occurring. This is to ensure that the organs are in the most favourable condition for retrieval and therefore in the best condition for the transplant recipient. Families need a lot of support from the critical care nurse as this can be a distressing time for them (Australian government organ and tissue donation authority, 2019). Consent is obtained from the senior available next of kin and the designated officer usually the DSN. The DSN approaches and obtains consents from families for donation in all cases where donation is feasible. In the instance of a Coroners Case, consent must also be obtained from the Forensic Pathologist and Coroner.

Conclusion

Critical care nursing is presented with a range of challenges across ED, ICU and CCU. With an aging population and increasing complexity of patient presentations, nursing within critical care offers a unique opportunity to not only practice nursing, but be a pivotal component in an increasingly technical, multidisciplinary and skilled area. Through professional frameworks, skill development and awareness of the system issues that occur within critical care, critical care nurses are in a unique position to have a positive impact on patient and family outcomes.

Online resources

1   Agency for Clinical Innovation (ACI): https://www.aci.health.nsw.gov.au/
2   Australian College of Critical Care Nurses (ACCCN): https://www.acccn.com.au/
3   College of Emergency Nursing Australasia (CENA): https://www.cena.org.au/
4   Australian College of Nursing (ACN): http://www.acn.edu.au/education
5   Cardiac Society of Australia and New Zealand (CSANZ): https://www.csanz.edu.au/

References

Agency for Clinical Innovation. (2015). *Intensive care service model: NSW level 4 adult intensive care units.* Retrieved from https://www.aci.health.nsw.gov.au/__data/assets/pdf_file/0006/283452/ic-service-model-web-v1.pdf

Agency for Clinical Innovation. (2018). Establishment, governance and operation of a close observation unit. Retrieved from https://www.aci.health.nsw.gov.au/__data/assets/pdf_file/0007/430837/Close-Observation-Units-Key-Principles.pdf

Agency for Clinical Innovation. (2019). Intensive Care Unit exit block project. Retrieved from https://www.aci.health.nsw.gov.au/__data/assets/pdf_file/0004/475177/Intensive-Care-Unit-Exit-Block-Project-Evidence-Review.pdf

Australian and New Zealand Intensive Care Society. (2019). The statement on death and and organ donation. Retreived from https://donatelife.gov.au/sites/default/files/anzics-statement-on-death-and-organ-donation-edition-4_1.pdf

Australian College of Emergency Medicine. (2019). *Triage.* Retrieved from https://acem.org.au/Content-Sources/Advancing-Emergency-Medicine/Better-Outcomes-for-Patients/Triage

Australian Government Organ and Tissue Authority. (2019). Donate Life. Retrieved from https://donatelife.gov.au/resources/clinical-guidelines-and-protocols/professional-statements

College of Intensive Care Medicine of Australia and New Zealand (CICM). (2013). Minimum standards for intensive care units seeking accreditation for training in intensive care medicine. (2011). Retrieved from https://www.cicm.org.au/CICM_Media/CICMSite/CICM-Website/Resources/Professional%20Documents/IC-1-Minimum-Standards-for-Intensive-Care-Units.pdf

College of Intensive Care Medicine of Australia and New Zealand (CICM). (2013). Minimum standards for intensive care units seeking accreditation for training in intensive care medicine. Retreived from http://www.cicm.org.au/CICM_Media/CICMSite/CICM-Website/Resources/Professional%20Documents/IC-3-Minimum-Standards-for-Intensive-Care-Units-Seeking-Accreditation.pdf

Cummings, E., Ellis, L., Georgiou, A., Keen, E., Showell, C., & Turner, P. (2012). *An evidence-based review and training resource on smooth patient flow.* Retrieved from https://www.health.nsw.gov.au/pfs/Documents/evidence-based-review.pdf

Department of Health Queensland Government. (n.d). *Cardiac services.* Retrieved from https://www.health.qld.gov.au/__data/assets/pdf_file/0022/444271/cscf-cardiac.pdf

Fairman, J., & Lynaugh, J. (1998). *Critical Care Nursing: A history.* Retrieved from https://books.google.com.au/books?id=gQE69t0cbrMC&printsec=frontcover&source=gbs_ge_summary_r&cad=0#v=onepage&q&f=false

Garry, L., Rohan, N., O'Conner, T., Patton, D., & Moore, Z. (2018). Do nurse led critical care outreach services impact inpatient mortality rates? *British Association of Critical Care Nurses, 21*(1): 40-46.

Mason, S., Knowles, E., Boyle, A. (2016). Exit block in emergency departments: A rapid evidence review. *Emergency Medicine Journal, 34*(1), 46–51.

NSW Health Department. (2002). Guide to the Role Delineation of Health Services. Retrieved from https://www.health.nsw.gov.au/services/publications/guide-role-delineation-health-services.pdf

NSW Health Department. (2019). *NSW Health guide to the deliniation of clinical services.* Retreived from https://www.health.nsw.gov.au/services/Publications/role-delineation-of-clinical-services.PDF

Organisation for Economic Cooperation and Development. (2011). *A skilled workforce for strong sustainable balanced growth.* Retreived from https://www.oecd.org/g20/summits/toronto/G20-Skills-Strategy.pdf

Sandeep, S., Hashmi, M., & Friede, R. (2019). *Multidisciplinary Rounds in the ICU.* Retrieved from https://www.ncbi.nlm.nih.gov/books/NBK507776/

Sharma, S., Hashmi, MF., & Friede, R. (2019). *Interprofessional rounds in the ICU.* Retrieved from https://www.ncbi.nlm.nih.gov/books/NBK507776/

South Western Sydney Local Health District. (2016). *Advanced Care Planning, End of Life and Palliative Care Strategic Plan 2016-2021.* Retrieved from https://www.swslhd.health.nsw.gov.au/pdfs/ACP_StratPlan.pdf

Williams, G., Kleinpell, R., & Alberto, L. (2018). *Global issues in critical care nursing.* Retrieved from wfccn.org/wp-content/uploads/2018/01/WFCCN_Chapter_9.pdf

10 Neonatal nursing

Critically sick babies require unique nursing skills

Evalotte Mörelius and Mandie Jane Foster

Chapter objectives

This chapter will offer the reader:

- A brief overview of nursing sick babies.
- A description of the key concepts directing nursing of sick babies.
- An outline of the most important neonatal nursing practices to prevent developmental consequences for the baby.
- A brief overview of challenges to neonatal nursing and nurses who practice in the neonatal intensive care unit.

Life outside the womb is completely new and unpredictable for newborn babies who rely on adults for protection in order to survive. Newborn babies are able to experience emotions such as positive touch or pain and they can signal their needs but need help to meet these needs. Their behavioural signals can be vague and difficult to detect and interpret, especially if the baby is born preterm or is sick. For instance, such signals can be a yawn, finger splay or drowsy eyes. Working as a nurse with newborns who are critically ill and/or born preterm requires special education, training and skills to care for the vulnerable baby for several weeks or months as well as parents in crisis.

Preterm birth and sick babies

Prevalence

A newborn baby's health, weight, Apgar score and gestational age (GA) at birth are key determinants of health and wellbeing throughout life (Australian Institute of Health and Welfare, 2019).

> An Apgar score measures a baby's appearance, pulse, grimace (reflex irritability), activity (muscle tone) and respiration out of 0–2 at 1 and 5 minutes following birth with a total score of 10 indicating a good overall status (American Academy of Pediatrics Committee on Fetus Newborn & American College of Obstetricians Gynecologists Committee on Obstetric Practice, 2015).

Approximately 15% of all babies need care in a neonatal unit (Liu et al., 2016). Some of the reasons relate to transition into the life outside the womb, for instance respiratory adaptation, jaundice or hypoglycaemia. Other reasons are congenital diseases/defects, birth complications, infections, or neonatal abstinence syndrome where the newborn baby needs extensive care to withdraw from drugs taken by the mother during pregnancy.

Preterm births are still the leading cause of newborn mortality (5%–13%) in developed countries (Liu et al., 2016)

Preterm is defined as babies born alive before 37 weeks of pregnancy with sub-categories of extremely preterm (less than 28 weeks), very preterm (28 to 32 weeks) and moderate to late preterm (32 to 37 weeks).

In Australia, 8.7% of all babies born are preterm with 14–15% of live newborn babies being admitted to one of the 23 newborn/neonatal intensive care units (NICU), special/intensive care nurseries or special care baby units around Australia. During 2017, 31,723 preterm babies were admitted to an Australian neonatal critical care setting (Australian Institute of Health Welfare, 2019). Longer hospital stays were associated with a lower GA and birth weight (Li et al., 2013).

Risk factors associated with a preterm birth

Risk factors can be internal or external; internal relate to the mother and/or baby, external relate to all other factors. Maternal risk factors for a preterm birth include cervical and placenta incompetence, infections, age (<18–20yrs or >35–40yrs), pre-eclampsia and other maternal complications or diseases.

Cervical incompetence means that the cervix is dilating too early, which increases the risk for preterm birth. Placenta incompetence means insufficient blood flow to the placenta, which causes insufficient nutrition to the foetus. Pre-eclampsia is a disorder developed during pregnancy, including high maternal blood pressure.

Risk factors for the preterm baby *at birth* include a low GA, birth weight, gender (male), growth restriction whilst in the womb (low weight for GA) and comorbidities. Preterm births are more prevalent in multiple pregnancies (69% twins; 94% triplets or more), mothers who smoke (13.6%), live in remote/very remote areas (13.5%), are Indigenous (14.2%), or live in a low socioeconomic area (Australian Institute of Health and Welfare, 2019).

External risk factors include poor maternity care, expertise of the staff team, hospital resources, organizational systems, and transportation time or mode from the referring to receiving NICU facility (Bolisetty, Legge, Bajuk, & Lui, 2015; The Royal Australian and New Zealand College of Obstetricians and Gynaecologists, 2017).

Risk factors associated with being born preterm

Preterm babies with a low GA (23–26 weeks) and very low birth weight (<1500g) are significantly more at risk of developing major neonatal morbidities (Bolisetty et al., 2015).

Neonatal morbidity is the risk of death during the first 28 days of the newborn's life.

The brain of a preterm baby is especially vulnerable for changes in the surrounding environment (Bergman, 2019). Therefore, babies in neonatal intensive care are at risk of a wide range of life-long developmental delays due to events including neonatal hypoxia, brain haemorrhage, distress and infection. These injuries, dependent on the degree of insult, can cause ongoing sensory, perceptual and motor disorders (Bergman, 2019; Boardman & Counsell, 2019). However, most of the consequences from brain complications are not evident until after discharge from the NICU.

Being born preterm also includes several immediate risks due to immaturity. Particular attention needs to focus on normal physiological development of the lungs. An early birth increases the risk of respiratory disorders with the need for oxygen therapy and ventilation support. Moreover, the gastrointestinal and renal systems are immature and need special considerations concerning the introduction of parenteral nutrition, oral feeding and medications, which increases the risk of hypoglycaemia. The immune system lacks a functional skin barrier and an existing or potential infection can be life threatening within minutes. The preterm baby's dermatological conditions are very different from full-term babies, with risk for water loss, pressure wounds, infections, fungus and difficulties in temperature regulation (Li et al., 2013; Webb et al., 2014; Australian Institute of Health Welfare, 2019).

Babies born preterm possess the functional nociceptive system required to feel pain. In fact, due to the preterm babies' undeveloped nervous system and their inability to inhibit noxious stimuli, they are more sensitive and experience more pain from a stimulus than full-term babies do. There is also evidence showing that newborn babies acquire implicit memories of pain, and this is why it is important to protect the baby from pain (Anand et al., 2017; Field, 2017).

Key considerations in the delivery of neonatal care

The potential and actual risks, consequences, management, and neuroprotective developmental care of preterm babies in Australia is complicated and multifactorial especially when 25% of Australian births occur in rural or remote areas where access to efficient maternity care is limited (The Royal Australian and New Zealand College of Obstetricians and Gynaecologists, 2017). Some of the key considerations to prevent developmental consequences for the baby are described below.

Promote parental involvement

A baby needs a warm, intimate, and continuous relationship with the parent, or a permanent substitute, to have the best chance of growing up without mental health issues related to insecure attachment (Bretherton, 1992). John Bowlby initiated the development of the attachment theory, defined as any form of behaviour that results in a baby attempting to retain proximity to the parent (Bretherton, 1992). If the child receives security and protection when seeking the parent, the attachment pattern is defined as secure. However, what sometimes happens in many NICUs is that separation between parents and their preterm baby is common, making it difficult for parents to interact with the baby thus affecting the parent-baby relationship and attachment negatively.

Hence, nurses need to enable parents to stay around the clock in the NICU and be involved in the care of their baby to facilitate a secure attachment. Family integrated

---

Box 10.1 - Case study (Julia)

Julia was born preterm at gestational week 26. Her parents were unprepared for the sudden, preterm birth and the immediate intensive care that followed. When they first met Julia, she was in an incubator with ventilatory support, a nasogastric tube for feeding and an umbilical cord line providing glucose solution. They were both shocked and scared by the unfamiliar environment and situation they now found themselves in. They tried to look at Julia through the incubator wall but could not comprehend that she was their daughter, both parents just wanted to leave the NICU. Knowing this moment is critically important for parents and the baby to develop a healthy bond and attachment, the nurse devoted all of her focus on the parents. Gradually, she helped them to look at Julia, open the incubator door, touch and talk to her, hold her hand and count her fingers and toes. Eventually the parents were able to open up and embraced the moment, which allowed them to express their emotions, fears, shock and distress.

Reflective questions:

1 Why is it important to encourage parents to bond with their preterm baby as early as possible?
2 What specific skills or examples did the nurse use in this case study?

---

care is a progression of family centred care where the family/parents are forefront to care delivery and carers are provided with ongoing education and opportunities to become confident independent primary carers of their baby under the supervision of the neonatal team (Als & McAnulty, 2011; Foster & Shields, 2019).

In line with what parents report as important and stressful in the NICU, it is essential that nurses orientate and inform parents of the NICU routine, services, facilities, monitors, tests, terminology, medications, ventilators and ways parents can communicate and care for their baby. Interventions for parental bonding and involvement include watching (looking, listening, responding to interaction behaviours), comforting (touching, skin-to-skin contact), talking/singing, performing routine care (temperature taking, changing nappies, bathing, weighing) and feeding. Guiding parents in what signs to watch for when their baby is happy and ready to interact (eyes open, relaxed posture, steady breathing and heart rate) or tired and needing to rest (looking away, squirming, grimaced facial expressions) will help parents understand their babies' needs and promote the parenting role (Als & McAnulty, 2011; Li et al., 2013; Healy & Fallon, 2014).

It is important for nurses to encourage closeness and interaction between the parent and baby immediately after birth. One way to do that is to take the baby out of the incubator and practice Kangaroo Mother Care (KMC). The main components of KMC include continuous Skin-to-Skin Contact (SSC) between a parent and the low-birth weight baby, exclusive breastfeeding, early discharge and follow-up care (Kostandy & Ludington-Hoe, 2019).

When practicing SSC, the baby is placed on the parent's naked chest, in an up-right position, securely attached with a binder. To maximise the area of SSC, the baby only wears a nappy, hat and socks. Preterm babies in SSC display less physiological stress, are more likely to be calm, settle without fussing and have a greater mature sleep organization compared to when in the incubator (Kostandy & Ludington-Hoe, 2019). Nurses supporting the parent-baby dyad in SSC need to make sure the baby keeps their airway open by ensuring a good head position whilst also monitoring the baby's temperature and oxygen levels.

Reduce the baby's stress and pain

When babies are in need of intensive care, they may be affected by the constant stimuli within the NICU being lighting, temperature, smell, touch, sound, movement, pain and stress. In order to protect the development of the brain, it is important to prevent negative consequences of intensive care therapy by avoiding over-stimulation, stress and pain (Als & McAnulty, 2011). Compared to healthy full-term babies, preterm babies are at a greater risk of consequences raised from an acute stress response. For instance, a painful procedure or a sudden high-pitched sound can cause a raised blood pressure in the preterm baby, risking brain haemorrhage.

Babies in pain show signs of an increased heart and respiratory rate, decreased oxygen saturations, and if possible, they cry. Typical facial signs of neonatal pain are eye squeezing, grimacing, brow furrowing, nasal-labial lines and an open mouth. The baby may also have an increased muscle tone and portray vigorous body movements (Field, 2017). Methods to reduce pain for babies during procedures include the use of oral sweet solutions, breastfeeding, non-nutritive sucking and parental support through SSC (Field, 2017).

Monitor deep sleep

Sleep plays a critical role in synaptic development, learning, and memory, and as such, it is imperative that sleep is supported and protected during the hospital stay. To avoid interruptions to the babies' deep sleep, all procedures need to follow the babies' individual rhythm and should be managed by two people, one whom performs the procedure and one (preferably the parent) who provides individualised support, including pain relief. The number of procedures performed on babies in the NICU need to be restricted to include only the most necessary interventions (Anand et al., 2017). Quiet times to promote rapid eye movement sleep are essential to facilitate brain development.

Support breastfeeding

Feeding is an opportunity for closeness and interaction between the parent and baby. This is a time that allows the parent to provide comfort, show affection and bond with their baby, whether that is through breastfeeding or feeding from a bottle or cup. The World Health Organization (WHO) recommends human breast milk exclusively until the baby is six months of age. Thereafter, the recommendation is to start with food along with breast milk and continue breast milk feeding until the child is at least two years of age. Some of the documented benefits of human breast milk include a lower risk of infection, fever and diarrhoea (Khan, Vesel, Bahl, & Martines, 2015). Some of the long-term benefits for the baby include protection against overweight/obesity (Horta, Loret de Mola, & Victora, 2015), diabetes type 2 (Horta & de Lima, 2019) and increased intelligence scores (Horta, de Sousa, & de Mola, 2018). For the preterm baby, the first step for feeding from the breast is SSC and sensing the warmth, connection and olfactory response where the ability to coordinate sucking, swallow and breathe develops with maturation. Besides maturation, other factors such as keeping the mother-baby dyad together around the clock in the NICU and opportunities to practice SSC have been shown to have a positive impact on breastfeeding outcomes (Bergman, 2019) and should be encouraged by all nurses working within a NICU.

It may take many weeks before the preterm baby can be fully breastfeed. In the meantime, nutrition is met through a combination of parenteral solutions, tube feeding and feeding from a cup with expressed breast milk. If the family's wish is to breastfeed, the nurse needs to actively encourage the mother to stimulate lactation through early and regular milk expression (Maastrup et al., 2014).

An understanding of the unique breastfeeding situation that comes with giving birth to a preterm or sick baby is crucial. NICU nurses need to be able to develop individualized feeding care plans to mothers and babies to limit the likelihood of breastfeeding cessation. Guiding parents of preterm babies in breastfeeding and lactation has to be performed with the utmost delicacy as mothers have expressed feelings of guilt and grief in not being able to provide enough milk for their babies (Ikonen, Paavilainen, & Kaunonen, 2015). Breastfeeding guidance and plans need to be in accordance with the mother's wishes, the development and competence of the baby, individualized, carefully followed and adjusted accordingly.

In 1991, the United Nations children's fund and WHO launched the Baby Friendly Hospital Initiative (BFHI), in order to support breastfeeding. The BFHI describes ten steps that health facilities should utilise for successful breastfeeding. The original steps did not completely comply with neonatal intensive care, therefore minor adjustments were suggested and subsequently incorporated (Nyqvist et al., 2013).

Box 10.2 - Case study (William)

William was born full-term and diagnosed with hypoglycaemia. William received emergency and ongoing treatment being intra-venous glucose therapy along with supplementary cup feeding. He is now three days old, off all intra-venous therapy and ready for discharge home once breastfeeding is successfully established. However, William appears reluctant to latch onto the breast, which has caused William's mother to become very distressed. The nurse came across William's mother whom was seen to be crying. On further inquiry, she stated that she felt confused with all of the nurses' recommendations in breastfeeding and although she had tried all of these different techniques, nothing was working and she was worried about how she would be able to manage breastfeeding at home. She said, William only gets upset, cries or falls asleep and she does not know what to do, she said that she just wanted to give up breastfeeding. Immediately, the nurse sensed that the mother felt disempowered, burdened, confused and at a loss with the information and advice given to her about breastfeeding. She immediately reassured the mother and encouraged the mother to relax and forget about the advice she had received and to trust her own maternal instincts and feelings. She asked the mother to find a comfortable position and practice SSC with William without feeling the pressure to breastfeed. The nurse left the room and let the mother-baby dyad settle together. An hour later, when the nurse returned they were both asleep in the SSC position. When the nurse returned after an additional hour, the mother was breastfeeding William and they both seemed happy, relaxed and ready to go home.

Reflective questions:

1 What interventions did the nurse execute?
2 In this case, what was the main reason/rationale for a successful breastfeeding outcome?

Take care of parents

Parents in the NICU are especially vulnerable to postpartum depression and post-traumatic stress disorders due to their experiences. On top of this, many families struggle with socioeconomic challenges and live in rural areas far from hospitals with neonatal intensive care facilities. In Australia, parents have reported high levels of stress experienced when they saw their baby limp, weak and in pain as they felt helpless and could not protect their baby. For these parents, the most important aspects of the neonatal care journey was to know their babies' medical treatment and transfer/discharge plans, have open honest communication, be able to help with the physical care and have open visitation times (Sweet & Mannix, 2012). Similarly, nurses relayed the importance in getting to know parents' wishes, involving them in care and transitioning with parents through the care continuum (Trajkovski, Schmied, Vickers, & Jackson, 2012). Yet the nurses were challenged by a lack of time, knowledge, experience or pressure to enact family integrated care and at times had inadvertently forced parents into engaging with their babies when they weren't ready (Skelton, Dahlen, Psaila, & Schmied, 2019). An overarching theme evident in the literature is the need for staff to be aware of the most important needs and situations that cause stress in parents inclusive of good communication, empathy and information sharing (Green, Darbyshire, Adams, & Jackson, 2015; Skelton et al., 2019; Sweet & Mannix, 2012; Trajkovski et al., 2012).

Ethics

Advanced life sustaining technology within neonatal critical care settings have resulted in an increased survival rate for preterm critically ill babies (Healy & Fallon, 2014). Ethical considerations to treat or not based on viability of life as indicated by a low birth weight and GA, challenge nurses globally because of the treatment, pain and risks for consequences that these babies face (Green et al., 2015; Green, Darbyshire,

---

Box 10.3 - Case study (Sarah)

Sarah was born at gestational week 24, weighing less than 500 grams. Sarah's parents had experienced several miscarriages whilst trying to conceive over the past ten years and thanks to in-vitro fertilisation, Sarah was finally born. Her parents were overwhelmed with joy and happiness. Unfortunately, Sarah was very sick during her first week of life and required intensive medical care including medications, ventilatory support, oxygen therapy and continual invasive painful procedures. During this intensive treatment regime, Sarah developed a severe brain haemorrhage, which had the potential to lead onto developmental delay. She also risked blindness because of complications with the retina due to the preterm birth. Despite the staff team continually informing the parents about Sarah's health status, risks, prognosis and choice of treatment – the reality of this unknown outcome was a daily-lived experience for Sarah's parents.

Reflective questions:

1 NICU nurses may experience conflicting feelings in situations like this, what ethical considerations comes to your mind?
2 Parents in such situations need a lot of support (friends, families, relatives, and staff) but what kind of support do you think NICU nurses require when confronted with situations like this?

Adams, & Jackson, 2016; Webb et al., 2014). The impact on how neonatal critical care issues are addressed and resolved in practice requires further inquiry to direct theory, research, practice, education, legislation and organisational systems.

Nurses working in the NICU face ethical dilemmas on a daily basis. For instance, when parents are not able to meet their newborn baby's needs due to disease, depression, or neglect albeit due to drug, alcohol or situations out of the mothers' or healthcare professionals' control.

Conclusion

Monitoring for the consequences of a preterm birth requires a holistic multi-systems multi-disciplinary collaborative team approach where treatment, support and care correlate to the gestational and developmental age, characteristics of the newborn and family that is aligned to the baby's normal developmental growth albeit within an external environment. The joy and challenges of being a nurse in the NICU includes working together with the whole family, supporting them through successes as well as reversion and eventually guiding them through their transition to home.

Online resources

1 Australian College of Neonatal Nurses: https://www.acnn.org.au/
2 Miracle Babies Foundation: https://www.miraclebabies.org.au/families/in-hospital/prematurity/
3 UNICEF, Ten steps to successful breastfeeding: https://www.unicef.org/nutrition/files/Baby-friendly-Hospital-Initiative-implementation-2018.pdf
4 World Health Organisation, Kangaroo Mother Care: A practical guide: https://apps.who.int/iris/bitstream/handle/10665/42587/9241590351.pdf; jsessionid=62FEBBFC834C4D7F1C045DBA0CE01739?sequence=1

References

Als, H., & McAnulty, G. (2011). The newborn individualized developmental care and assessment program (NIDCAP) with kangaroo mother care (KMC): Comprehensive care for preterm infants. *Current women's health reviews, 7*(3), 288–301. doi:10.2174/157340411796355216

American Academy of Pediatrics Committee on Fetus Newborn, & American College of Obstetricians Gynecologists Committee on Obstetric Practice. (2015). The Apgar Score. *Pediatrics, 136*(4), 819–822. doi:10.1542/peds.2015-2651

Anand, K. J. S., Eriksson, M., Boyle, E. M., Avila-Alvarez, A., Andersen, R. D., Sarafidis, K., ... Consortium, E. s. w. g. o. t. N. (2017). Assessment of continuous pain in newborns admitted to NICUs in 18 European countries. *Acta Paediatr, 106*(8), 1248–1259. doi:10.1111/apa.13810

Australian Institute of Health Welfare. (2019). Australia's mothers and babies data visualisations. Retrieved from https://www.aihw.gov.au/reports/mothers-babies/australias-mothers-babies-data-visualisations

Bergman, N. J. (2019). Birth practices: Maternal-neonate separation as a source of toxic stress. *Birth Defects Res, 111*(15), 1087–1109. doi:10.1002/bdr2.1530

Bolisetty, S., Legge, N., Bajuk, B., & Lui, K. (2015). Preterm infant outcomes in New South Wales and the Australian Capital Territory. *Journal of Paediatrics and Child Health, 51*(7), 713–721. doi:10.1111/jpc.12848

Boardman, J. P., & Counsell, S. J. (2019). Factors associated with atypical brain development in preterm infants: Insights from magnetic resonance imaging. *Neuropathol Appl Neurobiol.* doi:10.1111/nan.12589

Bretherton, I. (1992). The Origins of Attachment Theory - Bowlby, John and Ainsworth, Mary. *Developmental Psychology, 28*(5), 759–775. doi:Doi 10.1037/0012-1649.28.5.759

Field, T. (2017). Preterm newborn pain research review. *Infant Behavior & Development, 49*, 141–150. doi:10.1016/j.infbeh.2017.09.002

Foster, M., & Shields, L. (2019). Bridging the child and family centred care gap: Therapeutic conversations with children and families. *Comprehensive Child and Adolescent Nursing*, 1–8. doi:10.1080/24694193.2018.1559257.

Green, J., Darbyshire, P., Adams, A., & Jackson, D. (2015). Looking like a proper baby: Nurses' experiences of caring for extremely premature infants. *Journal of Clinical Nursing, 24*(1-2), 81–89. doi:10.1111/jocn.12608

Green, J., Darbyshire, P., Adams, A., & Jackson, D. (2016). It's agony for us as well. *Nursing Ethics, 23*(2), 176–190. doi:10.1177/0969733014558968

Healy, P., & Fallon, A. (2014). Developments in neonatal care and nursing responses. *British Journal of Nursing, 23*(1), 21. doi:10.12968/bjon.2014.23.1.21

Horta, B. L., & de Lima, N. P. (2019). Breastfeeding and Type 2 Diabetes: Systematic Review and Meta-Analysis. *Curr Diab Rep, 19*(1), 1. doi:10.1007/s11892-019-1121-x

Horta, B. L., de Sousa, B. A., & de Mola, C. L. (2018). Breastfeeding and neurodevelopmental outcomes. *Curr Opin Clin Nutr Metab Care, 21*(3), 174–178. doi:10.1097/MCO.0000000000000453

Horta, B. L., Loret de Mola, C., & Victora, C. G. (2015). Breastfeeding and intelligence: A systematic review and meta-analysis. *Acta Paediatr, 104*(467), 14–19. doi:10.1111/apa.13139

Ikonen, R., Paavilainen, E., & Kaunonen, M. (2015). Preterm Infants' Mothers' Experiences With Milk Expression and Breastfeeding An Integrative Review. *Advances in Neonatal Care, 15*(6), 394–406. doi:10.1097/Anc.0000000000000232

Khan, J., Vesel, L., Bahl, R., & Martines, J. C. (2015). Timing of breastfeeding initiation and exclusivity of breastfeeding during the first month of life: Effects on neonatal mortality and morbidity–a systematic review and meta-analysis. *Matern Child Health J, 19*(3), 468–479. doi:10.1007/s10995-014-1526-8

Kostandy, R. R., & Ludington-Hoe, S. M. (2019). The evolution of the science of kangaroo (mother) care (skin-to-skin contact). *Birth Defects Res, 111*(15), 1032–1043. doi:10.1002/bdr2.1565

Li, Z., Zeki, R., Hilder, L., & Sullivan, E. A. (2013). *Australia's mothers and babies 2011.* (Perinatal statistics series no. 28 Cat. no. PER 59). Canberra: AIHW National Perinatal Epidemiology and Statistics Unit. Retrieved from https://www.aihw.gov.au/reports/mothers-babies/australias-mothers-babies-2012/contents/summary

Liu, L., Oza, S., Hogan, D., Chu, Y., Perin, J., Zhu, J., et al. (2016). Global, regional, and national causes of under-5 mortality in 2000-15: An updated systematic analysis with implications for the Sustainable Development Goals. *Lancet, 388*(10063):3027–35.

Maastrup, R., Hansen, B. M., Kronborg, H., Bojesen, S. N., Hallum, K., Frandsen, A., … Hallstrom, I. (2014). Factors associated with exclusive breastfeeding of preterm infants. Results from a prospective national cohort study. *PLoS One, 9*(2), e89077. doi:10.1371/journal.pone.0089077

Nyqvist, K.H., Häggkvist, A.P., Hansen, M.N., Kylberg, E., Frandsen, A.L., Maastrup, R., … Haiek, L.N. (2013). Expansion of the Baby-Friendly Hospital Initiative ten steps to successful breastfeeding into neonatal intensive care: Expert group recommendations. *Journal of Human Lactation, 29*(3):300–309.

Skelton, H., Dahlen, H., Psaila, K., & Schmied, V. (2019). Facilitating closeness between babies with congenital abnormalities and their parents in the NICU: A qualitative study of neonatal nurses' experiences. *Journal of Clinical Nursing, 28*(15/16), 2979–2989. doi:10.1111/jocn.14894

Sweet, L., & Mannix, T. (2012). Identification of parental stressors in an Australian neonatal intensive care unit. *Neonatal, Paediatric & Child Health Nursing, 15*(2), 8–16.

The Royal Australian and New Zealand College of Obstetricians and Gynaecologists. (2017). Maternity care in Australia: A framework for a healthy new generation of Australians. Retrieved from https://ranzcog.edu.au/RANZCOG_SITE/media/RANZCOG-MEDIA/About/Maternity-Care-in-Australia-Web.pdf

Trajkovski, S., Schmied, V., Vickers, M., & Jackson, D. (2012). Neonatal nurses' perspectives of family-centred care: A qualitative study. *Journal of Clinical Nursing, 21*(17-18), 2477–2487. doi:10.1111/j.1365-2702.2012.04138.x

Webb, M., Passmore, D., Cline, G., & Maguire, D. (2014). Ethical issues related to caring for low birth weight infants. *Nursing Ethics, 21*(6), 731–741. doi:10.1177/0969733013513919

11 Paediatric nursing in the acute care setting

Peter Lewis, Deborah Ireson and Deborah Brooke

Chapter objectives

This chapter will offer the reader:

- An overview of paediatric nursing care in acute care settings
- A description of family-centred care: the dominant model of care in paediatrics
- An introduction to challenges for nurses caring for children and their families in hospital
- A discussion about how to support young people and their families in transition between paediatric and adult health care services

Introduction

Children undergo various transitions as their bodies grow and mature and as their social domains expand away from the family home and into school, community, and ultimately to independent living. In this linear narrative, children's interactions with the health care system and nurses in particular are limited to primary preventive contexts, such as when they receive vaccinations against infectious diseases or when they experience an acute illness or injury that can be managed by the general practitioner (GP). However, some young Australians also need the support of specialist paediatric services for a variety of reasons: they have a serious but acute illness or injury, they have an acute exacerbation of a condition that is chronic and complex, or they have chronic and complex conditions that require ongoing care both in the community and in hospital.

An acute illness or injury is one that occurs in the short term and can be cured or repaired without any ongoing adverse effects. Chronic and complex conditions are those that a child is born with or acquires that have life-long implications for a child's development, health, or wellbeing.

Health services for the care of acute illnesses or injury currently provided within Australian hospitals cease when a child turns eighteen years of age. For many children and their families who have had a long history of engagement with children's services, the transfer of care from paediatric to adult hospital can be a challenging and emotional time. Transfer of care to adult services shifts the focus onto the individual patient and parents can feel left out or redundant when this happens. Young people who have extensive and evolving care needs require careful management as they transition into adult services. Early support and preparation for young people, their families and services on both sides of the age divide becomes a necessary skill for many paediatric nurses.

This chapter introduces family-centred care as the dominant model of care delivery to children and young people hospitalised in Australia. It will discuss how children and their families can be affected by hospitalisation and the role of nurses working in that context. Finally, we discuss the process of transition between paediatric and adult services for children with chronic and complex conditions.

Paediatric nursing in context

The term paediatric nursing usually applies to nursing care of children under the age of 18 years. Paediatrics is a broad category that refers to the care of children with illnesses or conditions involving any bodily system, that are acute, chronic, or life limiting, congenitally diagnosed or acquired later in life. All major cities in Australia provide specialist paediatric services to care for children with a vast range of paediatric conditions. It is important to recognise that nurses who work there can gain experience in caring for children with rare illnesses or serious conditions that might not be cared for elsewhere. Children whose conditions are serious and/or complex are likely to be referred to one of the large paediatric centres where expertise in paediatric care is concentrated. These large specialist centres also receive children referred from rural and remote areas of Australia which can make life difficult for families who are removed from their community supports because of their child's hospitalisation. Some general hospitals provide paediatric services to children in their local community whose conditions are not difficult to manage, such as acute illnesses that can be relatively easily resolved with a short period of hospitalisation.

In Australia, completion of an undergraduate course leading to registration qualifies a nurse to work in paediatrics and several universities offer degrees up to Masters level to enable nurses to specialise in paediatrics. An interest in caring for children is imperative for paediatric nurses. The ability to establish rapport and develop relationships with children and their families is also highly desirable and these skills can be developed on-the-job in an acute care setting. Caring for children who are critically unwell and/or who require lengthy periods of hospitalisation that can last for years can be emotionally draining for nurses working in this area. In addition, establishing and maintaining relationships with parents and extended family members can be time-consuming and emotionally taxing especially for new graduate nurses who are simultaneously learning how to establish new relationships with colleagues and the complexities of an unfamiliar system. Paediatric nursing care is not only provided to children, but is also negotiated in partnership with families within an established model of family-centred care.

Family-centred care

A model of care provides a theoretical perspective of care upon which care delivery can be based in practice.

Family-centred care is a model of care delivery that dominates paediatric services. Family-centred care positions family members as constants in the child's life and experts in matters of the child's health and wellbeing. Within this model, nurses are to care for hospitalised children as members of a family unit that is integral to a child's wellbeing, rather than treat the child as an isolated individual (Arabiat, Whitehead, Foster, Shields, & Harris, 2018). It is a partnership model because it enables parents to participate actively in making decisions around and delivering care to a hospitalised child (Coyne, 2015). Central to the notion of partnership is respectful negotiation. Parents are not expected to be nursing assistants who undertake tasks delegated by the nurse caring for their child. Instead, family-centred care privileges the needs and preferences of the family over those of service providers rather than vice versa. Advantages of family-centred care for children include reducing adverse effects arising from parental separation, promotion of the bond between parent and child, increasing service transparency by enhancing communication and empathy, increased participation in health care by children and parents and enhanced satisfaction with the experience of hospitalisation for children and their families (Coyne, 2015).

The ideal of family-centred care has been notably difficult to achieve in practice (Dennis et al., 2017). Lack of an agreed definition and inconsistencies in implementation can create confusion for health professionals, children and their families about what family-centred care is and how it is meant to operate (Shields, 2015). This means that new graduate nurses might experience tensions around the aspirational goal of delivering family-centred care and the reality of having to accommodate the, at times competing, interests of the family and the health care service. Implementation of family-centred care is complicated by multiple factors including recent findings by Shields (2015) that there is limited evidence that family-centred care works consistently to achieve positive outcomes for patients. This is not to deny that the advantages of family-centred care that are based on respect for human dignity are not valuable, but to point out that the process of negotiation and the development of partnerships with children and their families in hospital, can at times be difficult to undertake.

Box 11.1 - Case study (Emma)

Emma is 3 month-old girl admitted with bronchiolitis. She requires respiratory support of humidified high flow nasal prong oxygen and nutritional support with nasogastric feeding, due to her increased work of breathing and marked respiratory distress. She was born at term and has no other significant medical history. She is very unsettled and irritable. She has been accompanied to hospital by her mother who appears tired and is becoming increasingly frustrated by Emma's unsettledness. Emma's mother feels that Emma would be more settled if she was able to feed orally on demand, however, it is most important to restrict Emma's intake in order to manage her respiratory distress.

Reflective questions:

1 What might be some of the contributing factors to Emma's mother's tiredness and frustration?
2 How could the nursing team caring for Emma and her mother communicate the importance of Emma's medical needs while respecting Emma's mother's desire to care for her daughter as best she can?
3 Why is it likely that nurses and mother will experience conflict during Emma's hospitalisation?

Acute hospitalisation

Family-centred care is based on partnership and the negotiation of care between nurses, parents and children in hospital. However, a one-off admission to hospital lasting a few days rarely provides adequate opportunity for meaningful partnerships to develop. Presentation to hospital because of acute illness or injury requires nurses to take charge of the admission and to reassure parents and children that 'someone' is in control of an unfamiliar and potentially frightening situation. Under these circumstances, partnership and negotiation are very difficult to achieve with parents and children who simply want the ordeal to end and to return to a normal life. However, as a hospital admission lengthens, nurses and families are likely to encounter challenges to the development or maintenance of therapeutic relationships.

> Therapeutic relationships comprise three elements – partnership, intimacy and reciprocity – that intersect at the point of encounter between the nurse and the patient (Richardson et al., 2015).

One challenge is the experience for a parent of being under surveillance, scrutinised and judged by ward nurses. This source of tension between parents and nurses can undermine the development of a trusting and therapeutic relationship. For therapeutics relationships to flourish between nurses and parents, nurses need to demonstrate their respect for parents' knowledge and skill at caring for their child and empathy for the families' situation. Tensions around the experience of parenting in public arise when the roles of the nurse and parent are unclear and centre on the questions over who has primary responsibility for the hospitalised child (Molloy et al., 2015).

To decrease tensions between nurses and families, it is necessary for nurses to use language that promotes collaboration rather than competition. For example, some parents might be offended if a nurse refers to a child as 'my child' or 'my patient' (Molloy et al., 2015). Superficially, this might appear to be a trivial point when parents are secure in their roles and relationships with their child. Nevertheless, such language might be interpreted negatively when parents feel ambivalent about their role, insecure about their relationship, or scrutinised or judged by nurses using the language of ownership. To reinforce the parents' role, nurses could consider referring to 'your child' to ensure that parents are constantly reminded of the special relationship that they have.

Another challenge pertains to feelings of boredom for parents especially when there has been limited negotiation with nurses of active roles for them while hospitalised (Arabiat et al., 2018). Parents of children might feel bored when hospitalisation necessitates that they spend more time with their child than they are used to or that they would like (Shields, 2016). Symptoms of boredom can include expressions of frustration, inability to settle, and paying constant attention to mobile electronic devices and it can be difficult for a nurse to negotiate roles and responsibilities when a parent is distracted (Erkoboni & Radesky, 2018). Boredom can be alleviated, and sociability promoted, for parents by providing patient accommodation in shared rather than single rooms. This can have the additional effect of reducing demands on the nurses' time (Curtis & Northcott, 2016).

Finally, boredom is one of a variety of stressors experienced by children who are hospitalised (Foster, Whitehead, & Arabiat, 2019). Young children between 16 and 30 months old can experience separation anxiety if their parents are absent from hospital. Older children can feel stressed when they feel disempowered or vulnerable as a result of their illness or hospitalisation and this can challenge nurses' ability to negotiate care. It is important for children to be able to play for developmental reasons – play is how children make sense of the world – to promote resilience and to help children cope with adverse feelings of stress attributable to hospitalisation (Williams et al., 2019). To facilitate the development of therapeutic relationships with children it might be necessary for nurses to interact with them through age appropriate play. This will necessarily mean having access to toys or other play things that can help children to interact and express themselves. This can also mean consulting with play therapists, building play rooms, and consulting with occupational therapists for children who need intensive support to engage in play.

Hospitalisation of children with extended care needs

Hospitalisation disrupts the familiar routines of a family (Oulton et al., 2015), however familiarity naturally develops with frequent admissions or lengthy periods of hospitalisation. Genuine partnership in these circumstances can create opportunities to deliver effective care to children and families that respect and accommodate the families' values, beliefs and preferences. This can be rewarding for nurses who take a genuine interest in and develop a genuine relationship with the patient and

---

Box 11.2 - Case study (Mary)

Mary is a 5 year old girl with a complex medical background, comprising of an undiagnosed neurological condition resulting in hypotonia and the need for nocturnal non-invasive respiratory support as well as nutritional support via a long term nasogastric tube. She has been admitted to the ward for management of left lower lobe pneumonia. On arrival to the ward she is febrile, tachycardic and tachypnoeaic with moderate work of breathing and is complaining of abdominal pain.

IV antibiotics and IV fluids have been commenced at full maintenance as she is not tolerating her usual feed regime of oral purees, thickened fluids as tolerated and 4 bolus NGT feeds/day of Ensure formula. Regular chest physio is ordered as well as a review of her existing respiratory support and guidelines for the addition of supplemental oxygen as needed. Mary is accompanied to hospital by her mother Sue, who is her primary carer. Sue is extremely anxious about Mary's deteriorating respiratory function and overall condition. She is wanting to have significant input in the management of Mary's feeding regime as well as make adjustments to her respiratory support, which have not been ordered by the medical team. Mary is also extremely anxious, becomes distressed quickly and is reluctant to allow any nursing care unless she is familiar with the nurse undertaking the care.

Reflective questions:
1   How might you initiate family-centred care for Mary and her mother?
2   Which health professionals will be involved in Mary's care during her hospitalisation and how might you go about coordinating them?
3   What do you imagine to be the optimal outcome of Mary's admission for (1) Mary, (2) her mother, and (3) you?

family. One example of this can be found in the frequent and repeated admission to hospital of children and young people with intellectual disability and complex health needs. Children and young people with intellectual disability can be reassured and their capabilities maximised by adherence to routine in daily life. For more information about nursing people with intellectual disability, please refer to Section 2.2.2.

Challenges when developing therapeutic relationships

During frequent and/or prolonged periods of hospitalisation, several complications can arise that challenge the capacity for nurses and families to develop meaningful therapeutic relationships. One is that it is possible for nurses to send mixed messages to children and families. On one hand, encouraging families to adhere to familiar routines, and to participate in or take responsibility for the care of their child and, on the other, by working in a system that can impose institutional constraints on family participation in care, the reasons for which are often opaque to parents. For example, it is common for accommodation to be provided for only one adult accompanying a child to hospital, which might limit opportunities for a child's care to be shared by either parents or members of their extended family. This can foster misunderstanding and undermine the trust of parents in nurses, the individual institution, or the health care system in general.

For partnerships that are respectful of parents' and families' willingness and capacity to participate in care, there also has to be genuine opportunity for parents to withdraw from caring for their child in hospital if they want to (Coyne, 2015). For example, parents who are particularly burdened by the care of a child with a chronic or complex illness might welcome the opportunity for respite that hospitalisation

---

Box 11.3 - Case study (Marcus)

Marcus is a 14-year old boy who is a planned admission to paediatric ward for a 2-week tune up as part of the ongoing management of his cystic fibrosis. Marcus was diagnosed with cystic fibrosis as an infant, is known to the respiratory team, and has regular outpatient follow up. His symptoms have always been well controlled, he and his family have been compliant with treatment and he has had infrequent hospital admissions. His development is age appropriate. Marcus' treatment during this admission will include a course of IV and nebulised antibiotics as well as continuing all of his regular oral medications (enzymes and vitamin supplements). Allied health input will include review by the dietician, physiotherapy and social work. Marcus was brought to the hospital by his mother who is his primary carer. When he is transferred to the ward however, he is accompanied by a family friend who states that his mother has left the hospital to pick up Marcus's siblings, aged 8yrs and 6yrs from school. She is unsure what time his mother will return. She informs you that Marcus's parents have recently separated and that Marcus's father is not allowed to visit him due to his history of substance abuse. She states that his mother works full time and has limited family support.

Reflective questions:

1 Given Marcus's age, is this admission an appropriate time to open a discussion about transition to adult services? How can this be facilitated?
2 What is the role of the new graduate nurse in this discussion and how can this be negotiated given the change in social circumstances for Marcus and his family?

offers. Hospitalised children are considered to be in a safe environment where care is available on a 24 hour basis. Parents will often take advantage of the opportunity for respite, however, only if they have developed a trusting relationship with ward nursing staff over a period of time. Discussion and negotiation are unlikely to be sufficient on their own for trust to develop to the extent that parents will be willing to leave their child in the care of ward nurses. If trust fails to develop, they will stay in hospital, sometimes to the detriment of their own health and to the development of effective partnerships in care.

Transition between paediatric and adult health care institutions

Family-centred care provides consistent partnership nursing support for children and families that responds to childhood cognitive and developmental stages. However, in the long term this can create a reliance on family focussed services which may leave young people and their families unprepared for feelings of isolation when this is not replicated in adult services (Kingsnorth, Gall, Beayni, & Rigby, 2011; Paton & Hiscock, 2019). Complex conditions persisting into adulthood, and children who are surviving life limiting disorders not previously seen in adult services, eventually face transition to adult care settings, which have less flexibility than paediatric settings that use a model of family-centred care.

Transition has been defined as 'the purposeful, planned movement of adolescents and young adults with chronic physical and medical conditions from child-centred to adult-oriented health care systems' (Blum et al., 1993, p. 570).

Children and families need adequate preparation for transition as moving away from paediatric services can be traumatic for some adolescents beginning to take responsibility for their healthcare, sometimes for the first time in their life. This may also be challenging for parents who have been responsible for meeting their child's complex healthcare needs (McLoughlin, Matthews, & Hickey, 2018). The potential outcome of this at the time of transition is that adolescents may disconnect from services with adverse effects on their health and well-being (Brooks et al., 2017). Seamless transition requires systematic approaches embedded early in the child's care in order to scaffold the process and prevent transition shock (Crowley, Wolfe, Lock, & McKee, 2011; Reiss, Gibson, & Walker, 2005). During a three or four-year period of transition, children gradually accept more responsibility for their healthcare. This can enhance the child's capability and willingness to accept responsibility for their care at the time of transfer to adult services. However, adolescents who are cared for by members of multiple services are more likely to fall through the gaps between paediatric and adult services requiring vigilance by nursing staff to identify the strategies to ensure successful transition (Razon et al., 2019).

Transition shock is a term used to describe the sense of disorientation and discomfort associated with the move from paediatric to adult focused services.

Specialised services may also offer tailored support where families are included in the transition process and where young people are encouraged to engage with condition specific social media groups and monitored websites, for example, 'myD' (my diabetes) and Trapeze, both of which are developed specifically for transitioning youth where relevant information can be sourced. Trapeze.org is a not for profit organisation operating throughout Australia that supports children with chronic conditions through developing stages of self-care and personal management. Trapeze aids the transition process by identifying areas of health care where participation in transition can be achieved for young people of transitioning age until young adulthood (24yrs). While there are various points to at which commence the transition process, in recognition of existing challenges, several states have developed strategies for the successful preparation and transfer of care from paediatric to adult services for young people with chronic and/or complex conditions. Ultimately, new graduate nurses can participate in the transition process in collaboration with and under the guidance of more experienced and specialised nurses in this aspect of care.

Conclusion

Paediatric nursing in the acute care setting is about caring for children within the context of their family unit. Specialist paediatric services are provided in paediatric hospitals and it is in these settings that the widest variety and the most unusual of experiences can be gained. However, paediatric services are provided at many peripheral hospitals as well and opportunities exist for nurses to care for children in these settings. Hospitalisation can be stressful for children and their families. Nurses in this context need to strive towards establishing meaningful therapeutic relationships that value the families' preferences and priorities.

Web resources

1 Association for the Wellbeing of Children in Healthcare: https://awch.org.au/
2 Australian Association for Adolescent Health: https://www.aaah.org.au/
3 Australian College of Children & Young People's Nurses: https://www.accypn.org.au/
4 Trapeze: A supported leap into adult health: http://www.trapeze.org.au/

References

Arabiat, D., Whitehead, L., Foster, M., Shields, L., & Harris, L. (2018). Parents' experiences of Family Centred Care practices. *Journal of Pediatric Nursing, 42*, 39–44. doi: 10.1016/j.pedn.2018.06.012.

Blum, R. W. M., Garell, D., Hodgman, C. H., Jorissen, T. W., Okinow, N. A., Orr, D. P., & Slap, G. B. (1993). Transition from child-centered to adult health-care systems for adolescents with chronic conditions: A position paper of the Society for Adolescent Medicine. *Journal of Adolescent Health, 14*(7), 570–576.

Brooks, A. J., Smith, P. J., Cohen, R., Collins, P., Douds, A., Forbes, V., Lindsay, J. O. (2017). UK guideline on transition of adolescent and young persons with chronic digestive diseases from paediatric to adult care. *Gut, 66*(6), 988–1000.

Coyne, I. (2015). Families and health-care professionals' perspectives and expectations of family-centred care: Hidden expectations and unclear roles. *Health Expectations, 18,* 796–808. doi: 10.1111/hex.12104.

Crowley, R., Wolfe, I., Lock, K., & McKee, M. (2011). Improving the transition between paediatric and adult healthcare: A systematic review. *Archives of Disease in Childhood, 96*(6), 548–553.

Curtis, P., & Northcott, A. (2016). The impact of single and shared rooms on family-centred care in children's hospitals. *Journal of Clinical Nursing, 26,* 1584–1596. doi: 10.1111/jocn.13485.

Dennis, C., Baxter, P., Ploeg, J., & Blatz, S. (2017). Models of partnership within family-centred care in the acute paediatric setting: a discussion paper. *Journal of Advanced Nursing, 73,* 361–374. doi: 10.1111/jan.13178.

Erkoboni, D., & Radesky, J. (2018). The elephant in the examination room: Addressing parent and child mobile device use as a teachable moment. *The Journal of Pediatrics, 198,* 1–6. https://doi.org10.1016/j.jpeds.2018.03.063.

Foster, M., Whitehead, L., & Arabiat, D. (2019). Development and validation of the needs of children questionnaire: An instrument to measure children's self-reported needs in hospital. *Journal of Advanced Nursing, 75*(10), 2246–2258. doi: 10.1111/jan.14099.

Kingsnorth, S., Gall, C., Beayni, S., & Rigby, P. (2011). Parents as transition experts? Qualitative findings from a pilot parent-led peer support group. *Child: Care, Health and Development, 37*(6), 833–840.

McLoughlin, A., Matthews, C., & Hickey, T. M. (2018). "They're kept in a bubble": Healthcare professionals' views on transitioning young adults with congenital heart disease from paediatric to adult care. *Child: Care, Health and Development, 44*(5), 736–745.

Molloy, R., Smyth, W., & Shields, L. (2015). Protocol for a study of who owns the child in hospital. *Working Papers in the Health Sciences, 1,* 1–6.

Oulton, K., Sell, D., Kerry, S., & Gibson, F. (2015). Individualising hospital care for children and young people with learning disabilities: It's the little things that make the difference. *Journal of Paediatric Nursing, 30*(1), 78–86. doi: 10.1016/j.pedn.2014.10.006.

Paton, K., & Hiscock, H. (2019). Strengthening care for children with complex mental health conditions: Views of Australian clinicians. *PLOS ONE, 14*(4), e0214821.

Razon, A. N., Greenberg, A., Trachtenberg, S., Stollon, N., Wu, K., Ford, L., Szalda, D. (2019). A multidisciplinary transition consult service: Patient referral characteristics. *Journal of Pediatric Nursing, 47,* 136–141.

Reiss, J. G., Gibson, R. W., & Walker, L. R. (2005). Health care transition: Youth, family, and provider perspectives. *Pediatrics, 115*(1), 112–120.

Richardson, C., Percy, M., & Hughes, J. (2015). Nursing therapeutics: Teaching student nurses care, compassion, and empathy. *Nurse Education Today, 31,* e1–e5. http://dx.doi.org/10.1016/j.nedt.2015.01.016.

Shields, L. (2015). What is "family-centred care"? *European Journal for Person Centred Healthcare, 3,* 139–144.

Shields, L. (2016). Family-centred care: the 'captive mother' revisited. *Journal of the Royal Society of Medicine, 109,* 137–140. doi: 10.1177/0141076815620080.

Williams, N., Brik, A., Petkus, J., & Clark, H. (2019). Importance of play for young children facing illness and hospitalisation: rationale, opportunities, and a case study illustration. *Early Child Development and Care,* 1-10 doi.org/10.1080/03004430.2019.1601088.Published online 5th April 2019.

12 Nursing and acute mental health settings

Richard Lakeman, Iain Graham, Lucy Nuzum, Diane Russ and Stephen Van Vorst

Chapter objectives

This chapter will offer the reader:

- Insight into the history and current context of responding to acute mental health and behavioural disturbances in Australian health services.
- An overview of crisis theory and how psychosocial crisis manifests in emotional and behavioural dysregulation.
- An outline of common mental health and related problems and how they manifest in presentations to emergency and crisis services.
- A discussion about the complexities involved in responding to suicidal and self-injurious behaviour.
- Discussion about the purpose of mental health acute inpatient units and their place in the continuum of care for people presenting with acute mental health issues.
- An overview of current challenges, concerns, and competing discourses that impact on service responses to people with acute mental health issues.

Introduction

Acute mental health problems, psychosocial crises and dysregulated behaviour are highly prevalent in people who present to health services. This chapter discusses these issues and signposts particular contemporary issues of relevance to all nurses, not just those who are specialist *Mental Health Nurses* (MHNs). The Australian health system is comprised of a range of services to assist in addressing crisis, including phone counselling services, services in primary care settings, emergency or first responders, emergency departments and specialist acute care teams, and inpatient services. This chapter will commence with a discussion of the context of mental health care in Australia and how the present configuration of services and responses to mental distress and crisis has evolved.

A Mental Health Nurse is a registered nurse who holds a recognised specialist qualification in mental health. Taking a holistic approach, guided by evidence, the mental health nurse works in collaboration with people who have mental health issues, their family and community, towards recovery as defined by the individual. (ACMHN, 2010, p.5)

Context

The evolution of acute mental health care has resulted in new structures and services being created in an attempt to meet the complexities and challenges found in Australian health services. The aims of acute mental health nursing care have been described as being about establishing and maintaining a therapeutic ward atmosphere, facilitating individually focused care plans for patients and their significant others, and ensuring compliance with the medical prescription of care while providing physical and emotional safety. However, there are contemporary views that see mental health services as being in a state of crisis (Hickie, 2019) and mental health nursing expertise as having been eroded and undervalued (Lakeman & Molloy, 2018).

Historically the framework of mental health care was custodial (Barnes & Bowl, 2000), where the person with mental distress was managed by incarceration behind asylum walls. However, this system of care was challenged from the late 1950s onwards, leading to a movement of asylum closure and the provision of community-based services (Richmond, 1983). This movement can be understood as a means to provide more humanistic care and personal attention to those with mental distress. Services were transferred to general hospitals with an assumption that this would lead to better integration with primary and social care. The model to be adopted was to be the same as other hospital disciplines namely inpatient and outpatient provision, which in turn would be supported by group homes, hostels, day hospital services and community mental health teams of nurses, social workers and allied health (Corney, 1999). However, there have been many criticisms of this model with those with both acute and long-term mental health problems receiving less than desirable care. Today there is more correctional service and police involvement with mental health clients. There are calls for more services to be better integrated and the role of those providing care to be broader and at the same time more specialised in order to deal with the challenges and complexities people presenting with acute mental health issues deserve.

Crisis or psychiatric emergency?

There are various ways to access acute mental health services in Australia. However, presentation to emergency departments (EDs) is a common pathway to assessment and care. The number of mental health-related presentations to EDs was around 3.6% of all ED presentations in 2017-2018, but the number of presentations per 10,000 of the population had increased by 10% in the previous five years (Australian Institute of Health and Welfare, 2019). Most people who attended ED with a mental health problem in 2017–2018 were diagnosed as having a mental or behavioural disorder due to psychoactive substance use, or an anxiety or stress-related condition (Australian Institute of Health and Welfare, 2019).

Police and ambulance personnel are often the first responders to an acute crisis or emergency and often refer people for further assessment via EDs. These referrals are generally involuntary, and people are most likely to be diagnosed with a mental disorder due to substance misuse (Maharaj, 2007). Intoxication with alcohol or methamphetamine is implicated in the majority of patients with aggressive behaviour in Australian EDs and often leads to sedation being administered against the person's will (Oliver et al., 2019). Some State Services have adopted a co-responder model, whereby MHNs or allied health professionals accompany police and undertake an assessment of people in the field. There is little evidence to date that this approach reduces presentations to EDs (Puntis et al., 2018). People that attend EDs with mental health problems have been found to wait longer, experience longer stays, and leave before treatment is completed than those with primarily physical problems (Australian College for Emergency Medicine., 2018).

> A crisis occurs when a person faces an obstacle to important life goals that at least for a time are insurmountable using customary methods of problem-solving (Caplan, 1964).

Crisis

Many people who present to emergency services are in *crisis*. According to Caplan (1964), people generally live their lives in a state of homeostasis; when this homeostasis is disrupted by challenging events (which may be physical, psychological, emotional, or social), balance is disrupted, and when not restored quickly enough, a state of crisis occurs. A crisis may be categorised as developmental (related to the transition from one life stage to another), situational (related to an unforeseen or overwhelming event), or existential (related to life's purpose).

Crisis intervention aims to ensure the safety of people, define and assist the person in solving the problem, assist the person to view the problem or situation more reasonably and mobilise or provide the right kind of support. There are many theories of crisis intervention and models of treatment (James & Gilliland, 2001). In some places, crisis resolution teams that assist people at home are considered a crucial part of some mental health services (Wheeler et al., 2015). In Australia, the person in crisis will often be referred to community mental health teams or non government organisations (NGOs) for a brief follow-up until the crisis is resolved and then referred to services in primary care.

> A psychiatric emergency is an acute problem of behavioural control or imminent dangerousness to self or others (Claassen et al., 2000).

Psychiatric emergency

A *psychiatric emergency* calls for immediate and sometimes continuing containment or treatment. It may be manifested as a deterioration or relapse of a mental illness, e.g. mania, suicidal and self-injurious behaviour, delirium or unexplained neurological or

---

Box 12.1 - Case study (Jason)

Jason, a 45-year-old male who presented to the ED after texting a suicide note to his partner. Police responded and found him intoxicated. He reportedly stated, 'I can't think straight; I can't do this; I need help'. He reported that he got recently separated from his partner of many years who had immediately re-partnered. He had subsequently started drinking excessive amounts of alcohol and had recently lost his license and his job as a courier as a result of drinking. Consider what assistance Jason might need to be safely discharged home.

acute psychotic symptoms, adverse drug effects, poisoning, or other toxic states, e.g. Lithium toxicity. All registered nurses should be able to recognise a psychiatric emergency and intervene or refer to appropriate services.

Acute behavioural disturbance

People commonly present to acute services in a state of *emotional or behavioural dysregulation* often manifested by extremes in emotions, anger and sometimes irrational behaviour. It is a feature of disrupted equilibrium in crisis, drug and alcohol intoxication, acute relapse in bipolar affective disorder, and is a feature of borderline personality disorder (BPD) (Bayes, Parker, & McClure, 2016). Trauma and invalidating environments in early life can lead to later difficulties with the regulation of emotions and the development of mental health problems (Kezelman & Stavropoulos, 2012).

> Emotional dysregulation may be defined as impaired processes in evaluating, modifying and monitoring emotional reactions (Bayes et al., 2016).

Trauma-informed care is a new approach to care and requires a reconceptualisation of traditional approaches to health and human service delivery whereby all aspects of services are organised around the prevalence of trauma throughout society (particularly as complex trauma is not always recognised). Services that are 'trauma-informed' are aware of and sensitive to the dynamics of trauma, as distinct from directly treating trauma per se (the appropriate term in the latter case is 'trauma-specific' treatment). (Kezelman & Stavropoulos, 2012, p. 112)

People may also present with acute behavioural disturbances related to *psychosis*. Psychosis may arise as a consequence of stress in a person who may be vulnerable to psychotic illness, in people who may be under the influence of illicit substances or in states of drug withdrawal, and in those who may be sleep deprived or experiencing a metabolic disturbance. Psychosis may be manifested by grandiosity, paranoia, suspiciousness, and potentially dangerous behaviour. Psychosis can challenge the capacity of health professionals to empathise and respond in a helpful way (Lakeman, 2020).

Often a busy ED or ward environment is far from the ideal environment to address behavioural disturbances, the environment may exacerbate symptoms, or worsen dysregulated behaviour. The following reflect the ideal features of an environment

---

Box 12.2 - Case study (Sheryle)

Sheryle is an 18-year-old woman brought into the ED by ambulance. Sheryle had attended a party and had locked herself in the bathroom and threatened suicide. The first responders were unable to make much sense of Sheryle's story. She screamed and appeared inconsolable. She reluctantly attended ED and on arrival, screamed at the triage nurse that she just wanted a smoke and was verbally abusive. How would you provide trauma-informed care to Sheryle?

conducive to safely engaging with and assessing a person with an acute behavioural disturbance or mental health problem:

- Low background noise, and bright lighting to reduce the potential for misinter-preting stimuli;
- Privacy to disclose fears or concerns and to enable assessment or brief interven-tions (if indicated);
- Few people or crowds;
- Opportunities to pace, walk and otherwise sublimate energy;
- Warm empathic, congruent and unambiguous communication from all staff;
- The establishment or maintenance of rapport with one or more people with whom to receive reassurance and assist with emotional coping;
- The identification of unmet needs and facilitation of the services;
- Clear and unambiguous communication about what to expect from helpers (including time frames);
- A means of escape (flight) should one feel threatened;
- Opportunities to utilise existing, established or self-identified coping strategies to reduce anxiety (e.g. Smoking for some people)

Suicide and self-harm

Suicide is a pressing concern to the Australian population. Standardised death rates for suicide ranged between 11.9 and 12.9 deaths per 100,000 people between 2014 and 2018 and was the leading cause of death for people aged between 15 and 54 (Australian Bureau of Statistics., 2019). Not every person who completes suicide has a mental illness. Mood disorders are most prevalent, followed by mental and behavioural dis-orders due to psychoactive substance use and anxiety and stress-related disorders (Australian Bureau of Statistics., 2019). These disorders are also the most prevalent mental health problems in the population. For every completed suicide, many more people attempt suicide (over 65,000 each year), and deliberate self-harm is a leading cause of presentation to emergency departments (Krysinska et al., 2015).

Suicidal thoughts and behaviour are common, but the nomenclature can be confusing. O'Carroll et al. (1996) suggest that there are three types of suicidal behaviour: (1) Risk taking thoughts and behaviour with immediate risk (e.g., speeding in a motor vehicle) or remote risk (e.g., smoking cigarettes); (2) Suicidal thoughts, which might be casual or serious, persistent or transient; and (3) Suicide Related Behaviours, which can include sui-cidal acts (completed suicide or attempts), and instrumental suicidal behaviours, threats (e.g., writing suicide notes) or gestures (e.g., sitting on ledges).

Nurses will encounter suicidal individuals and people who self-harm (often without suicidal intent) in many hospital and community settings. The suicidal crisis is com-plex and idiosyncratic, and despite considerable investment in services, research and greater numbers of people seeking help via the medical system, this has made little dif-ference to the disturbing statistics in Australia. At a population level, reducing access to the means of suicide and providing assertive follow-up and treatment as appro-priate to those who present with suicidal behaviour has been proposed as the most

---

Box 12.3 - Case study (Juanita)

Juanita had several presentations to the ED during her teens with deliberate self-harm. She was usually quite difficult to engage with in the ED as the focus of care is the management of medical emergencies. After a medically serious overdose of medication following a breakdown in a relationship, the ED nurse referred her to a dialectical behavioural therapy (DBT) programme for youth where she learned skills to regulate her emotions, tolerate distress and build better relationships. Though she occasionally continued to have thoughts of suicide she did not engage in self-harm or suicidal behaviour.

---

likely way to reduce mortality and hospital presentations (Krysinska et al., 2015). This means providing tailor made care, treatment and response to people at the earliest opportunity and for as long as needed. For individuals and families, nurses can make a difference. The surprisingly limited research on how people resolve suicidal crisis and keep on living suggests that even brief encounters with nurses and others can be personally significant, promote hope and a shift towards living and recovery (Chan, Kirkpatrick, & Brasch, 2017; Lakeman & FitzGerald, 2008).

Nursing the person in a suicidal crisis and assisting them to re-engage with the world positively is a highly skilled interpersonal activity (Cutcliffe, Stevenson, Jackson, & Smith, 2007). The response to suicide and self-harm in inpatient units has often been to lock doors and increase observations to minimise risk. However, what suicidal people report is that they want to feel safe, connected with others, protected and they wish to re-establish control (Berg, Rørtveit, & Aase, 2017). There needs to be a balance between the institutional need for surveillance and observation, and the individual's need for engagement and connection (Bowles, Dodds, Hackney, Sunderland, & Thomas, 2002). These roles can be experienced as conflicting and create a dilemma for the nurse.

Acute inpatient settings

People are admitted to acute mental health units because they need specialist nursing care. In 2017–18 there were over 260,000 overnight mental health-related hospitalisations with 4 in 5 occurring in public hospitals and 1 in 5 in private hospitals (Australian Institute of Health and Welfare, 2019). The average length of stay is around two weeks. Some State Services also provide or broker out 'Step-Down' services where people may be supported in residential care facilities

After an initial mental health assessment, if a person is deemed to have a significant mental illness or mental disorder that may require admission for the safety of the person or others. Reasons for admission are varied (diagnosis tells only part of the story), but most commonly are: acutely disturbed behaviour, dangerousness either to self or others, and poor self-care (Bowers, 2005). In Australia almost half of all hospital stays are involuntary (Australian Institute of Health and Welfare, 2019).

Inpatient units are mandated to provide a safe and secure environment for the consumer and the community. However, inpatient units can be unpredictable, highly emotional and busy environments for consumers to enter (Cleary, Hunt, Horsfall, & Deacon, 2011). The experience of hospitalisation can be potentially traumatic and people may not receive the help they need. Theoretically, a patient is observed, diagnosed and commences treatment (whether psychological or pharmacological), along with a comprehensive physical and medical assessment to determine any co-morbidities (Bowers, 2005).

Multidisciplinary teams within acute units are positioned to provide a comprehensive range of support and inclusive care to the consumer and their family/carers. A whole team approach can and ought to support the consumer towards planning their discharge with a *recovery* focus and is recognised to improve consumer outcomes (Marynowski-Traczyk et al., 2019).

> The concept of mental health recovery is a contested one, which is often contrasted to clinical recovery, or the absence of symptoms of illness. It usually refers to a personal process of finding meaning and realising goals and potential regardless of the presence of symptoms.

Discharge planning is ideally commenced as soon as practicable from admission with the consumer and significant others concerned for the consumers' health and wellbeing: This can be family, case managers, allied staff, or support workers. When considering discharge and recovery, nurses and consumers benefit from using a *strength-focused and goal-orientated* plan (Reid, Escott, & Isobel, 2018).

Challenges facing the field

Goffman (1968) famously described the experience of life in the asylums which he described as a 'total institution' and the process of institutionalisation which occurred, for both patients and staff. Today's inpatient facilities tend to be located on general hospital campuses, are more accessible to the public, and length of stay is brief. They do, however, develop their own cultures, and service reform agendas often seek to influence the culture of inpatient services, which are often resistant to change (Lakeman, 2013).

Traditionally, nursing has shaped the culture of mental health units and nursing models of care. Models such as the 'Tidal Model' (Barker & Buchanan-Barker, 2004) have provided a theoretical and moral foundation for practice in acute settings. Today centralised government, both State and Commonwealth exert greater influence on local practices, and biomedical models of mental distress predominate in policy and practice. Mental Health Nursing has had little influence over the public discourse about mental health and illness, what services are needed, or indeed what nurses might offer. For example, in Queensland all acute mental health units are required to be locked to prevent absconding despite robust evidence that this does not prevent absconding or aggression (Lakeman, 2017; Schneeberger et al., 2017).

> Seclusion and restraint are restrictive practices that are arguably used for reasons of safety and when all other options have been explored. 'Seclusion is defined as the confinement of a patient at any time of the day or night alone in a room or area from which free exit is prevented' and 'restraint is defined as the restriction of an individual's freedom of movement by physical or mechanical mean.'. This would include 'chemical restraint' the use of sedative medications.

One long-standing view of Mental Health Nursing is that it is primarily concerned with the facilitation of the conditions for mental health to flourish (Barker, 1989). Coercive or *restrictive practices* such as seclusion, restraint, forced medical treatment and arbitrarily locking people up, do not sit easily with mental health nursing theory or practice. It is now widely acknowledged that restrictive practices are not therapeutic. It is a part of the national reform agenda to reduce incidents leading to seclusion and restraint (see: The Australian Mental Health Commission). MHN's have extensively researched the factors which contribute to minimally coercive practices in inpatient environments, and this research has given rise to a programme of care called 'safewards' (Bowers et al., 2014). Safewards includes a set of 10 key interventions which primarily include changing the way health professionals talk with and about service users. The Australian College of Mental Health Nurses has also provided guidelines to improve the safety of all people accessing acute mental health services (ACMHN, 2019).

Violence and aggression towards health professionals is a pressing and growing concern for nurses in acute care settings. Most workplaces have a 'Zero Tolerance Approach' to violence policy and associated procedures. However, it is noteworthy that there have been an increasing number of people brought to EDs with behavioural dysregulation and increasing rates of involuntary treatment in Australia. Australia has the highest rates of involuntary treatment in the world at 282 hospitalisations per 100,000 individuals compared to a median of 106.4 per 100,000 across 22 countries (Sheridan Rains et al., 2019). Meeting aggression or behavioural dysregulation with coercive transportation, assessment and treatment may exacerbate the problem. Nurses ought to be involved in critically considering alternative non-coercive pathways to care and treatment.

Conclusions

Acute mental health presentations pose a challenge to health professionals in many health and welfare settings and every health professional needs to be equipped to respond in a containing and helpful way. The specialist skills of MHNs need to be recognised and mobilised in the service of addressing acute manifestations of mental illness and importantly to be engaged in the ongoing work to coach, health and assist in the resolution of problems.

Nurses are the largest and only continuously present professional workforce in acute inpatient services and have developed the capacity to be with and assist people in acute and sometimes extreme states of distress. They also have a pivotal role to play in assisting people to resolve problems in community teams, in primary care and in other health care settings.

Online resources

1 Australian Bureau of Statistics: Causes of Death: https://www.abs.gov.au/Causes-of-Death
2 Up to date information about the provision of mental health services in Australia: https://www.aihw.gov.au/reports-data/health-welfare-services/mental-health-services/overview
3 The National Mental Health Commission: https://www.mentalhealthcommission.gov.au/

References

ACMHN. (2019). Safe in Care, Safe at Work (SICSAW): Ensuring safety in care and safety for staff in Australian mental health services. Retrieved from Canberra: https://www.mentalhealthcommission.gov.au/getmedia/aec947de-3c06-462e-bb73-51e37e810180/Safe-in-Care-Safe-at-Work-Full-version

Australian Bureau of Statistics. (2019). *3303.0 - Causes of Death*, Australia, *2018*. Retrieved from Canberra: https://www.abs.gov.au/ausstats/abs@.nsf/Lookup/by%20Subject/3303.0~2018~Main%20Features~Intentional%20self-harm,%20key%20characteristics~3

Australian College of Mental Health Nurses (2010). Standards of Practice for Mental Health Nurses. Canberrra. ACMHN

Australian Institute of Health and Welfare. (2019). *Mental health services-in brief 2019*. (Cat. no. HSE 228). Canberra: Australian Institute of Health and Welfare Retrieved from https://www.aihw.gov.au/reports/mental-health-services/mental-health-services-in-australia-in-brief-2019/contents/table-of-contents

Barker, P. (1989). Reflections on the philosophy of caring in mental health. *International Journal of Nursing Studies, 26*(2), 131–141.

Barker, P. J., & Buchanan-Barker, P. (2004). *The Tidal Model: A guide for mental health professionals*. Routledge.

Barnes, M., & Bowl, R. (2000). *Taking over the asylum - Empowerment and mental health*. Basingstoke, UK: Palgrave.

Bayes, A., Parker, G., & McClure, G. (2016). Emotional dysregulation in those with bipolar disorder, borderline personality disorder and their comorbid expression. *Journal of Affective Disorders, 204*, 103–111.

Berg, S. H., Rørtveit, K., & Aase, K. (2017). Suicidal patients' experiences regarding their safety during psychiatric in-patient care: a systematic review of qualitative studies. *BMC Health Services Research, 17*(1), 73. doi: 10.1186/s12913-017-2023-8.

Bowers, L. (2005). Reasons for admission and their implications for the nature of acute inpatient psychiatric nursing. *Journal of Psychiatric and Mental Health Nursing, 12*(2), 231–236. doi: 10.1111/j.1365-2850.2004.00825.x.

Bowers, L., Alexander, J., Bilgin, H., Botha, M., Dack, C., James, K., Stewart, D. (2014). Safewards: The empirical basis of the model and a critical appraisal. *Journal of Psychiatric and Mental Health Nursing, 21*(4), 354–364. doi: 10.1111/jpm.12085.

Bowles, N., Dodds, P., Hackney, D., Sunderland, C., & Thomas, P. (2002). Formal observations and engagement: A discussion paper. *Journal of Psychiatric and Mental Health Nursing, 9*(3), 255–260.

Caplan, G. (1964). *Principles of preventive psychiatry*. New York: Basic Books.

Chan, K. J., Kirkpatrick, H., & Brasch, J. (2017). The Reasons to Go On Living Project: Stories of recovery after a suicide attempt. *Qualitative Research in Psychology, 14*(3), 350–373. doi: 10.1080/14780887.2017.1322649

Claassen, C. A., Hughes, C. W., Gilfillan, S., McIntire, D., Roose, A., Lumpkin, M., & Rush, A. J. (2000). Toward a redefinition of psychiatric emergency. *Health services research, 35*(3), 735–754. Retrieved from https://www.ncbi.nlm.nih.gov/pubmed/10966093

Cleary, M., Hunt, G. E., Horsfall, J., & Deacon, M. (2011). Ethnographic research into nursing in acute adult mental health units: A review. *Issues in Mental Health Nursing, 32*(7), 424–435. doi: 10.3109/01612840.2011.563339.

Corney, R. (1999). Mental health services in primary care: The overlap in professional roles. *Journal of Mental Health, 8*(2), 187–194.

Council of Australian Governments. (2017). *The fifth national mental health and suicide prevention plan*. Commonwealth of Australia Canberra, ACT Retrieved from https://www.coaghealthcouncil.gov.au/Portals/0/Fifth%20National%20Mental%20Health%20and%20Suicide%20Prevention%20Plan.pdf

Cutcliffe, J. R., Stevenson, C., Jackson, S., & Smith, P. (2007). Reconnecting the person with humanity: How psychiatric nurses work with suicidal people. *Crisis, 28*(4), 207–210.

Goffman, E. (1968). *Asylums: Essays on the social situation of mental patients and other inmates*: AldineTransaction.

Hickie, I. (2019). Time for structural reform in mental health: who is up for the challenge? *Australian Health Review, 43*(4), 361–362. doi: https://doi.org/10.1071/AHV43N4_ED.

James, R. K., & Gilliland, B. E. (2001). *Crisis Intervention Strategies* (4th ed.). Belmont, CA: Wadsworth/Thompson Learning.

Kezelman, C., & Stavropoulos, P. (2012). *Practice guidelines for treatment of complex trauma and trauma informed care and service delivery.* Retrieved from https://www.childabuseroyal-commission.gov.au/sites/default/files/IND.0521.001.0001.pdf

Krysinska, K., Batterham, P. J., Tye, M., Shand, F., Calear, A. L., Cockayne, N., & Christensen, H. (2015). Best strategies for reducing the suicide rate in Australia. *Australian & New Zealand Journal of Psychiatry, 50*(2), 115–118. doi: 10.1177/0004867415620024.

Lakeman, R. (2013). Talking science and wishing for miracles: understanding cultures of mental health practice. *International Journal of Mental Health Nursing, 22*(2), 106–115.

Lakeman, R. (2017). Mandated locked wards and mental health nursing. *ACMHN News*, Summer, 18–10.

Lakeman, R. (2020). Advanced empathy: A key to supporting people experiencing psychosis or other extreme states. *Psychotherapy and Counselling Journal of Australia*, 8(1). Available: http://pacja.org.au/?p=5379

Lakeman, R., & FitzGerald, M. (2008). How people live with or get over being suicidal: a review of qualitative studies. *Journal of Advanced Nursing, 64*(2), 114–126. doi: 10.1111/j.1365-2648.2008.04773.x.

Lakeman, R., & Molloy, L. (2018). Rise of the zombie institution, the failure of mental health nursing leadership, and mental health nursing as a zombie category. *International Journal of Mental Health Nursing, 27*(3), 1009–1014.

Maharaj, R. (2007). A comparison of the use of coercive measures between patients referred by the police and patients referred by other sources to a psychiatric hospital in Australia. *BMC Psychiatry, 7*(S1), S127. doi: 10.1186/1471-244X-7-S1-S127.

Marynowski-Traczyk, D., Broadbent, M., Kinner, S. A., FitzGerald, G., Heffernan, E., Johnston, A., … Crilly, J. (2019). Mental health presentations to the emergency department: A perspective on the involvement of social support networks. *Australasian Emergency Care, 22*(3), 162–167. doi: https://doi.org/10.1016/j.auec.2019.06.002.

O'Carroll, P. W., Berman, A. L., Maris, R. W., Moscicki, E. K., Tanney, B. L., & Silverman, M. M. (1996). Beyond the Tower of Babel: a nomenclature for suicidology. *Suicide and Life-Threatening Behavior, 26*(3), 237–252.

Oliver, M., Adonopulos, A. A., Haber, P. S., Dinh, M. M., Green, T., Wand, T., Chalkley, D. (2019). Impact of acutely behavioural disturbed patients in the emergency department: A prospective observational study. *Emergency Medicine Australasia, 31*(3), 387–392. doi: 10.1111/1742-6723.13173.

Puntis, S., Perfect, D., Kirubarajan, A., Bolton, S., Davies, F., Hayes, A., Molodynski, A. (2018). A systematic review of co-responder models of police mental health 'street' triage. *BMC Psychiatry, 18*(1), 11.

Reid, R., Escott, P., & Isobel, S. (2018). Collaboration as a process and an outcome: Consumer experiences of collaborating with nurses in care planning in an acute inpatient mental health unit. *International Journal of Mental Health Nursing, 27*(4), 1204–1211. doi: 10.1111/inm.12463.

Richmond, D. (1983). Inquiry into health services for the psychiatrically ill and developmentally disabled. *New South Wales: Department of Health, NSW Division of Planning and Research.*

Schneeberger, A. R., Kowalinski, E., Fröhlich, D., Schröder, K., von Felten, S., Zinkler, M., Huber, C. G. (2017). Aggression and violence in psychiatric hospitals with and without open door policies: A 15-year naturalistic observational study. *Journal of Psychiatric Research, 95*, 189–195. doi: https://doi.org/10.1016/j.jpsychires.2017.08.017.

Sheridan Rains, L., Zenina, T., Dias, M. C., Jones, R., Jeffreys, S., Branthonne-Foster, S., Johnson, S. (2019). Variations in patterns of involuntary hospitalisation and in legal frameworks: an international comparative study. *The Lancet Psychiatry*, 6(5), 403–417. doi: 10.1016/S2215-0366(19)30090-2.

Wheeler, C., Lloyd-Evans, B., Churchard, A., Fitzgerald, C., Fullarton, K., Mosse, L., Johnson, S. (2015). Implementation of the Crisis Resolution Team model in adult mental health settings: A systematic review. *BMC Psychiatry*, 15(1), 74.

Part II: Section II: Nursing in the community and home-based contexts

13 Community nursing

Lisa Whitehead and Kylie McCullough

Chapter objectives

This chapter will offer the reader:

- Insight into the roles of nurses when working with communities.
- An outline of the philosophy of Primary Health Care as it relates to nursing and midwifery.
- An overview of health promotion principles and activities.
- A detailed example of a health promotion activity in practice.
- Working with communities and families.
- The scope of home-based care.

Introduction

Nurses and midwives work in a variety of roles and settings outside of the hospital environment. This chapter considers community nursing practice as working with communities and not just in the community. This approach includes both the provision of clinical care within people's homes and community settings as well as community development, health promotion and advocacy. Practical strategies for working with communities based on the principles of Primary Health Care will be described.

What is a community?

A community is defined as '...a group of people who share common interests, who interact with each other and who function collectively within a defined social structure to address common concerns' (Clarke, 2008). Community is commonly defined both by geographical area and by a set of relationships. The geographical locations where we live and/or work provide important sources for connections with others beyond immediate family and friends. Common interests may include inhabiting a particular geographical area, kinship or extended family relationships, common identity or lifestyle activities or a particular ideology or belief system. Membership of a community may provide protection, reassurance, social support, employment and a means of maintaining identity, values, beliefs and practises. Furthermore, healthy communities are characterised by wide participation in decision-making and provide opportunities for learning and skill development. The community can play an important role in developing and sustaining networks of reciprocal relations that strongly influence our health, happiness and wellbeing (Australian Institute of Family Studies, 2016). Nurses and midwives work across a range of community settings in a myriad of diverse roles.

A community setting means a location outside of a hospital inpatient, acute care setting or a hospital clinic setting. A community setting may include, but is not limited to, a home, group home, assisted living facility, correctional facility, hospice, long-term care facility, schools, community-based health care clinics such as general practice, immunisation services, child health and community midwifery services, sexual health and comprehensive primary health care services.

How do nurses work with communities?

In addition to clinical care such as wound and medication management, palliative care, client assessment and provision of in-home care and support; community health nursing is focussed on prevention and health promotion across the lifespan. The role includes: education, advocacy, counselling, management, screening and surveillance, collaboration and research.

Schools are an important health promoting community where nurses manage acute health care needs as well as education and screening particularly in regards to immunisation, sexual health, mental health and healthy lifestyle interventions. Child and maternal health care roles as well as care of the aging in both residential facilities and independent living situations are fundamental to the health of the population at large. Community nurses are autonomous practitioners and often require advanced practice skills and knowledge. Nurses working in rural and remote communities have a broad, generalist scope of practice and may be the only resident health care workers in a community.

Community nurses are employed by local governments, community organisations, Aboriginal Medical Services, General practices clinics, and large employers such as mining companies. Care provided in the community setting can be ongoing rather

---

Box 13.1 - Case study (Jane)

Jane is a community nurse in a rural town. Jane has noticed that many children in the town appear to be above healthy weight and this has also been raised as an area of concern by a number of community members. Jane undertakes a community assessment that involved reviewing the national and local data in addition to available data at the clinic. These data revealed that not only were a high proportion of children above a healthy weight but this was also an issue for adults in the community. Jane reviewed the services and resources available locally and found that there were limited health and education programmes to raise awareness, support behaviour change and promote early intervention. Jane plans to bring together a group of key members in the community to define health goal/s for the community, brainstorm community options and resources and select interventions which will be developed into a project action plan. The project action plan will include health promotion activities and Jane will include opportunities for objective evaluation over time to assess the effectiveness of the community driven interventions.

than episodic such as care requiring hospitalisation. Community based nurses have the opportunity to establish networks and relationships that facilitate inter-professional collaboration and client-centred care over time and long-term. It is vital that nurses have a good understanding of the demographic characteristics, health needs and social factors that relate to the communities they work in.

Determining community health needs

It is important that care reflects the needs of the community and knowledge about the community develops over time and through contact with the community. General population health needs are described in a range of publications including the Australian Institute of Health and Welfares' bi-annual health report Australia's Health (Australian Institute of Health and Welfare, 2018) and information about Aboriginal and Torres Strait Islander peoples can be sourced from the Indigenous Health Info net resources (Australian Indigenous HealthinfoNet, 2019). Basic demographic information that describes population numbers, age distribution, gender and ethnicity for specific suburbs, towns and regions are available from the Australian Bureau of Statistics (Australian Bureau of Statistics, 2019) as well as some socio-economic data such as income and education which is important when considering the health needs of a community (Australian Bureau of Statistics, 2011). Data may be available in health records or through health service evaluations and reports. Where possible, a community assessment of health needs should be conducted in order to prioritise and plan health services and health promotion activities. In addition to medical health needs, the social determinants of health must be considered as modifiable factors that impact on the health of communities.

The Social Determinants of Health (SDoH) are a well-established construct for understanding and examining the causes of ill health (Liamputtong, 2019). The SDoH recognise that people's lifestyles, social world and environments strongly influence their health. The SDoH include factors such as social support, food, education, work, early life and addiction (Talbot & Verrinder, 2018; Wilkinson & Marmot, 2003). Inequalities in health are strongly correlated with income and education. Better health outcomes and a longer life expectancy are linked to higher income and access to education (Rosling, Rosling, & Rosling Ronnlund, 2018). Access to health services varies across Australia and is a fundamental factor in the health of communities. People living in rural and remote areas face particular health challenges, with reduced health outcomes on almost all indicators and measures, including a burden of disease for those living in very remote areas 1.7 times the rate of those living in urban environments (AIHW, 2018). A higher proportion of Aboriginal and Torres Strait Islander peoples live in very remote areas (21%), compared to approximately 2% of the non-Indigenous population (AIHW, 2018). In rural and remote Australia, the complexity of delivering healthcare is magnified by unique characteristics and challenges, including distance, access and resources (Paliadelis, Parmenter, Parker, Giles, & Higgins, 2012).

Primary health care

An important element in addressing health inequalities is access to health care services that recognises and work toward addressing the SDoH. This requires a reorientation of the health system away from the 'medical' model of treating the disease or infirmity at an individual level to a Primary Health Care (PHC) approach. A PHC approach includes the social and psychological aspects of a health problem as well as the medical diagnosis and treatment. PHC activity and services within a community are driven by the needs of a community and include both the prevention and management of those needs identified.

PHC first gained recognition as an approach to health care at the International Conference on PHC in Alma Ata, Russia, in 1979. Representatives from many of the member nations of the WHO and other global health bodies came together in an attempt to address global health inequalities and urge Governments to reorient their health services to a social justice model of health (WHO, 1978). The declaration reaffirmed the WHO definition of health as not just being the absence of disease but a state of physical, mental and social wellbeing that is a basic human right and provided a definition of PHC as follows;

> PHC is an essential health care based on practical, scientifically sound and socially acceptable methods and technology made universally accessible to individuals and families in the community through their full participation and at a cost that the community and country can afford to maintain at every stage of their development in the spirit of self-reliance and self-determination. It forms an integral part both of the country's health system, of which it is the central function and main focus, and of the overall social and economic development of the community. It is the first level of contact of individuals, the family and community with the national health system bringing health care as close as possible to where people live and work, and constitutes the first element of a continuing health care process (WHO, 1978, p. 1,2).

PHC has a focus on how care is provided rather than what just what services are provided (Australian Nursing Federation, 2009; McMurray & Clendon, 2010; WHO, 1986) and emphasises community participation and empowerment, social justice and equity, cultural safety, trust and accountability (Talbot & Verrinder, 2018). This is in contrast to the term primary care which usually refers to General Practice as the first level of access into the health system, with secondary care relating to outpatient specialist services and tertiary meaning hospital level care.

Barriers to the adoption of the Declaration have been reported as including: resistance to change (particularly where additional funding is needed); a lack of research with community as a focus rather than a specific disease or process; lack of well-prepared workforce to put PHC into action; and competing political and professional interests which maintain the flow of health funding to tertiary level care (Gillam, 2008).

In an effort to progress the aims of the Declaration, conference delegates in Ottawa created the Ottawa charter to guide health promotion policies and programs. The Ottawa charter described Health Promotion as actions that develop personal skills and strengthen community action to enhance self-reliance, create supportive environments, build healthy public policy and reorientate health services to a collaborative and holistic approach to health service provision (WHO, 1986). The Declaration of Alma Ata and the Ottawa charter form the foundation of modern PHC philosophy.

PHC in Australia

In 2009, The Australian Nursing Federation (ANF) released a report outlining the consensus between Nurses and Midwives in supporting the philosophy and implementation of PHC in Australia (ANF, 2009). The report outlines several areas where nurses and midwives can make a significant contribution to PHC objectives such as in health promotion, management of chronic disease, aged care, child and family care and mental health. The generalist role of nurses in working with disadvantaged communities such as Indigenous and, Culturally and Linguistically Diverse (CALD) communities and those living in rural and remote areas was explicitly described.

> Disadvantaged communities refers to groups within society that have difficulty accessing health services due to geographical, financial, language, education or cultural barriers.

The importance of a PHC approach to health service delivery is also evident in the Australian codes of conduct for Nurses; where principle seven states, 'Nurses promote health and wellbeing for people and their families, colleagues, the broader community and themselves and in a way that addresses health inequality' (Nursing and Midwifery Board of Australia, 2018, p.14). PHC is a model of health service delivery that has the potential to address the issues related to the spiralling costs and burden of chronic disease through preventative care and the potential to bring about significant health improvements within communities through the reduction in health inequalities (Talbot & Verrinder, 2018).

Health promotion in practice

Once the health needs of a community are identified and the root causes of health issues examined, planning health promotion interventions can begin. Many models of health behaviour change are available including the Trans-theoretical Model and Health beliefs model (Talbot & Verrinder, 2018).

Often education is the focus of health behaviour change with the expectation that if people know the consequences of their behaviour is poor health, that they will use that information to improve their own health. However, increasing health literacy and supporting behaviour change is more complex than providing education alone (Kelly & Barker, 2016). The Ottawa charter describes developing personal skills as activities that empower people to make healthy choices through knowledge. Nurses need skills in undertaking community assessments, understanding the data and working with communities in addition to the ability to develop educational programs and resources to support health literacy through the practical application of health knowledge.

Health behaviour change requires supportive environments and community involvement in developing interventions to be successful. An example of community involvement in a nurse-led health screening program is described by Byers, Michell, & McCullough (2018). Their aim was to increase access to screening mammograms for women living in several remote desert communities. The nurse and midwife worked closely with the women in organising the logistics of travelling to a regional centre and provided the link to resources and organisations for education and access to screening services.

Nurses working with communities also have a responsibility to advocate for healthy public policy and the reorientation of health services from acute hospital care to health promotion and the prevention of ill health. Furthermore, strengthening community action through facilitating community development activities is an important strategy decreasing health and social inequalities. The key principle of community development is involvement of the community throughout the whole project, from identification of an issue, through understanding the extent and cause of the issue, identifying strategies to address the issue, implementing interventions and evaluation. Skills and knowledge are developed through the process of prioritising, planning, implementing and evaluating health promotion activities and projects are more likely to succeed if they meet the needs of the community in a way that is acceptable, affordable and accessible to that community.

Health promotion activities in practice

Box 13.2 - Case study (Jane II)

Jane is a nurse working in a small rural community with a high proportion of Aboriginal and Torres Strait Islander residents. Jane has been speaking with the school principal about opportunities for health education. She knows that Type 2 diabetes and obesity are significant health issues for her community. Jane also understands that to address community wide issues, it is imperative that the community is engaged, that the community and services work in partnership and a joint sense of ownership is generated. Jane runs a number of community consultations to build engagement, partnership and ownership. Through the consultations, the community identified the main issue as being the quantity of high-sugar drinks being consumed by teenagers in the town.

Jane researched health promotion activities aimed at reducing the consumption of high-sugar drinks and used the Ottawa charter as a framework for considering different approaches:

Developing personal skills by increasing health literacy: Jane could provide education about the health effects of high sugar drinks and teach the teenagers how to read a food label and determine the health risks and benefits of a variety of drinks. She found a range of audio-visual materials and activities online which she can adapt to the needs of her community.

Create supportive environments by reducing access to high-sugar drinks: Jane could work with the school and local store to assess the availability of high sugar drinks and source healthier alternatives. Her knowledge of social marketing strategies enables her to recommend a ban on advertising in the school and community spaces of high-sugar drinks.

Strengthen community action: Jane recognises that teenagers are often influenced by their peers when choosing health behaviours. She could spend time with teens at the school establishing a rapport and working with them to develop a health resource. A music video or similar project could provide an opportunity to learn about healthy drinks as well as meet the teenager's needs for autonomy and social connection.

Reorienting health services: Jane's understanding of the social causes of ill health and the role of nurses in preventing health promotion aids her in negotiating that time away from the clinic necessary to work at the school on this project.

Building healthy public policy: Jane's knowledge about health means she can advocate on behalf of the community for changes in policy. She may be motivated to contribute to national-level policy development but can also advocate at a local level and write a brief article in the school newsletter calling for a ban on high-sugar drinks being sold at the local school.

Working with families

Providing care in a community based setting creates the potential for nurses to build relationships that go beyond the client alone to building connections with family and the wider community. The nature of the work that community based nurses undertake increasingly involves managing a long-term relationship and complex care needs with individuals, families and communities. Examples include long-term condition management and end of life care in the home setting.

The number of people living with one or more chronic conditions continues to increase worldwide (Forouzanfar et. al., 2016) and includes a wide range of health problems such as heart disease, diabetes, asthma, dementia and depression. Whilst a number of definitions of chronic illness exist, the common features of many definitions are that chronic conditions require a multifaceted approach to management over an extended time period and a coordinated input from a wide range of health professionals. The majority of the management of chronic conditions takes place in the community setting and family can be highly influential in promoting positive health outcomes (Ory, Ahn, & Jiang, 2013). Positive family functioning can lead to greater levels of motivation and confidence to self-manage conditions (Stamp et al., 2015). Evidence on how families can specifically support the self-management of chronic conditions is emerging and includes adaptation within the family to maintain cohesion between family members, normalisation and contextualisation of the chronic condition (Whitehead, Jacob, & Towell, 2017). Family adaptability to living with chronic conditions has been found to be a powerful determinant of carer health where change in roles and subsequent adaptation can be stressful (Whitehead et al., 2017). Nurses working in community settings can play an important role in assessing how families are adapting to living with chronic illness and to explore strategies to cope with challenges in the home setting (Corry, While, Neenan, & Smith, 2015; Deek et al., 2016). However, the ability to work with families as a unit, in a collaborative, non-hierarchical way requires support and skills (Bell, 2014). An approach that focuses on strengths rather than pathology is recommended (Wright & Bell, 2009) and nurses are encouraged to explore the family's experience of health and illness, identify meanings, and support clinical reasoning and judgment to implement family nursing interventions (Duhamel, Dupuis, Turcotte, Martinez, & Goudreau, 2015). Guidelines developed by the International Family Nursing Association (IFNA) highlight the fundamental assumptions for nurses working with families and these can be located on the International Family Nursing Association website (IFNA, 2015; IFNA, 2017).

Home-based care

The provision of nursing care and support in the home has been recommended as an area that needs to expand to promote more sustainable approaches to healthcare (Department of Health, Western Australia, 2019). Services already offered but remain limited include palliative care, wound management and chronic condition management.

Although palliative care is commonly associated with end-of-life cancer care, there is increasing recognition of the role of palliative care in managing symptoms such as chronic pain, nausea and fatigue experienced by people with life-limiting conditions in the final stages of their disease, which may be a year or more before their death (AIHW, 2019; Wilkinson, Slatyer, McCullough, & Williams, 2014). A challenge for nurses in home-based care is to overcome the misconception that palliative care is only for those whose death is imminent and advocating for patients with conditions other than cancer to have access to palliative care services. The goal of enabling patients to die in their preferred place is a key performance indicator for end of life care services. For those people who wish to die at home support requires planning and development to facilitate this choice (Hoare, Morris, Kelly, Hun, & Barclay, 2015).

Summary

The role of the nurse working in the community setting is diverse and requires an understanding of the wider drivers of health and wellbeing as well as the ability to work with communities and families. Nurses have the potential to improve health outcomes through prevention and management, especially of chronic disease. Nurses are well positioned, due to their education, skills and values, to address the need for holistic care that acknowledges the social determinants of health. By being embedded within communities, nurses are able to promote public health and disease prevention to make healthier choices, and empower individuals and families through the provision of support and working alongside local populations. Nurses can create knowledge, skills and confidence within communities around ownership of health, and help to build health resilience in their communities. In the current climate of increasing health burden related to chronic conditions and multi-morbidity, the nurse's role as a culturally attuned promoter of health, as provider, are invaluable.

Online resources

1 IFNA Generalist competencies for family nursing: https://internationalfamily nursing.org/2015/07/25/ifna-position-statement-on-generalist-competencies-for-family-nursing-practice-2/
2 The Australian Primary Health Care Nurses Association: https://www.apna.asn.au/
3 The International Family Nursing Association: https://internationalfamily-nursing.org/

References

Australian Bureau of Statistics. (2011). Socio-economic indexes for areas. Retrieved from https://www.abs.gov.au/websitedbs/censushome.nsf/home/seifa
Australian Bureau of Statistics. (2019). Data by region. Retrieved from https://itt.abs.gov.au/itt/r.jsp?databyregion
Australian Institute of Family Studies. (2016). Community engagement: A key strategy for improving outcomes for Australian families (CFCA Paper No. 39). Retrieved from https://aifs.gov.au/cfca/publications/community-engagement/what-community
Australian Indigenous HealthinfoNet. (2019). Retrieved from https://healthinfonet.ecu.edu.au/
Australian Institute of Health and Welfare. (2018). *Australia's health 2018*. Retrieved from https://www.aihw.gov.au/reports/australias-health/australias-health-2018/contents/table-of-contents

Australian Nursing Federation. (2009). Primary Health Care in Australia. A nursing and midwifery consensus view. Retrieved from http://www.rcna.org.au/WCM/Images/RCNA_website/Files%20for%20upload%20and%20link/policy/documentation/position/consensus_statements_PHC_Australia.pdf

Bell, J. M. (2014). Family centred care and family nursing: Three beliefs that matter most. *Pfledge, 27*, 213–217. https://doi.org/10.1024/1012-5302/a000369

Byers, L., Michell, K., & McCullough, K. (2018). Awareness, acceptability and access to screening mammography for remote Aboriginal women. *Health Promotion Journal of Australia, 29*, 366–367. doi: 10.1002/hpja.40.

Clarke, M. (2008). *Community Health Nursing.* (5th ed.). New Jersey: Pearson Education.

Corry, M., While, A., Neenan, K., & Smith, V. (2015). A systematic review of systematic reviews on interventions for caregivers of people with chronic conditions. *Journal of Advanced Nursing, 71*(4), 718–734. https://doi.org/10.1111/jan.12523

Deek, H., Hamilton, S., Brown, N., Inglis, S. C., Digiacomo, M., Newton, P. J... Davison, P. M. (2016). Family-centred approaches to healthcare interventions in chronic diseases in adults: a wuantitive systematic review. *Journal of Advanced Nursing. 72*(5), 968–979. https://doi.org/10.1111/jan.12885

Department of Health Western Australia. (2019). Sustainable Health Review: Final Report to the Western Australian Government. Department of Health, Western Australia. Retrieved from https://ww2.health.wa.gov.au/Improving-WA-Health/Sustainable-health-review

Duhamel, F., Dupuis, F., Turcotte, A., Martinez, M., & Goudreau, J. (2015). Integrating the illness beliefs model in clinical practice: A family systems nursing knowledge utilization model. *Journal of Family Nursing, 21*(2), 322–348. https://doi.org/10.1177/1074840715579404

Forouzanfar, M., Afshin, A., Alexander, L., Anderson, H., Bhutta, Z., Biryukov, S., Murray, C. J. (2016). Global, regional, and national comparative risk assessment of 79 behavioural, environmental and occupational, and metabolic risks or clusters of risks, 1990–2015: A systematic analysis for the Global Burden of Disease Study 2015. *The Lancet, 388*(10053), 1659–1724. https://doi-org.ezproxy.cdu.edu.au/10.1016/S0140-6736(16)31679-8

Gillam, S. (2008). Is the declaration of Alma Ata still relevant to Primary Health Care? *British Medical Journal, 336*(7643), 536.

Hoare, S., Morris, Z. S., Kelly, M. P., Hun, I., & Barclay, S. (2015). Do patients want to die at home? A systematic review of the UK literature, focused on missing preferences for place of death. *PLoS ONE, 10*(11). https://doi.org/10.1371/journal.pone.0142723

IFNA. (2015). *IFNA Position Statement on Generalist Competencies for Family Nursing Practice.* Retrieved from https://internationalfamilynursing.org/wordpress/wp-content/uploads/2015/07/GC-Complete-PDF-document-in-color-with-photos-English-language.pdf

IFNA. (2017). *IFNA Position Statement on Advanced Practice Competencies for Family Nursing.* Retrieved from https://internationalfamilynursing.org/2017/05/19/advanced-practice-competencies/

Kelly, M. P, Barker, M. (2016). Why is changing health-related behaviour so difficult? *Public Health, 136,* 109–116. doi: 10.1016/j.puhe.2016.03.030.

Liamputtong, P. *Social determinants of health,* (Ed.), (2019). Oxford University Press.

McMurray, A., & Clendon, J. (2010). *Community health and wellness: Primary Health Care in practice.* Chatswood: Mosby.

Nursing and Midwifery Board of Australia. (2018). Code of conduct for nurses. Retrieved from http://www.nursingmidwiferyboard.gov.au/Codes-Guidelines-Statements/Professional-standards.aspx

Ory, M. G., Ahn, S, & Jiang, L. (2013). Success of a national study of the chronic disease self-management program: Meeting the triple aim of health care reform. *Medical Care, 51*(11), 992–998. Retrieved from http://www.jstor.org/stable/42568848

Paliadelis, P., Parmenter, G., Parker, V., Giles, M., & Higgins, I. (2012). The challenges confronting clinicians in rural acute care settings: a participatory research project. *Rural and Remote Health 2012; 12:* Retrieved from: www.rrh.org.au/journal/article/2017

Rosling, H., Rosling, O., & Rosling Ronnlund, A. (2018). *Factfulness: Ten reasons we're wrong about the world- and why things are better than you think*. Great Britain: Hodder & Stoughton.

Stamp, K. D., Dunbar, S. B., Clark, P. C., Reily, C. M., Gary, R. A., Higgins, M., & Ryan, R. M. (2015). Family partner intervention influences self-care confidence and treatment self-regulation in patients with hearing failure. *European Journal of Cardiovascular Nursing, 15*(5), 317–327. https://doi.org/10.1177/1474515115572047

Talbot, L., & Verrinder, G. (2018). *Promoting health: The Primary Health Care Approach*, (ed.). Chatswood: 6thElsevier Australia.

Whitehead, L., Jacob, E., Towell, A., Abu-qamar, M., & Cole-Heath, A. (2017). The role of the family in supporting the self-management of chronic conditions: A qualitative systematic review. *Journal of Clinical Nursing, 27*(1–2), 22– 30. https://doi.org/10.1111/jocn.13775

WHO. (1978). The Declaration of Alma Ata. Retrieved from http://www.who.int/publications/almaata_declaration_en.pdf

WHO. (1986). The Ottawa Charter for Health Promotion. Retrieved from http://www.who.int/healthpromotion/conferences/previous/ottawa/en/

Wilkinson, A., Slatyer, S., McCullough, K., & Williams, A. (2014). Exploring the quality of life at the end of life (QUAL-E) instrument with Australian palliative care hospital patients: hurdles and directions. *Journal of Palliative Care, 30*(1), 16–23.

Wilkinson, R., & Marmot, M. (2003). *Social determinants of health: The solid facts*. Retrieved from Copenhagen: http://www.euro.who.int/__data/assets/pdf_file/0005/98438/e81384.pdf

Wright, L. M., & Bell, J. M. (2009). *Beliefs and illness: A model for healing*. Calgary, Alberta Canada: 4th Floor Press.

14 Nursing and people with intellectual disability

Nathan J. Wilson, Virginia Howie and Gail Tomsic

Chapter objectives

This chapter will offer the reader:

- Insight into the history and current contexts of nursing and people with intellectual disability.
- An outline of the key health issues facing people with intellectual disability.
- A description of contemporary contexts where the nursing of people with intellectual disability occurs.
- An opportunity to build a knowledge base and develop nursing skills specific to people with intellectual disability.
- An overview of future challenges to nursing and nurses who practice in this area.

Introduction

People with Intellectual Disability (ID) represent about 3% of the population (AIHW, 2012). Many of the issues facing people with ID in relation to health and illness reflect those of the general population, although there are some important differences of which nurses need to be aware. In order to provide quality nursing care, it is important to have an understanding of the challenges faced by people with ID when accessing health care. However, evidence suggests that many nurses who encounter people with ID often feel under-prepared, overwhelmed, struggle to understand the role of family and paid caregivers, and find communication barriers difficult to overcome (Lewis et al., 2017). These issues can lead to delayed treatment and/or misdiagnosis and contribute to increased morbidity and, in some cases, mortality. This chapter offers nurses an overview of the health issues facing people with ID and some insights into strategies to promote better outcomes for people with ID.

Historical and current contexts of support

In Australia, the internationally accepted term - *intellectual disability* – is used; however, around the world terms such as mental retardation (now very outdated), learning disability, intellectual developmental disorder, or developmental disability are also found. By definition, people with ID have both a *cognitive and an adaptive behaviour disability* that originated before the age of 18 years (Schalock et al., 2010). This means that people with ID find it difficult to understand and learn as well as having a reduced ability to manage their lives independently. In previous decades it was common for people with ID to live in mental health institutions to be cared for by mental health nurses across Australia and/or went to segregated schools. From the 1960s, it was accepted that placing people with ID in mental health institutions was inappropriate and so ID-specific services were developed that required ID-specific trained nurses. From the 1970s onwards, a national policy of deinstitutionalisation set a goal to close all large residential institutions (Young & Ashman, 2004) and only a small number remain operational today. Currently, many people with ID live at home with family or in shared accommodation, and many live on their own with support strategies in place.

A cognitive disability means a person has problems with memory, learning, attention, reading, writing, mathematics and comprehension. An adaptive behaviour disability means a person has problems with the age-appropriate living, functional, communication and social skills that you need to live independently.

The goals of deinstitutionalisation have mirrored changing societal attitudes towards the full inclusion of people with ID in society and it is not uncommon for the general population to have experience of interacting with people with ID. Today, large numbers of children with ID attend mainstream schools and many adults with ID work in the open employment market. Most importantly, this also means that it is common for people with ID to access mainstream health services. The recently legislated National Disability Insurance Scheme (NDIS) in Australia means that people with ID have a funding package, that provides choice and control over which services they receive to meet their individual needs. (Collings, Dew, & Dowse, 2016). This is important for nursing as there are many health-related support needs that will become a part of the NDIS as the policy evolves over the coming decade.

Key health issues facing people with ID

In this section, the key areas to be covered are: Co-morbidities associated with intellectual disability, mental health conditions and ID, and health behaviours associated with ill health.

Co-morbidities and ID

Although people with ID should never be referred to or labelled by their diagnosis, it is important to establish what might have caused the diagnosis as these are often associated with specific health issues of which nurses need to be aware in order to provide appropriate nursing care. The most common cause of ID is a genetic disorder (Peterlin & Peterlin, 2016). There are more than 700 genetic syndromes, the most common associated with ID being Down syndrome (Vissers, Gilissen, & Veltman, 2015). Other causes include prenatal problems (e.g., diabetes), problems at birth (e.g., hypoxia), and illnesses or injuries during early childhood that impact the developing brain (Australian Bureau of Statistics, 2014). When nursing a person with ID, consideration must also be given to the co-morbidities that are often associated with genetic conditions. For example, people with Down syndrome are at greater risk of congenital

---

Box 14.1 - Case study (Jasseke)

Jasseke was 27 when she died from kidney failure due to high calcium blood levels. She had severe ID, autism and no verbal communication. Jasseke became ill with a high BP and was taken to her GP by her carers who said that she was perfectly fit and not to worry. Jasske continued to deteriorate and was taken back to her GP by her carers, no action was taken. Two months later, Jasseke collapsed and was admitted to hospital – her kidneys had failed and she died (MENCAP, 2012).

Reflective questions:
1 What role do you think that Jasseke's impaired communication played in her illness and death?
2 What factors might have contributed to Jasseke's misdiagnosis?
3 If nurses were involved in Jasseke's care, what nursing interventions might have identified the cause of the problem earlier?

---

heart defects, early onset dementia and endocrine problems when compared to the general population (Wilson & Charnock, 2017). Although ID can occur in isolation, it can be accompanied by other problems such as sensory impairment, epilepsy, neuromuscular deficits and autism spectrum disorders (Peterlin & Peterlin, 2016). One of the most common co-morbidities for people with ID is a mental health condition.

Mental health conditions and ID

The coexistence of ID and mental illness is referred to as a dual diagnosis (Werner & Stawski, 2012). Dual diagnosis affects approximately 30–40% of people with ID, which is 2–3 times greater than the general population (Tonge, Torr, & Trollor, 2017). Common severe mental health conditions associated with ID are schizophrenia, obsessive compulsive disorder and bipolar disorder (Manohar et al., 2016). In addition, the rates of common mental health problems such as anxiety and depression are higher for people with ID than the general population (Davis, Saeed, & Antonacci, 2008; Weise & Trollor, 2018). Difficulties arise with the identification of dual diagnoses for a variety of reasons such as variations in intelligence quotient (IQ) levels, inability to communicate feelings of anxiety or depression, individual behavioural problems, and lack of resources, knowledge and confidence by staff (Tua, Neville and Scott, 2017). The risk of *diagnostic overshadowing* is also prevalent.

The term diagnostic overshadowing refers to a tendency to attribute the presenting symptoms to a person's ID and therefore to risk failing to diagnose an underlying health disorder (Geiss et al., 2018).

Nurses are an integral part of the diagnostic and therapeutic processes within the mental health interdisciplinary team. In a review of the literature, Bakken and Sageng (2016) found that treatment in dual diagnoses was more effective when nurses targeted mental health symptoms rather than behaviours. It is important that people with ID are adequately screened in order to receive appropriate and equitable treatment. The use of mental health screening tools specifically designed for the use of people with ID serve as an assessment so people with ID are referred to appropriate services (Bates, Priest, & Gibbs, 2004).

Sedentary behaviour, overweight and underweight

People with ID are less physically active compared to the general population (Lante et al., 2014) and problems with sedentary behaviour, being overweight or underweight are well documented. Being female with ID, having Down syndrome, taking medications and living more independently are factors that are strongly associated with obesity (Hsieh, Rimmer, & Heller, 2014). By contrast, being a male with ID and having cerebral palsy are associated with being underweight (Bhaumik et al., 2008). Nurses need to be aware of the differences within the ID population in order to accommodate varying healthcare needs. In addition, some behavioural challenges, such as those associated with a diagnosis of Autism, can also present issues when the person has significant food sensitivity related to a sensory problem. For example, some people might have an aversion to certain food textures creating dietary imbalances that affects the person's weight.

Key considerations in the delivery of care

Key issues covered in this section are: the transition from child to adult health services, health literacy and ID, capacity, consent and supported decision making, and communicating health needs.

Transition from child to adult health services

Transition from paediatric to adult care is a stressful time for children with special health care needs and their families (Bloom et al., 2012). The Australian adult and paediatric health systems work very differently. In the paediatric system, family are central to care and parents play an important role in how care is directed to the child with ID. In addition, the paediatrician is often a constant in the life of the child and the family and will understand the child's needs and the family's priorities. By contrast, in the adult health system, an adult with ID is likely to have a multitude of medical specialists over time with no primary physician providing the overall care in the same way that a paediatrician does for a child with ID. The adult health system is more individually-focussed; this is not sufficient for a person with ID who requires support in order to navigate the healthcare system.

Health literacy and ID

People with ID have lower levels of health literacy and are more prone to health risk behaviours that may contribute to the development and exacerbation of chronic disease (Scott & Havercamp, 2016). Low health literacy influences how people seek support, navigate healthcare systems, understand nutrition and medical instructions, organise health care appointments, complete paperwork and analyse the risk and benefits of information provided by health care professionals (Australian Commission on Safety and Quality in Health Care, 2019). Health literacy is challenging for people with ID due to problems with memory, attention, information processing and communication. People with ID are often overlooked in health education programs (McIlfatrick et al., 2011) and health professionals fail to make *reasonable adjustments* in the delivery of health information.

> The key elements of making reasonable adjustments are: (1) Identifying the person and not their carer, (2) Focus on the things that are important to the person, (3) creating a safe and comfortable space, (4) Planning of care, (5) Creating accessible resources, (6) Increase health staff knowledge about ID and (7) adjusting your communication approach (Oulton, Sell, Kerry, & Gibson, 2015)

Examples of reasonable adjustments that nurses can make include allowing more time for and during health appointments, using appropriate language during communication with the person with ID and their careers, adapting health education activities and information, and making information accessible by using plain English (Oulton, Sell, Kerry, & Gibson, 2015). There are a number of tools in the wider literature that can assist with these key steps including hospital passports, personalised disability profiles and an *All About Me* booklet. Such resources assist nurses to personalise the hospital journey, and make reasonable adjustments to reduce anxiety and improve health outcomes.

Capacity, consent and supported decision making

Patient consent to treatment is a legal requirement as well as an ethical and a human rights issue in healthcare (Bird, 2011). Consent to medical treatment for people with ID can be complicated by communication problems as well as negative and disablist assumptions by health professionals. For example, some nurses may incorrectly assume that a person with ID is unable to consent and then fails to provide them with adequate information about a procedure. By contrast, when a person with ID does lack the capacity to understand, some nurses may give information and treatment options that are too difficult for them to understand (Bernal, 2019). Both instances are professionally problematic for the nurse and do not reflect best practice. Bird (2011) offers two criteria when deciding if a person with ID is able to consent: (1) an ability to comprehend and retain information, and (2) weigh that information in the balance to arrive at a choice (p. 250). Sometimes, despite the best efforts of the nurse, gaining proxy consent from a substitute decision maker is needed. Each state and territory in Australia has different legislation relating to capacity to consent; nurses need to understand and know about these differences. Even where a person with ID cannot consent, a process of *supported decision-making* between the person, their family and/or carers, is identified as best practice.

> Supported decision making is 'a system in which people work together to understand an individual's desires and choices and then provide means for that person to exercise their legal capacity…as opposed to someone else's decision made on their behalf' (Devi, 2013, p. 795).

Communication and symptoms of ill health

According to the AIHW (2012), almost 60% of people with ID have severe communication limitations distinguishing them from other major disability groups. Having a communication disability is strongly associated with increased risk of preventable and multiple adverse events in hospital due to communication difficulties associated with people with ID in the time-limited setting of a hospital ward (Hemsley, Balandin, & Worral, 2012). Some people with ID have problems with receptive communication (difficulty understanding abstract concepts and complex language); others have expressive communication problems (difficulty expressing concerns, symptoms, feelings); and some have difficulties with both (Centre for Developmental Disability Health [CDDH], 2016). Another major communication issue for many people with ID is *acquiescence*. Many nurses are unaware of this issue and thus are unaware of the negative impact it can have on the care of a person with ID.

> Acquiescence is where a person with ID does not actually understand what is being asked of them and so they typically respond 'yes' so that they feel they are pleasing the nurse by giving the answer they think that the nurse wants.

Sometimes a person with ID is unable to verbally communicate their health needs due to their disability, and behaviour is the only way of communication. For example, a person with ID experiencing a headache may bang their head; a person with ID and a stomach ache may scream and bang the walls; or a person with ID and a gastric ulcer may suck their hand. Each case is an example where the individual cannot verbally communicate their pain symptoms and therefore communicate through, what appears to be, maladaptive behaviour. de Knegt et al. (2013) identified a range of behavioural-based pain indicators that nurses should be aware of when assessing pain behaviours in people with ID: different motor and facial activity, unusual social-emotional indicators and nonverbal communication that is out of the ordinary for the person. In this instance, enlisting the support of carers when undertaking assessment of the person is a useful strategy for nurses.

Role of family and carers

Carers, particularly family, usually have extensive knowledge of the health and life history of the person with ID. In addition, they will have insight into their personality and behavioural responses, and are fundamental to facilitating positive communication interactions during client interactions. In addition, reliance on carer knowledge of the individual, sometimes serves to bridge the gap in nurses' own knowledge and skills of care to the person with ID (Lewis, Gaffney, & Wilson, 2017). While tapping into carer knowledge is essential, nurses also need to be prepared for family members and carers to advocate, sometimes strongly, for the person with ID and not be intimidated by this *advocacy*. Nurses also need to be mindful and respectful of parents' and carers' vigilance as an important strategy to minimise fear, anxiety, and ensure adequate care and safety. The online resources section at the end of this chapter offers an interesting insight from the parents' perspective and provides some useful tips on how to promote positive parent-health professional interactions.

> Advocacy means speaking in support of or on behalf of another person who may not be able to speak independently on his/her own behalf.

Cultural considerations

Cultural considerations add a further dimension to patient-nurse-carer interactions when working with people with ID and their families across Australia. Australia is a multicultural nation; therefore, nurses will find themselves caring for people from a non-English speaking background (NESB) as well as First Nation Australians. There is a higher incidence of ID in the Aboriginal and Torres Strait Islander populations requiring nurses to be cognisant of the history of Australia's First Nations people in order to provide culturally safe care. More information about nursing and Aboriginal and Torres Strait Islander health can be found in Chapter 6. Many families from a NESB already face many societal barriers and the addition of having a child with ID can overtly add to these problems when accessing healthcare services (O'Hara, 2003). Disability may be viewed differently in other cultures. For example, some families will refuse certain types of assistance for their child with ID stating it is 'God's will' that the child has a disability, whereas other families may view disability as a 'gift' to the family based on cultural beliefs. Nurses should respect and support the cultural health belief systems of all clients from differing cultural backgrounds, and at the same time, offer information in a culturally appropriate manner. Consider also, the use of inter-preter services or engaging Aboriginal Liaison Officers to facilitate communication, both of which are available in most healthcare organisations across Australia.

Australian practice contexts

Nurses who specialise in caring for people with ID do so across a range of differ-ent contexts. Most nurses who specialised in caring for people with ID previously worked within larger residential institutions. Following the closure of most of these institutions, there has been a steady decrease in the number of nurses who provide this type of care. However, a small number of these facilities remain, particularly in NSW where services in the Hunter region continue due to delays in the building of more contemporary accommodation. Nurses need to be cognisant that most people with ID who still live at these sites will find transitioning to smaller residential style settings a major challenge, sometimes requiring multidisciplinary input to facilitate a smooth changeover. Similarly, nurses who worked in these institutions for decades face significant change to their working environment as professional roles and career

---

Box 14.2 - Case study (Sam)

Sam is a 14-year-old boy who recently arrived in Australia as a refugee from Syria and speaks Arabic. Sam has severe ID with challenging autistic behaviours and only recently started to attend a special school where everyone speaks English. Sam has presented to the Emergency department accompanied by his parents; he has sustained a large lacera-tion on the bottom of his left foot. Sam has long unkempt hair, long finger and toe nails, is vocalising in an incoherent manner, and is pacing around and pushing people away.

Reflective questions:

1 What issues come to mind that impact Sam's ability to accept nursing care?
2 What type of information do you need from Sam's parents to plan his care?
3 What would Sam's nursing care plan look like?
4 What strategies do you need to consider regarding care at home?

Box 14.3 - Clinician's story

I work as an RN with young adults with intellectual disability who also have chronic and complex health problems and live in 24-hour staffed group homes. Most of these young adults also have a physical disability. My day at work involves working directly with the clients to provide personal care and grooming, tube-feeding, respiratory support, daily physiotherapy, positioning and postural drainage. In addition, I also oversee health care planning, attend specialist medical appointments, train support workers in health procedures, and also respond to emergency situations. The work with each client is in partnership with families and services. It is one of the most rewarding nursing jobs I have ever had and I believe it is one of the few areas where you truly practice holistic nursing

---

pathways disappear and new practice models in ID care are formulated such as in GP practices, acute care settings and community contexts.

Different ways of working have already evolved in smaller residential services, and in community-based group homes. Examples of nursing roles include those of nurse specialists who oversee health care plans for every person with ID in the service; nurses who work in 24-hour residential settings who provide direct and complex nursing care (e.g. people with ID who have a tracheostomy or gastrostomy); and roving roles where the nurse provides drop-in support once or twice across a 24-hour period (Wilson et al., 2018). The key issue faced is that nurses are often working in isolation as the sole practitioner when leading health care planning processes. Managing chronic health conditions associated with ID are core business, although such nurses need to be adaptable in order to respond during acute health care situations.

During deinstitutionalisation there was an expectation that people with ID would access mainstream healthcare services. Unfortunately, this resulted in many people with ID falling through the gaps. In recognition of the need to improve services and care, some governments saw the need to adopt ID specific policy, for example, the NSW government policy *A Service Framework for Health Care of People with ID* (NSW Health, 2012). In NSW, there is currently a small number of specialised ID health assessment services involving nurses with ID expertise in a team leadership role within the interdisciplinary environment. It is imperative that these specialist roles continue with an expectation that the roles will further develop over time, and that other states and territories also take this initiative. Adopting an ID specific model of care has been apparent in other countries around the world for some time.

Practice exemplars from overseas

In the UK, the role of the specialist learning disability nurse (LDN) receives professional recognition, which is not currently reflected in Australia or elsewhere in the world (Jaques et al., 2018). The UK LDN role incorporates three major tasks: (1) providing ID education across all disciplines and settings; (2) acting as advocate in acute care settings; and (3) brokering between services as well as between clients, their families and healthcare professionals to ensure better health outcomes (Jaques et al., 2018). However, it is evident that current ID healthcare needs in Australia are not being met. Recent research highlighting that people with ID die on average 27 years earlier than the general population and that 38% of deaths are potentially avoidable (Trollor, Srasuebkul, Xu, & Howlett, 2017) suggests that the role of an LDN in Australia is well-warranted. The UK government recently launched an inquiry into the value of mandatory training of all nurses in the care of a person with ID. Although in early consultation phase, it is emblematic of the underlying global issue: that nurses need specific knowledge in how to care for a person with ID and how to make reasonable adjustments that promote positive experiences and improve health outcomes for this vulnerable group.

Challenges facing the field

Current Australian research shows that nurses who work within disability services are vital in leading the direct provision of quality care to people with ID and chronic and complex needs – a model of care referred to as *being nurse-led and relationship-centred* (Wilson, Wiese, Lewis, Jaques, & O'Reilly, 2018). At some stage, this will need to be acknowledged in more explicit terms by the NDIS as no other group of health professionals has the skills to provide this level and type of care. The next decade will be a critical time for nurses who work with people with ID as the NDIS policy framework adjusts to the realities of individual's support needs. For nurses who either work with people with ID or are looking to do so, this policy adjustment presents both opportunities and risks. This is because the NDIS currently funds allied health supports and the cost to train support workers to implement health care plans, however does not fund diagnostic, assessment and general medical services, hospital care, or discharge planning. These are all under the domain of state funded mainstream health services. This leaves nurses who are currently employed by disability services, which are not health-funded, in a state of employment and career limbo. Although the NDIS has a cost category for complex care, this currently does not specifically refer to the role of nurses. There are, however many potential opportunities for nurses. For example, the NDIS framework now has evolved to include a category for continence nurses to provide support as well as specialised mental health nurses. This suggests that at a policy level, the NDIS framework is adapting to what people with ID actually need rather than defining every health need as a state-based health department issue.

Conclusion

This chapter explored a range of issues about the role of nurses in supporting the health of people with ID. People with ID are more likely to have additional health problems, greater health risks and face numerous barriers when accessing mainstream health system. Nurses are uniquely positioned to be at the forefront of improving health outcomes for people with ID across Australia. By adopting a relationship-centred approach to nursing care with the person as the focal point of the care, and guided by the professional nursing codes of practice, positive outcomes will result. The future role/s of the nurse who specialises in nursing people with ID will be complex and will require different approaches as the policy settings of the NDIS evolve and the responsibilities of the health system and disability services become clearer.

Online resources

1　Professional Association of Nurses in Developmental Disability, Australia Inc. (PANDDA): http://www.pandda.net/
2　Working with people with intellectual disabilities in healthcare settings: http://www.cddh.monashhealth.org/wp-content/uploads/2016/11/2016-working-with-people-with-intellectual-disabilities.pdf
3　Books Beyond Words; making information accessible to people with ID: https://booksbeyondwords.co.uk/
4　Parents perspectives of what they want from nurses: http://www.intellectualdisability.info/how-to-guides/articles/through-our-eyes-what-parents-want-for-their-children-from-health-professionals

References

Australian Bureau of Statistics (ABS). (2014). *Intellectual Disability, Australia, 2012.* Catalogue number 4433.0.55.003. Retrieved from http://www.abs.gov.au

Australian Commission on Safety and Quality in Health Care. (2019). Safe and high-quality care for patients with cognitive impairment: Cognitive impairment. Retrieved from https://www.safetyandquality.gov.au/our-work/cognitive-impairment/

Australian Institute of Health and Welfare (AIHW). (2012). *Disability in Australia: Intellectual Disability* (Cat No: 4433.0.55.003). Canberra, Australia: AIHW.

Bakken, T. L., & Sageng, H. (2016). Mental health nursing of adults with intellectual disabilities and mental illness: A review of empirical studies 1994–2013. *Archives of Psychiatric Nursing, 30*(2), 286–291. doi: 10.1016/j.apnu.2015.08.006.

Bates, P., Priest, H., & Gibbs, M. (2004). The education and training needs of learning disability staff in relation to mental health issues. *Nurse Education in Practice, 4*, 30–38. doi: 10.1016/S1471-5953(03)00016-7.

Bernal, J. (2019). *Consent and people with intellectual disabilities: The basics.* University of Hertfordshire. Retrieved from http://www.intellectualdisability.info/how-to-guides/articles/consent-and-people-with-intellectual-disabilities-the-basics

Bloom, S. R., Kuhlthau, K., Van Cleave, J., Knapp, A., Newacheck, P., & Perrin, J. M. (2012). Health care transition for youth with special health care needs. *Journal of Adolescent Health, 51,* 213–219.

Bhaumik, S., Watson, J. M., Thorp, C. F., Tyrer, F., & McGrother, C. W. (2008). Body mass index in adults with intellectual disability: Distribution, associations and service implications: A population-based prevalence study. *Journal of Intellectual Disability Research, 52,* 287–298.

Bird, S. (2011). Capacity to consent to treatment. *Australian Family Physician, 40*(4), 249–250.

Centre for Developmental Disability Health. (2016). *Working with people with intellectual disabilities in healthcare settings.* Melbourne, Victoria: Monash Health.

Collings, S., Dew, A., & Dowse, L. (2016). Support planning with people with intellectual disability and complex support needs in the Australian national disability insurance scheme. *Journal of Intellectual and Developmental Disability, 41*(3), 272–276. http://dx.doi.org/10.3109/13668250.2016.1151864

Davis, E., Saeed, S. A., & Antonnaci, D. J. (2008). Anxiety disorders in persons with developmental disabilities: Empirically informed diagnosis and treatment. *Psychiatry Quarterly, 79*(3), 249–263. doi: 10.1007/s11126-008-9081-3.

De Knegt, N., Pieper, M. J. C., Lobbezoo, F., Schuengel, C., Evenhuis, H. M., Passcheir, J., & Scherder, E. (2013). Behavioral pain indicators in people with intellectual disabilities: A systematic review. *The Journal of Pain, 14*(9), 885–896. doi: 10.1016/j.jpain.2013.04.016.

Devi, N. (2013). Supported decision-making and personal autonomy for persons with intellectual disabilities: Article 12 of the UN convention on the rights of persons with disabilities. *The Journal of Law, Medicine & Ethics, 41*(4), 792–806. https://doi.org/10.1111/jlme.12090

Geiss, M., Chamberlain, M., Weaver, T., McCormick, C., Raufer, A., Scoggins, L., Petersen, L., Davis, S. & Edmonson, D. (2018).Diagnostic Overshadowing of the Psychiatric Population in the Emergency Department: Physiological Factors Identified for an Early Warning System. *Journal of the American Psychiatric Nurses Association, 24*(4), 327–331. https://doi.org/10.1177/1078390317728775

Hemsley, B., Balandin, S., & Worrall, L. (2012). Nursing the patient with complex communication needs: Time as a barrier and a facilitator to successful communication in hospital. *Journal of Advanced Nursing, 68*(1), 116–126. doi: 10.1111/j.1365-2648.2011.05722.x.

Hsieh, K., Rimmer, J. H., & Heller, T. (2014). Obesity and associated factors in adults with intellectual disability. *Journal of Intellectual Disability Research, 58*(9), 851–863. doi: 10.1111/jir.12100.

Jaques, H., Lewis, P., Wiese, M., O'Reilly, K., & Wilson, N. J. (2018). Understanding the contemporary role of the intellectual disability nurse: A review of the literature. *Journal of Clinical Nursing, 27*(21–22), 3858–3871. doi: 10.1111/jocn.14555.

Lante, K., Stancliffe, R., Bauman, A., Van Der Ploeg, H., Jan, S., & Davis, G. (2014). Embedding sustainable physical activities into the everyday lives of adults with intellectual disabilities: A randomised controlled trial. *BMC Public Health, 14*(1), 1–6.

Lewis, P., Gaffney, R. J., & Wilson, N. J. (2017). A narrative review of acute care nurses' experiences nursing patients with intellectual disability: Underprepared, communication barriers and ambiguity about the role of caregivers. *Journal of Clinical Nursing, 26*(11–12), 1473–1484. doi: 10.1111/jocn.13512.

McIlfatrick, S., Taggart, L., & Truesdale-Kennedy, M. (2011). Supporting women with intellectual disabilities to access breast cancer screening: A health professional perspective. *European Journal of Cancer Care, 20*, 412–420. doi: 10.1111/j.1365-2354.2010.01221.x.

Manohar, H., Subramanian, K., Kandasamy, P., Penchilaiya, V., & Arun, A. (2016). Diagnostic masking and overshadowing in intellectual disability: How structured evaluation helps. *Journal of Child and Adolescent Mental health Nursing, 29*, 171–176. doi: 10.101111/jcap.12160.

MENCAP. (2012). Death by Indifference: 74 deaths and counting, a progress report 5 years on. MENCAP, London.

NSW Health. (2012). Service Framework to Improve the Health Care of People with Intellectual Disability http://www.health.nsw.gov.au/disability/Pages/health-care-of-people-with-ID.aspx

O'Hara, J. (2003). Learning disabilities and ethnicity: Achieving cultural competence. *Advances in Psychiatric Treatment, 9*(3), 166–174. doi: 10.1192/apt.9.3.166.

Oulton, K., Sell, D., Kerry, S., & Gibson, F. (2015). Individualizing hospital care for children and young people with learning disabilities: It's the little things that make a difference. *Journal of Paediatric Nursing, 30*, 78–86.

Peterlin, A., & Peterlin, B. (2016). Contemporary approach to diagnosis of genetic causes of intellectual disability. *Journal of Special Education and Rehabilitation, 17*(3/4), 62–70. doi: 10.19057/jser.2016.10.

Schalock, R. L., Borthwick-Duffy, S. A., Bradley, V. J., Buntinx, W. H., Coulter, D. L., Craig, E. M., Shogren, K. A. (2010). *Intellectual disability: Definition, classification, and systems of supports.* Washington, DC: American Association on Intellectual and Developmental Disabilities.

Scott, H., & Havercamp, S. (2016). Systematic review of health promotion programs focused on behavioural changes for people with intellectual disability. *Intellectual and Developmental Disabilities, 54*(1), 63–76. doi: 10.1352/1934-9556-54.1.63.

Tonge, B., Torr, J., & Trollor, J. (2017). Mental health and wellbeing in people with intellectual disability. In S. Bloch, S. Green, A. Janca, P. Mitchell, & M. Robertson (Eds.), *Foundations of clinical psychiatry* (4th ed., pp. 401–417). Melbourne: Melbourne University Publishing.

Trollor, J. N., Srasuebkul, P., Xu, H., & Howlett, S. (2017). Cause of death and potentially avoidable deaths in Australian adults with intellectual disability using retrospective linked data. *BMJ Open, 7*(e013489). doi: 10.1136/bmjopen-2016-013489.

Tua, C., Neville, C., & Scott, T. (2017). Appreciating the work of nurses caring for adults with intellectual disability and mental health issues. *International Journal of Mental Health Nursing, 26*, 6, 29–638. doi: 10.1111/inm.12291.

Vissers, L., Gilissen, C., & Veltman, J. (2015). Genetic studies into intellectual disability and related disorders. *Nature Reviews: Genetics, 17*(0), 9–18. doi: 10.1038/nrg3999.

Weise, J., & Trollor, J. (2018). Preparedness and training needs of an Australian public mental health workforce in intellectual disability mental health. *Journal of Intellectual and Developmental Disability, 43*(4), 431–440. doi: 10.3109/13668250.2017.1310825.

Werner, S., & Stawski, M. (2012), Mental health: Knowledge, attitudes and training of professionals on dual diagnosis of intellectual disability and mental health disorder. *Journal of Intellectual Disability Research, 56*, 291–304. doi: 10.1111/j.1365-2788.2011.01429.x.

Wilson, N. J., & Charnock, D. (2017). Developmental and intellectual disability. In E. Chang & A. Johnson (Eds.), *Living with chronic illness and disability: Principles for nursing practice* (3rd ed., pp. 129–145). Sydney, Australia: Elsevier.

Wilson, N. J., Lewis, P., O'Reilly, K., Wiese, M., Lin, Z., Devine, L., Goddard, L. (2018). Reframing the role, identity and standards for practice for registered nurses working in the specialty area of intellectual and developmental disability in Australia: The NDIS and beyond. *Collegian.* doi: 10.1016/j.colegn.2018.06.002.

Wilson, N. J., Wiese, M., Lewis, P., Jaques, H, & O'Reilly, K. (2018). Nurses working in intellectual disability-specific settings talk about the uniqueness of their role: A qualitative study. *Journal of Advanced Nursing.* doi: 10.1111/jan.13898.

Young, L., & Ashman, A. F. (2004). Deinstitutionalization for older adults with severe mental retardation: Results from Australia. *American Journal on Mental Retardation, 109*(5), 397–412.

15 Child and family health nursing

Cathrine Fowler and Deborah Stockton

Chapter objectives

This chapter will offer readers:

- Insight into the history of child and family health nursing
- An awareness of the changing nature and complexity of child and family health nursing
- A comprehensive overview of the contemporary nursing approaches used to work with families and their young children (birth to 5 years)
- An opportunity to consider the depth and breadth of knowledge to work within this nursing speciality
- An overview of the future challenges for nurses working within the speciality of child and family health nursing

Introduction

Child and family health nursing is one of the oldest nursing specialities in Australia, providing essential nursing services to families with infants and young children (birth-to-five years). These free universal child and family health services are provided by Registered Nurses with postgraduate specialty qualifications based on care that is proportionate to the disadvantage and needs of a population (Schmied et al., 2014). The desired outcome is to reduce the gap in health inequities within and across populations enabling enhanced services to be available for the most disadvantaged populations while providing services to all families regardless of socioeconomic status.

> Universal child and family health services are provided by local Council or Health Districts. In areas with smaller populations, one child and family health service may cover several towns visiting each town on a weekly or fortnightly basis.

The main child and family health workforce are registered nurses with a child and family health nursing post-graduate qualification as a minimal requirement (Kruske & Grant, 2012). In most Australian child and family health services, the nurse works autonomously with a focus on well-child health. Well-child health community-based services provide: child physical and developmental surveillance and assessment programs, health promotion and parent education and support programs, psycho-social and perinatal mental health assessment and intervention; support to enhance parent — infant/child relationship development; and parental (main carer) physical and emotional health.

In recent decades the work of child and family health nurses has developed to mirror the changes and expectations of Australian society to include: an increased focus on the health and parenting support needs of men's role as fathers, same sex parents and their families and refugee families.

Historical and current contexts of clinical practice

Prior to and post the First World War, disease was a major cause of early childhood mortality (Armstrong, 1939). A lack of services for families and poor living conditions resulting in gastroenteritis was an outcome of inadequate sanitation and purity of food and milk supply (Fowler, Dickinson, & Brown, 2018). In the early 20th century, the provision of Australian public health nursing services was limited. State and territory governments started to identify and instigate plans for the establishment of maternal and child health services that used health promotion education and illness prevention strategies to ameliorate early child and maternal death and improve the health of mothers and young children (Fowler et al., 2018). In NSW from 1921, all registered nurses working in the baby health clinics were required to have completed mothercraft training (Armstrong, 1939).

> Baby Health Clinics were established in towns and suburbs, often in buildings provided by local councils or Country Women's Association of Australia (CWAA). These centres are now called by several different names depending on the Australian state or territory they are in. The service can be a stand-alone service managed by nurses or be located within a generalist community centre which increases the access to specialist intervention.

In recent years UNICEF has instigated a global initiative to improve the focus on the critical first 1,000 days (from conception to the end of the second year) of a child's life. This initiative is in recognition of the importance of the first 1,000 days and the critical need for an increased focus on supporting the parent child relationship and providing surveillance, early assessment and intervention (Lo, Das, & Horton, 2017). Nurses are playing a major role in implementing this initiative.

Becoming a child and family health nurse

To become a child and family health nurse you must be a registered nurse and have completed a recognised qualification in child and family health nursing. There are inconsistencies with the nomenclature between states, but overall there are similarities in the role of these nurses. Nomenclature include: child and family health nurse (NSW, South Australia, Northern Territory and Tasmania); maternal child health nurse (Victoria and Australian Capital Territory); child health nurse (Queensland); and community child health nurse (Western Australia).

Child and family health services

Australia is one of the few countries with a free and comprehensive universal health service for parents and children under school-age. Importantly, these are all nurse-led services with nurses taking major responsibility for assessment and/or surveillance of the children and their families, providing parent education and providing referrals to other health professionals or services. These services provide a continuum of care appropriate to the level of need and complexity of vulnerability and risk factors experienced by families. Services at the primary level include primary child and family health nursing services and telephone helplines. The nurses working in these services are able to refer families with presenting issues that are unable to be resolved at a primary level. These parents and/or their children are often in need of intensive assessment and interventions that is provided within the context of an extended centre based service, home-visiting consultation or 24×7 residential service setting. Residential care is not currently available to parents in Tasmania or the Northern Territory. Services Australian parents (families) and their young children can access are listed in Table 15.1.

Table 15.1 Child and family health services

Clinical services	
Primary level services	
Digital Technology supported parenting advice and support	Access to parenting advice from nurses and referral to other services.
Universal centre-based services	Child health centres are located in most Australian communities. A free service for parents with children 0 to school age children.
Short-term home visiting	Offered by universal services as an initial contact with a nurse and when parents are unable to attend centre-based services due to multiple births or other issues that make attendance difficult.
Parent education groups	Range of education programs with a health promotion focus e.g. preparation for parenthood, new mothers groups, sleep and settling groups, infant feeding, toddler behaviour management and transition to school.
Secondary level services	
Mobile clinic services	Improve access to populations that are disadvantaged due to cultural issues or living within isolated area.
Telehealth parenting services	Increasing access via video-conferencing
Extended centre based	Consultation 4 hours to 6 hour with a nurse and if necessary allied health professional.
Therapeutic parenting groups such as: • Postnatal Depression Therapy groups • Circle of Security program	Groups with a therapeutic focus offered to mothers and their partners experiencing postnatal depression and anxiety; and parent infant relationship challenges.
Tertiary level services	
Residential programs	Parents stay for several days to gain 24 hour support to access intensive assessment and support.
Sustained home visiting programs	Often commence in the antenatal period and extending until child is 2 years old.

For many parents a visit to a child and family health centre to see a nurse remains a central access point. As an outcome of the visit the nurse may refer the parent to other specialist services or health professionals.

The changing nature and complexity of child and family health nursing

The complexity and focus of child and family health nursing has changed over the decades from a main focus on reducing infant and maternal mortality at the beginning of the 20th century through improving mothercraft skills and child health, health promotion, child protection, surveillance and assessment (Armstrong, 1939). Since the 1980s the role has been enhanced to include perinatal and infant mental health assessment and interventions. The constant during the past 100 plus years has been the strong foundation of primary health care that continues to underpin child and family health nursing.

Traditionally, a well-accepted part of Australian culture identified and promoted the mother as the main caregiver of infants and young children. Even though women remain the main carers there is now increasing acknowledgement, acceptance and celebration of the diverse family formations and roles in Australia. In growing numbers families are now attending child and family health services as they proudly identify their role as parents and the increased acceptance within Australian society that includes same sex couples and 'stay at home' fathers while the mother returns to paid work. Critically, there are groups of parents that require additional support to enable them to parent safely. For example, parents with an intellectual disability, parents with a child who has a chronic illness or a disability, parents with a mental illness and parents who have experienced traumatic events during childhood or as adults such as child abuse or family violence. Further, a growing cohort of carers is grandparents who have responsibility for their grandchildren while parents do paid work. Some grandparents have fulltime custody of their grandchildren due to parental incarceration, drug or alcohol misuse or death of the parent (Qu, Lahausse, & Carson, 2018).

In the 2016, the National Framework for Health Services for Aboriginal and Torres Strait Islander Children and Families was developed (Department of Health, 2016). Within this document there is a call for health services to move from a focus on Organisational policies and procedures to focusing on the needs and preferences of Aboriginal and Torres Islander children and families (Department of Health, 2016). New services and approaches have started to be developed, for example in the Mid North Coast of NSW Tresillian Family Care Centres in partnership with the Local Health District and Durri Aboriginal Corporation Medical Service have implemented a Tresillian 2 U mobile van service – bringing the service to towns of lower population density often isolated due to transport and socio-economic challenges. This service is staffed by child and family health nurses and Aboriginal health workers to enable a culturally appropriate approach for the local Aboriginal community including the co-design of localised group programs with Aboriginal Elders and health workers.

Working within such diverse communities can be challenging as having a set routine approach to solving parenting and infant behaviour issues and concerns is no longer acceptable or effective. An increase in flexibility is required in the way the nurses work with families, this includes an enhanced understanding of cultural and social issues. Child and family health nurses are becoming skilled at using a strengths and relationship-based approach for working with families.

Box 15.1 - Case study (Mae)

Mae is a mother of a much anticipated 2-week old daughter. The child and family health nurse arrives for the first home visit to do a routine assessment and to invite the mother to come for future visits to the clinic. Mae's mother-in-law is visiting from China to provide support in the early months of motherhood. It was impossible for the nurse to complete the psychosocial assessment because of grandmother's presence. The nurse makes an appointment for Mae to visit the clinic next week to complete the assessment.

During the follow-up appointment Mae's responses during the psychosocial assessment are of concern. She is experiencing feelings of panic and is concerned she is a terrible mother as she is regularly criticised by her mother-in-law. Mae and the nurse discuss strategies she can use to improve the situation and that will be acceptable to her family. Mae decides she will join the new mothers' group the nurse facilitates each week to expand her social network.

Reflective questions:

1   List potential differences in parenting approaches between Chinese parents and parents from English speaking backgrounds.
2   Why did the nurse postpone the psychosocial assessment until the next appointment with Mae?
3   What are some of the strategies the nurse could use to assist Mae make decisions about combining Chinese and western parenting approaches?
4   What other benefits other than expanding her social network can you identify for Mae when she joins a mothers' group?

Importantly, because of the foundation of knowledge and clinical skills as registered nurses with specialist nursing qualifications we are well placed to not only focus on the health of the new mother and her infant but when necessary provide nursing care for the often diverse and complex population that the nurse encounters on a daily basis. This places child and family health nurses in a unique position due to our scope of practice as registered nurses that other health, welfare and education disciplines cannot provide for families with children from birth to school age due to their less expansive scopes of practice. Nurses are often the non-threatening accessible entry point for families to the interprofessional colleagues who frequently work alongside us providing specialised assessment and intervention, and providing guidance, reassurance and support.

There are many misconceptions about the work of child and family health nurses that can reduce the value placed on our work by nursing, midwifery, other professional colleagues and the wider Australian community. A major misconception is that all child and family health nurses do is weigh babies and provide parenting advice as there is a lack of understanding about the hidden work of child and family health nurses (Shepherd, 2011). This perception for many of us causes a dilemma. While much of our work is focused on child health and parenting support and education this makes it safe for families to access the service. For example, if a caregiver or family member

---

Box 15.2 - Case study (Mathew)

The child and family health nurse receives a notification that Josie's and Andrew's son Mathew is being discharged from the Neonatal Intensive Care Unit (NICU). Matthew was born at term but was identified as having respiratory and cardiac problems that required surgery. At the first home visit the nurse identifies that both Josie and Andrew are terrified of managing Matthew's physical care requirements. After working with the nurse, Josie and Andrew are able to identify their additional support and education needs. The main priority is to learn how to manage the combination of Mathew's medical and physical care especially as he reaches new developmental milestones.

Reflective questions:

1   Identify the key issues for Josie and Andrew?
2   What general nursing knowledge and skills would supplement the child and family health nurse specialist knowledge and skills to work with Josie and Andrew?
3   As Josie is likely to have neglected her physical and emotional health due to the need to focus on Andrew's health challenges – what questions would you ask Josie before providing advice or making suggestions?
4   What other health and community services within your local community would you liaise with to provide additional support and services for Josie and Andrew?

---

is experiencing family violence, developing or have a mental or physical illness, they can safely visit a nurse to have their baby weighed as an accepted activity of parenting. However, in the privacy of the consultation room it is not uncommon for the carer to reveal their emotional distress and often associated physical health concerns and/or the abuse that is occurring within their home.

Our concern is particularly that carers experiencing family violence or mental illness continue to be allowed to attend their local child and family health service by their partner or family, without the stigma or risk that may occur when initially accessing mental health or domestic violence services. As a safe starting point and soft entry, the nurse can work with the carer to identify ways to access and engage with specialised health, support and intervention services. Frequently, the presenting issue of an infant's unsettled behaviour, difficult feeding or toddler and pre-schooler behavioural challenges are just the 'tip of the iceberg'. The role of the child and family nurse is to ensure there are no underlying physical or mental health issues with the child or the carer. In many instances these underlying problems are the cause, not the outcome of the young child's dysregulated behaviour. The nurse will then collaboratively work with the carer to both resolve and manage the identified issues. Frequently being able to uncover and manage these underlying health and/or social support issues resolves the child's behavioural issues.

A striking feature of child and family health nurses is the growing number with additional qualifications. Many nurses now have qualifications in: advanced clinical nursing; children's nursing; adult, infant, child and adolescent mental health; women's health; midwifery; education; management; and public health. An increasing number of child and family health nurses have research masters and doctoral degrees and are starting to make a significant contribution to child and family health nursing evidence and knowledge through research and knowledge translation.

For example, a student with a Master degree has investigated the critical thinking skills of child and family health nurses when conducting psychosocial assessments. Importantly, she found that the nurses in her sample had highly developed critical thinking ability (Sims & Fowler, 2018). While a doctoral student is exploring the therapeutic alliance between mothers and nurses during an admission to a residential early parenting service using both a therapeutic alliance questionnaire, the adult attachment interview and semi-structured interviews. Another student is using a participatory action research to explore the adaptation of metropolitan child and family health specialist (Level 2) service models for diverse contexts including rural and regional.

An area of opportunity for career advancement is as a nurse practitioner. From our investigations there does not seem to be any child and family health nurses who have registered as nurse practitioners in Australia although a small number have undertaken Masters studies towards this goal.

Contemporary nursing approaches for working with young children and their families

In the past two decades, child and family health nursing has seen a significant shift in the expectations of how we work with parents from an expert model to a more collaborative or co-productive model while maintaining our focus on the child (Fowler, Lee, Dunston, Chiarella, & Rossiter, 2012). This shift in practice is in line with other children's nursing specialities that use a child focused and family inclusive practice approach (Fowler et al., 2012). Central to working collaboratively with parents is the use of relationship and strengths-based approaches facilitating the need to work co-productively with parents to develop new knowledge and skills. This co-productive approach assists parents to take joint ownership of the problem-solving and decision-making that occurs within a consultation (Fowler et al., 2012).

Nurses are able to provide a safe base for parents to explore their parenting experience and build their confidence and skills enabling the parent in turn to provide a sense of security and a safe base for their child to explore their world. Critically the expertise of the nurse is not diminished but fully utilised as they provide guidance about safe parenting practice and when asked provide strategies that may assist the parent manage their identified problems. A positive outcome for the parents is often increased health literacy and self-efficacy or confidence in their ability to parent.

A co-production model of nursing practice requires that the nurse works with parents to co-produce knowledge, design interventions and review outcomes that are informed by the unique family context rather than immediately providing the 'right way' to improve the situation. This approach sends a crucial message to parents that they have existing knowledge and skills, and can build on these thereby contributing to the development of parental self-efficacy.

Different roles

The recognition of the importance of the early years of a child's life by governments has continued to provide new opportunities for nurses to expand their role. Specialist child and family health services play a pivotal role in the assessment, care and support provided for children and families with increasingly complex physical, developmental,

mental health, social and behavioural health needs (Australian Health Minister's Advisory Council, 2015). A critical role for the nurse is promoting child safety by identifying child protection risks and being an advocate for the child while balancing the building of a trusting therapeutic relationship with the parent.

The role of child and family health nurses has been acknowledged as a specialist practice role (Borrow, Munns, & Henderson, 2011). These specialist practice skills are demonstrated in parent child relationship development programs, early parenting intensive day services and residential units, as cofacilitators in postnatal depression therapy groups, working with families identified at significant risk that include refugee families, parents with a history of substance misuse and/or mental illness, domestic violence and incarcerated parents. The nurses work with the parent based on the findings of their history taking and assessments to design physical and psychosocial interventions that include: the Edinburgh Postnatal Depression Scale, NCAST Parent Child Interaction Assessment Scale, HOME Inventory, and the Ages and Stages Assessment. They are able to use the outcomes as a pre- and post-test of the effectiveness of their work with a family.

Box 15.3 - Case study (Sue)

Sue is a 25 year old mother with an 18 month old son and 2 month old daughter living in a rural town, 1 hour away from her nearest regional centre. Sue sought assistance from her local nurse for breastfeeding difficulties with her daughter. Sue discloses that she has been having trouble sleeping and is feeling quite desperate trying to care for both her children. Her husband is working in a mine as a fly-in, fly-out worker as they have not been able to plant crops for the past 2 years due to the drought.

A psychosocial assessment identified that Sue was likely to be experiencing postnatal depression further compounded by sleep deprivation. The nurse referred Sue to a secondary level Family Care Centre for more intensive support regarding her baby's feeding and sleeping difficulties. During the consultation Sue discussed the challenges she was experiencing both in settling her baby and her toddler, who was now waking overnight. Sue's lack of confidence in making positive parenting decisions was explored. Small achievable goals were identified by Sue in collaboration with the nurse. Sue accepted a referral to a perinatal psychology service which could be accessed via telehealth. Follow-up support was provided through the use of telehealth virtual consultations by the nurse.

Reflective questions:

1   What evidence can you find that the nurse used a relationship-based approach to working with Sue?
2   Working with distressed parents can take an emotional toll on nurses. If you were this nurse what strategies would you use to maintain your emotional and physical health?
3   How can telehealth be used to enhance access to services to support families in the early parenting period?

While some of these opportunities are a re-establishment of past modes of engaging with families, others are newly developed. Child and family health nursing services are identified as working in either a primary, secondary or tertiary level service.

The opportunities for child and family health nurses continue to increase with the renewed recognition of the nurses' knowledge and skills. These positions include providing parenting assessment, advice, education and support within:

- Paediatric hospitals and wards for parents with a young child who has a chronic illness
- Aboriginal and Torres Islander health services
- Practice and pharmacy nurses
- Justice health and correctional services working with incarcerated mothers
- Drug and alcohol rehabilitation services
- Community service to assist parents with intellectual disabilities
- Child protection services.

Working often autonomously, frequently isolated and undertaking emotionally sensitive work with parents, their young children and families' requires nurses to develop and sustain professional reflective capacity and be well supported by their employers. This 'emotional work' undertaken daily in listening to the concerns and experiences of parents and seeking to support them through often complex circumstances while balancing being an advocate of the child can be distressing for the nurse. Regular clinical supervision and, if necessary, access to employee support services are essential to ensure the nurse is able to learn from these clinical experiences and to assist processing critical incidents.

Conclusion

Child and family health services currently rely strongly on child and family health nurses to provide services for parents with young children. Importantly, registered nurses have the breadth of knowledge and skills that go beyond the child's first five years to provide a comprehensive service for families.

The foundation knowledge gained through a comprehensive pathophysiology and psychosocial general nursing education in addition to their child and family health qualification allows the establishment of a scope of practice that positions them to offer high quality child health anticipatory guidance, child and family health surveillance, assessment and intervention, parenting education and parenting support. Other professional disciplines can have difficulty or are unable to provide such comprehensive care. In rural and remote areas in particular having this breadth of knowledge and skills allows the child and family health nurse to take on a dual role providing health care to the extended family. Importantly, the child and health nurse is able to offer opportunistic care, advice and advocacy regardless of the age of the family member.

Online resources

1 National standards of practice for maternal, child and family health nursing practice in Australia: https://www.mcafhna.org.au/Portals/0/PositionStmt-PDF/National%20Standards%20of%20Practice%20for%20MCaFHNA.pdf
2 UNICEF first 1000 days: http://1000days.unicef.ph

References

Armstrong, W. (1939). The infant welfare movement in Australia. *Medical Journal of Australia*, October 28, 641–648.

Australian Health Minister's Advisory Council (2015). *Healthy, Safe and Thriving: National Strategic Framework for Child and Youth Health*. COAG Health Council. Retrieved from: http://www.coaghealthcouncil.gov.au/Portals/0/Healthy%20Safe%20and%20Thriving%20-%20National%20Strategic%20Framework%20for%20Child%20and%20Youth%20Health.pdf

Borrow, S., Munns, A., & Henderson, S. (2011). Community-based child health nurses: An exploration of current practice. *Contemporary Nurse*, *40*(1), 71–86.

Department of Health. (2016). *National Framework for the Health Services for Aboriginal and Torres Strait Islander Children and Families, Australian Government*. Retrieved from: https://www.catsinam.org.au/static/uploads/files/national-framework-for-health-services-for-aboriginal-and-torres-strait-islander.pdf

Fowler, C., Dickinson, M., & Brown, N. (2018). Tresillian Family Care Centres: 100years of service for New South Wales Families. *International Journal of Birth and Parent Education*, *6*(1), 1–4.

Fowler, C., Lee, A., Dunston, R., Chiarella, M., & Rossiter, C. (2012). Co-producing parenting practice: learning how to do child and family health nursing differently. *Australian Journal of Child and Family Health Nursing*, *9*(1), 7–11.

Kruske, S., & Grant, J. (2012). Educational preparation for maternal, child and family health nurses in Australia. *International Nursing Review*, *59*, 200–207.

Lo, S., Das, P., & Horton, R. (2017). A good start in life will ensure a sustainable future for all. *The Lancet*, *389*(10064), 8–9.

Qu, L., Lahausse, J., & Carson, R. (2018). *Working Together to Care for Kids: A survey of foster and relative/kinship carers. (Research Report)*. Australian Institute of Family Studies. Retrieved from: https://aifs.gov.au/publications/working-together-care-kids

Schmied, V., Fowler, C., Rossiter, C., Homer, C., Kruske, S., & The CHoRUS team. (2014). Nature and frequency of services provided by child and family health nurses in Australia: results of a national survey. *Australian Health Review*, *38*(2), 177–185.

Shepherd M. (2011). Behind the scales: Child and family health nurses taking care of women's emotional wellbeing. *Contemporary Nurse*, *37*(2), 137–148.

Sims D., & Fowler C. (2018). Postnatal psychosocial assessment and clinical decision-making, a descriptive study. *Journal of Clinical Nursing*, *27*(19–20), 3739–3749.

16 The role of the Community Mental Health Nurse

Rhys Jones and Sheila Mortimer-Jones

Chapter objectives

This chapter will offer the reader:

- Insight into the general role of the Community Mental Health Nurse (CMHN).
- An understanding of some of the challenges and issues that nurses face in the community mental health setting.
- An overview of some of the more specialist community mental health nursing roles.

Introduction

The CMHN[1] has a wide variety of functions and roles. As a member of the multidisciplinary team (MDT), the major role of the CMHN is to manage the mental healthcare of clients in the community. Although there are no specific qualifications required for a registered nurse to hold the position of CMHN in Australia, nurses are usually required to have significant experience working in the field of mental health. Some employers may, however, demand postgraduate qualifications in mental health or evidence of credentialing by the Australian College of Mental Health Nurses (Australian College of Mental Health Nurses, 2017).

According to the Australian Institute of Health and Welfare (2019), 435,000 Australians had community mental healthcare contact between the years 2017 and 2018. CMHNs visit these Australians in their homes to assess and monitor their mental state and assist them in their recovery. Duties that are incorporated within the role of the CMHN include psychosocial interventions, mental state examinations and risk assessments, medication administration and liaison with family members or carers and representatives from other services. They are also involved in crisis intervention and the supervision of clients on Community Treatment Orders.

> A Community Treatment Order is an order under the Mental Health Act (MHA) for a person to receive compulsory treatment in the community.

The general role of the Community Mental Health Nurse

A typical working day commences with handover in the outpatient mental health clinic. This clinic may be located within the same building as the hospital, in a separate building within the hospital grounds or in a community mental health centre. During handover any overnight incidents involving known clients will be discussed and particular roles for the day are allocated. The CMHN is expected to manage the care of a large number of clients, typically between 20 and 30 (Heslop, Wynaden, Tohotoa, & Heslop, 2016). Community case management involves visiting the clients and families at home, arranging appointments with the psychiatrist, monitoring medication adherence and side effects, assessing the clients' mental state and risk, monitoring their physical state and general wellbeing, liaising with family members and carers and other community agencies and ultimately updating the client's management plan, as they work with the client towards the client's vision of recovery.

> Being in recovery refers to 'learning how to live a safe, dignified, full, and self-determined life, at times in the face of the enduring symptoms of a serious mental illness' (Davidson, Drake, Schmutte, Dinzeo, & Andres-Hyman, 2009).

There are other additional roles or duties that the CMHN may be allocated as part of their workload. For example, the Duty Officer takes calls from clients whose mental health professional key worker is not available. They will then triage their call. The results of the triage could be a written note for the mental health clinician to follow up on their return, or another member of the team could be asked to follow up the client in the meantime. The Duty Officer also takes calls from the police who may request a joint attendance with CMHNs at a client's home, which the Duty Officer will then organise. Another role of the Duty Officer may be to administer depot injections to clients who present at the clinic. Depot injections are intramuscular neuroleptic medications that are released slowly over a period of 2–4 weeks, depending on the drug and the dose. Alternatively, there may be a dedicated Depot Clinic in cases where the catchment area is large. The role of the Depot Nurse will be to keep records of depot medication they have administered, or that have been missed, conduct a brief mental state examination (MSE) and risk assessment on the clients and inform the client's mental health worker if there are any issues.

The multidisciplinary team

The MDT comprises the CMHNs, the Psychiatrist, the Clinical Nurse Specialist, an Occupational Therapist, a Social Worker, a Psychiatric Registrar, a GP Liaison Nurse and a Psychologist. In large community mental health clinics, a First Psychosis/Early Intervention Liaison Officer may also be present. The CMHN is a key member of the MDT. They have a great deal to offer, as they are often the only member of the team to visit the client in their home and thus have insight into how the clients are managing with their domestic affairs. Frequently a client may present quite well in an interview with the psychiatrist but are not managing at home. The CMHN is often in the best position to assess this. In addition, their close links with the family can provide a valuable source of information on the client's mental state, relationships and social functioning. Furthermore, the nature of the public mental health system and the manner in which psychiatrists are trained often means a high turnover of medical staff. As such, the CMHN is often a long-term and stable member of the team. Intimate knowledge of the clients and their treatment over medium and long term is extremely valuable as this can provide a check against unnecessary treatment changes, as well as first-hand knowledge of risk factors and signs of relapse.

> Signs of relapse are specific to the client and may include lack of sleep, distractibility, social isolation and risk-taking behaviours.

MDT meetings provide a good opportunity for each member of the team to discuss the care of any clients that they have concerns with and discuss plans for discharge. The CMHN acts as a consultant for other members of the MDT. For example, they may be engaged by other members of the team to do joint home visits, administer intramuscular injections, assist with assessments, provide information on the MHA and offer advice and expertise in nursing-related issues such as physical health problems, medication adherence and the management of side effects.

Intake meetings

Once or twice a week, it is a common practice for the MDT to hold an intake meeting. Intake meetings are where new referrals are discussed amongst the MDT members. Referrals arise from a variety of sources such as the Psychiatric Liaison Nurse based in the Emergency Department of the hospital, GPs, family or carers or other interested parties such as social workers. In this meeting, the MDT will discuss each referral and make a decision whether or not the person meets the criteria for follow-up with the team. The criteria for admission to the public mental health service in Australia is based on its capacity to provide care and treatment to people with severe mental illnesses, people whose psychological distress severely impacts on their ability to function or people with a mental disorder who are at risk. Additionally, the team will discuss the availability of the appropriate mental health professional within the team as well as their waiting lists. During these meetings there may be a formal process of checks to ensure that new clients have been followed up and that medical appointments have been arranged and attended. This is likely to include a brief handover of the assessment and treatment of the client to date.

If the criteria for admission to the community mental health service are not met, the referrer will be informed of the decision and given suggestions for follow-up. These suggestions could involve a range of options depending on the specific circumstances and may include the continuation of current treatment as best practice, referral to the private sector or non-government agency or referral to, or continuing care with, the client's GP. The latter may or may not involve input from the GP Liaison Nurse.

If the criteria for admission to the mental health service are met, the most appropriate person will make contact with the client for an assessment. This assessment may occur at the mental health outpatient clinic or it may take place at the client's home or at the client's GP surgery. If it is deemed appropriate for CMHN assessment, the nurse will examine past medical records and liaise with stakeholders who may be able to provide more background information. The CMHN will then interview the client. The purpose of the interview is to determine whether or not the person has a treatable mental disorder, to make an assessment of any risks that may be posed by the person to themselves or others, and to determine the client's attitude toward potential treatment. The client's attitude to treatment is important due to the possibility that the client may actively avoid treatment. This could be due to the nature of the illness, past history of treatment or due to the client's level of insight into their illness.

Initial assessment

The assessment will normally take the form of a semi-structured conversational style interview following the components of the MSE. Such an interview may be conducted in the presence of a support person for the client, often a family member or carer. Risk assessment is carried out routinely as a component of the MSE; however, both the risk assessment and MSE are regularly documented formally within the medical records and the online management system. Other electronic statistical input required by the CMHNs includes the Health of Nation Outcome Scales (HoNOS), which measures the health and social functioning of people with a mental illness. For more information about technology, critical issues associated with entering and using electronic patient information and the nurse's role, please refer to Chapter 3.

The first objective of the CMHN on meeting a new client for the first time is to establish rapport. Through the development of the therapeutic relationship, the client learns to trust the CMHN and become involved in decisions relating to their care. Although interpreters are routinely used at the clinic for clients for whom English is not their first language, there may be other supports available such as a Multicultural Liaison Officer. Support such as this can be extremely helpful in the provision of care. For instance, they may be able to link a Chinese client with a Chinese counsellor. A CMHN therefore should be aware of their own limitations and refer clients on to other services as required. The CMHN will liaise with family and other professionals involved in the client's treatment to determine a course of action. The approach taken is generally to work with the person and carers to find a course of action agreeable to the person that is likely to be effective in dealing with the issue at hand. The CMHN will be the leading decision maker; however, they will make this decision in conjunction with any other health professionals who are involved. Hence, the role of the CMHN involves a great deal of leadership and organisational and problem-solving skills.

CMHN follow-up

The CMHN and the client will decide on the psychosocial intervention required and the frequency of the home visits. These visits could be weekly initially depending on the acuity and will become less frequent as required. During the home visits, the client's mental state and risk and general wellbeing will be routinely assessed. The client will be provided with information about their illness and the treatments and resources available. Signs of relapse will be discussed and a management plan developed. The CMHN will ensure that the client has their required prescriptions and will monitor medication adherence and side effects such as metabolic syndrome. The CMHN may therefore take the client's blood pressure and monitor blood glucose, diet and weight during the home visits. Family and/or carer involvement is integral in providing the optimum care for the client. The CMHN will therefore ensure that when family is involved in the care they are educated about the mental illness and its impact. Signs of relapse, the importance of early intervention and the availability of resources are important components of this information.

Emergency assessment

The CMHN may be required to attend a client's home for an emergency assessment. The call is generally made by the police or by a family member. In the latter case, the CMHN may contact the police for a joint home visit. This is particularly the case where the client appears to be at high risk. On these occasions, CMHNs visit in pairs, and they will take the lead in decisions regarding the client's mental state. The CMHNs may decide that the client cannot be managed safely in the community and requires hospital admission. In circumstances when the client is unwilling to accept this, it becomes the CMHN's role to facilitate an involuntary admission. Australian states and territories have different MHAs with different official functions for clinicians.

> The aim of the MHA is to provide a framework for the involuntary assessment and treatment of people with a mental illness with the least possible restriction of their rights and freedoms.

If an authorised nurse operating under the MHA of their state or territory believes that the client meets the criteria for an involuntary admission, and they believe that no safe alternative exists, they may organise the transfer of the person to a mental health facility for assessment by a psychiatrist. This process usually involves liaising with the Nurse Unit Manager of the ward in order to organise a bed for the client. The CMHN will complete legal forms that order the person to attend the hospital – usually they will be transported in a hospital vehicle; however, on occasions an ambulance may be used. Family members may be recruited to assist with this process, the aim being to facilitate the process in the least restrictive manner and also maintaining the safety and reputation of the client and everyone else involved. After facilitating the transfer to hospital, the CMHN will liaise with the psychiatrist who will carry out the formal assessment under the MHA or with the team who will be assessing and treating the client in the hospital. They will also liaise with the referrer and family member to keep them up to date of events.

In the case where admission to a hospital is not considered necessary, a decision will be made about the most appropriate course of action. This may involve regular home visits from the CMHN, referral to specialist services such as Hospital in the Home and/ or a referral for an appointment with the psychiatrist. On occasions it may be that mental health services are not the appropriate agency to address the client's issues. It may be that the person's mental disorder is minor and does not pose a major risk. As such, it may be appropriate to refer them to their GP for advice and treatment. Other options may be community-based counselling, or perhaps the person would benefit from services such as the Alcohol and Other Drug Service. It would then be the CMHN's role to either refer the person on to the appropriate services or simply inform the person about the support services that are available in the community.

Challenges and issues

Mental health is one of the few areas of healthcare where people are sometimes treated against their will. This poses an obvious challenge for the CMHN as they attempt to develop a therapeutic relationship with people who do not want treatment, but may be obliged to receive it as a requirement of a Community Treatment Order (CTO). Conversely, there may be occasions when both the family and the client may request treatment or hospitalisation in circumstances where the clinician believes this is unwarranted. For example, for people with borderline personality disorder who are not acutely distressed (Mortimer-Jones et al., 2019) or for people with substance abuse issues in the absence of a mental illness. In cases such as these, the CMHN needs to have excellent communication and negotiation skills.

Internalised stigma, shame or embarrassment experienced by the client or by their family is another challenge that CMHNs face (Quinn, Williams, & Weisz, 2015). Internalised stigma can lead to a reluctance to engage with mental health services or indeed a lack of acknowledgement that there is a mental health issue at all. CMHNs must attempt to establish rapport and provide psychoeducation to people who are unwilling or unable to accept that there is an issue. Another challenge for the CMHN can be family dynamics. For example, parents may blame themselves for the disturbed mental state of their offspring (Cohen-Filipic & Bentley, 2015). This is an issue for the CMHN, as the family's behavioural and emotional functioning will also need to be addressed.

Although the majority of people with a mental illness pose no risk, on occasions people may become violent, for example, if they are experiencing their first episode of psychosis (Humphreys, Johnstone, MacMillan & Taylor, 1992). In situations such as this, the client may believe that the CMHN is a threat and hence they may feel the need to defend themselves with violence against the nurse who they may perceive as planning an attack on them. Substance abuse is another factor to be considered; when substance abuse is combined with a mental illness it has been found to be a predictor of violence (MacArthur Foundation, 2001). Access to weapons in the home environment and the lack of immediate assistance can also increase the risk to CMHNs (Godin, 2003). Furthermore, the presence of others in the home environment can also be an issue (Spencer & Munch, 2003). Indeed, family and friends may pose more of a risk to CMHNs than the client, especially when alcohol and other drugs are involved. Risk of violence can be assessed with the aid of standardised risk assessment instruments; however, CMHNs often tend to rely on their clinical judgement arising from their experience (Murphy, 2004).

The CMHN also needs to be aware of professional boundaries while working closely with clients in their home environment. The maintenance of professional boundaries while building a therapeutic relationship with the client requires a great deal of skill and mastery (Karanikola, Kaikoushi, Doulougeri, Koutrouba, & Papathanassoglou, 2018). It is important that the CMHN does not put themselves into any compromising situation. People with antisocial traits may claim malpractice, and there are generally no witnesses to support the CMHN, unlike in the ward situation. Maintenance of professional boundaries and clear documentation is therefore essential.

Another challenge for the CMHNs can be the shortage of resources. Inpatient mental health beds are often in high demand and short supply. The CMHN may find themselves making decisions based on resource availability including redirecting the client to an emergency department where the care and treatment of the client whilst available is unlikely to be optimal (Nordstrom et al., 2019),

Specialised roles

In addition to the general CMHN role, there are other specialised roles such as the GP Liaison Nurse and the First Psychosis/Early intervention Liaison Officer. CMHNs who hold these positions have their own specific functions within the MDT. The GP Liaison Nurse works closely with GPs – this may be in the form of sharing the care of a client (shared care). The role also involves providing information and advice to GPs on mental health and illness and treatment therapies. Another specialised role is the First Psychosis Liaison Officer or Early Intervention Officer. These specialists tend to have a small number of clients who have experienced psychosis for the first time. These clients therefore tend to be young adults generally, and the focus is on maintaining social networks, maintaining connection and commitment to work or college life, and providing education on mental health and illness. The overarching goal of the First Psychosis Liaison Officer therefore is to identify and strengthen protective factors such as good coping skills and a caring, stable family environment.

Conclusion

The CMHN needs to have a sound knowledge of mental illness, treatment modalities and psychosocial interventions, pharmacology, the MHA, knowledge of how the mental health system operates and knowledge of community resources available. In addition, they must have very strong communication, leadership and organisational skills and confidence in their ability. They frequently work alone and so must exercise sound judgement to maintain their own safety and strong assessment skills to maintain the safety of the client and others. Due to the intimate nature of the relationship with the client and their presence within the client's home environment, the CMHN must be culturally competent and have the ability to maintain professional boundaries. CMHNs face many issues and challenges; however, they are highly skilled, autonomous practitioners with the ability to effectively manage these situations. Furthermore, they have the flexibility and time to build therapeutic relationships with their clients, which is not always possible in the ward environment. For nurses who wish to upskill in the field of mental health, there are several postgraduate mental health courses available in Australia.

Online resources

1 Mind: https://www.mindaustralia.org.au/
2 Community Mental Health Australia: https://cmha.org.au/
3 Beyond Blue: https://www.beyondblue.org.au/
4 Embrace Multicultural Mental Health: https://embracementalhealth.org.au/
5 Flourish Australia: https://www.flourishaustralia.org.au/
6 SANE Australia: https://www.sane.org/
7 Australian Institute of Health and Welfare: https://www.aihw.gov.au/reports/mental-health-services/mental-health-services-in-australia/report-contents/community-mental-health-care-services
8 Mental Health Foundation Australia: https://www.mhfa.org.au/
9 Australian College of Mental Health Nurses: http://www.acmhn.org/
10 Helping Minds: https://helpingminds.org.au/

Note

1 The acronym CMHN, which stands for Community Mental Health Nurse, is also used as an acronym for Credentialed Mental Health Nurse. In the context of this chapter, CMHN refers to a Community Mental Health Nurse, who may or may not be credentialed with the Australian College of Mental Health Nurses.

References

Australian College of Mental Health Nurses. (2017, October 23). Applying for a mental health nurse credential. Retrieved from http://www.acmhn.org/credentialing/applying-for-credentialing

Australian Institute of Health and Welfare. (2019, October 9). Mental health services in Australia. Retrieved from https://www.aihw.gov.au/reports/mental-health-services/mental-health-services-in-australia/report-contents/community-mental-health-care-services

Cohen-Filipic, K., & Bentley, K. J. (2015). From every direction: guilt, shame, and blame among parents of adolescents with co-occurring challenges. *Child and Adolescent Social Work Journal, 32*(5), 443–454. doi:10.1007/s10560-015-0381-9

Davidson, L., Drake, R. E., Schmutte, T., Dinzeo, T., & Andres-Hyman, R. (2009). Oil and water or oil and vinegar? Evidence-based medicine meets recovery. *Community Mental Health Journal, 45*(5), 323–332. doi:10.1007/s10597-009-9228-1

Godin, P. (2003). Home alone in east London. *Mental Health Nursing, 23*(3), 12.

Heslop, B., Wynaden, D., Tohotoa, J., & Heslop, K. (2016). Mental health nurses' contributions to community mental health care: an Australian study. *International Journal of Mental Health Nursing, 25*(5), 426–433. doi:10.1111/inm.12225

Humphreys, M. S., Johnstone, E. C., MacMillan, J. F., & Taylor, P. J. (1992). Dangerous behaviour preceding first admissions for schizophrenia. *British Journal of Psychiatry, 161*(4), 501–505. doi:10.1192/bjp.161.4.501

Karanikola, M., Kaikoushi, K., Doulougeri, K., Koutrouba, A., & Papathanassoglou, E. D. E. (2018). Perceptions of professional role in community mental health nurses: the interplay of power relations between nurses and mentally ill individuals. *Archives of Psychiatric Nursing, 32*(5), 677–687. doi:https://doi.org/10.1016/j.apnu.2018.03.007

MacArthur Foundation. (2001). The MacArthur violence risk assessment study – Executive summary. Retrieved from http://www.macarthur.virginia.edu/read_me_file.html

Mortimer-Jones, S., Morrison, P., Munib, A., Paolucci, F., Neale, S., Hellewell, A., Hungerford, C. (2019). Staff and client perspectives of the Open Borders programme for people with borderline personality disorder. *International Journal of Mental Health Nursing, 28*(4), 971–979. doi:10.1111/inm.12602

Murphy, N. (2004). An investigation into how community mental health nurses assess the risk of violence from their clients. *Journal of Psychiatric and Mental Health Nursing, 11*(4), 407–413. doi:10.1111/j.1365-2850.2004.00727.x

Nordstrom, K., Berlin, J. S., Nash, S. S., Shah, S. B., Schmelzer, N. A., & Worley, L. L. M. (2019). Boarding of mentally ill patients in emergency departments: American Psychiatric Association resource document. *The Western Journal of Emergency Medicine, 20*(5), 690–695. doi:10.5811/westjem.2019.6.42422

Quinn, D. M., Williams, M. K., & Weisz, B. M. (2015). From discrimination to internalized mental illness stigma: the mediating roles of anticipated discrimination and anticipated stigma. *Psychiatric Rehabilitation Journal, 38*(2), 103–108. doi:10.1037/prj0000136

Spencer, P. C., & Munch, S. (2003). Client violence toward social workers: the role of management in community mental health programs. *Social Work, 48*(4), 532–544. doi:10.1093/sw/48.4.532

Part II: Section III: Nursing in other and cross-clinical contexts

17 Rehabilitation nursing

Julie Pryor and Murray Fisher

Chapter objectives

This chapter will provide the reader with:

- An understanding of rehabilitation as everybody's business
- An appreciation of the importance of rehabilitation in the Australian health system
- An understanding of the importance of starting rehabilitation early
- Identification of the skills nurses need to contribute to patient rehabilitation
- Key considerations for nursing in sub-acute rehabilitation
- Opportunities for nursing in relation to rehabilitation

Introduction

Rehabilitation is primarily about a person regaining control over their body and their life (Ozer, 1999). Following injury or illness, this journey can be long and require input from a diverse range of people and services to achieve the best outcomes. Health services are central to this, but for many people so are other services such as housing and community support. The following definition from the World Health Organization and World Bank (2011, p. 96) identifies rehabilitation as 'a set of measures that assist individuals who experience, or are likely to experience, disability to achieve and maintain optimal functioning in interaction with their environments.'

Internationally, the importance of rehabilitation as everybody's business is highlighted in England in their *Commissioning Guidance for Rehabilitation* (National Health Service England, 2016). This document identifies 'parks, cycle paths, outdoor gyms, swimming pools, leisure facilities, scouts/guides, play areas, smart phone apps' and 'structured peer support' as major contributors to rehabilitation (National Health Service England, 2016, p. 13). In Australia, a good example is in paediatric rehabilitation where schools as well as disability and social services are included across a child's lifespan.

An often-overlooked fact is that there are patients with rehabilitation needs in every healthcare setting. However, how well these needs are met depends on the ability of clinicians to identify those needs, to understand the importance of starting rehabilitation early and to possess the skills to do so. All health services should be rehabilitative so no matter where you work as a nurse it is essential to have rehabilitation skills in your toolkit (Pryor, 2002). For most patients, the ideal is for rehabilitation to start early (Wade, 2016a) and this may mean before the specialist rehabilitation team gets involved.

In Australia, rehabilitation is a type of specialised multidisciplinary sub-acute health service where 'the primary clinical purpose or treatment goal is improvement in the functioning of a patient with an impairment, activity limitation or participation restriction due to a health condition' (AIHW, 2013 p. 11).

> Other sub-acute care types include palliative care, geriatric evaluation and management and psychogeriatric care.

While sub-acute and non-acute (also referred to as maintenance) care account for only a small proportion of hospitalisations in Australia (5% in 2016–17), their significance is better understood in relation to patient days (14% in 2016–17) (AIHW, 2018) resulting from the longer lengths of stay associated with these care types. Rehabilitation is the most common type of sub-acute care.

Approximately 4.3 million (18%) people in Australians live with a disability (AIHW, 2019a). Dependence on others and reduced quality of life are often thought of as part of living with a disability, but this does not have to be the case. Rehabilitation can help as most rehabilitation inpatients return home (92% in 2017–18) (AIHW, 2019b), which makes rehabilitation an important part of the Australian healthcare system.

Rehabilitation is unique in its contribution to 'functioning', with 'functioning' being the third health indicator identified by the World Health Organisation (WHO) following mortality and morbidity (WHO, 2019).

> Human functioning is a process influenced by a wide range of environmental and personal factors in addition to health conditions as explained in the International Classification of Functioning, Disability and Health (WHO, 2001).

As noted by WHO (2019), 'for rehabilitation to realize its full potential by contributing to optimizing people's functioning of the population at large, it needs to be fully integrated into the health system'. For some patients, this starts with prehabilitation through pre-operative education and exercise programs.

> Prehabilitation is 'a proactive approach that enables patients to become active participants in their care' (Wynter-Blyth & Moorthy, 2017, p. 1).

The importance of active patient participation in rehabilitation cannot be overstated. For optimal rehabilitation outcomes, patients need to 'work'. This involves physical, emotional and biographical work (Pryor & Dean, 2012). Understanding this positions rehabilitation as 'a co-production between patients, their family and friends, and the treating clinicians' (Pryor, 2014, p. 3).

The context of rehabilitation

In Australia, rehabilitation as a type of sub-acute care is delivered as an inpatient service (including inreach and outreach) as well as ambulatory services (outpatients, day hospital, home-based and telerehabilitation) in public and private hospitals, with an increasing proportion provided by the private sector in recent years (AIHW, 2019a).

Private hospitals provide most of the inpatient rehabilitation for orthopaedic joint replacements, fractures or other orthopaedic conditions and for reconditioning (AROC, 2018). Public rehabilitation inpatient services provide most of the rehabilitation for spinal cord injury, acquired brain injury, stroke and multi trauma (AROC, 2018), where the length of stay is typically much longer.

Rehabilitation is provided for all age groups, but there are far more adult than paediatric rehabilitation services. Specialist inpatient and community services for adult brain injury and spinal cord injury rehabilitation are provided in all the mainland States. Stroke, another rehabilitation sub-speciality with evidence supporting the provision of specialist services and supported by national clinical guidelines (Stroke Foundation, 2019a) is less commonly catered for in stroke-specific rehabilitation services, but there is growing emphasis on starting rehabilitation early in acute stroke units (Stroke Foundation, 2019b). Rehabilitation services may be co-located with an acute hospital or stand alone; in Australia both models are used.

The rehabilitation patient is typically older, with just over 82% aged over 60 years in 2017–18 (AIHW, 2019a). While females accounted for more than half (57%) of all rehabilitation care separations in this period, there were more males than females in the age groups 0–4 years, 10–14 and 15–19 (AIHW, 2019a).

Characteristics of people needing rehabilitation can vary across the impairment groups, with people experiencing traumatic brain injury, spinal cord injury and multiple trauma being younger (mean age 55, 54.4 and 49.6 years, respectively), and more than two-thirds are male (McKechnie, Pryor, Fisher & Alexander, 2019). People who are undertaking rehabilitation for orthopaedic conditions (including fracture and replacement) or for reconditioning are generally over 70 years of age and only 30–44% are male (McKechnie et al., 2019).

Data on 16 impairment groups from sub-acute rehabilitation services are collected by AROC. This includes stroke (ischaemic and haemorrhagic), brain dysfunction (traumatic and non-traumatic), neurological conditions, spinal cord dysfunction (traumatic and non-traumatic), amputation of limb (traumatic and non-traumatic), arthritis, chronic pain, orthopaedic disorders (fractures, replacements, soft tissue injury and other), cardiac, pulmonary disorders, burns, congenital deformities, other disabling impairments, major multiple trauma, developmental disability and reconditioning/restorative.

Education is an important component of the rehabilitation process, 'learning by the patient and also often by family members of how to achieve wanted activities in the presence of altered or limited skills and abilities' (Wade, 2015, p. 1151), reinforcing that therapy is only part of rehabilitation. This is evident in the program logic model developed for rehabilitation in NSW (NSW Agency for Clinical Innovation Rehabilitation Network, 2019), where the core activities of rehabilitation service delivery are described as:

- person-centred assessment, treatment, education and care,
- coordinated goal-directed synergistic teamwork,
- therapeutic interventions promoting recovery, adaptation, compensation and prevention,
- enabling self-management, and
- providing a facilitatory environment.

Though rehabilitation is a multidisciplinary endeavour, nursing input is central to every one of the core activities listed above. This means nursing plays a significant role in the effectiveness of rehabilitation.

Key considerations for nursing in sub-acute rehabilitation

In this section we introduce and discuss three key considerations for nursing in sub-acute rehabilitation in Australia: (1) increasing complexity of rehabilitation patients, (2) meeting the diverse needs of a multi-cultural patient cohort with a multi-cultural nursing workforce and (3) inequity of access to rehabilitation.

Increasing complexity of rehabilitation patients

In English, the prefix 'sub' is associated with being inferior or less important, as in substandard or subordinate; therefore it is possible that sub-acute care is understood to be simpler or less important than acute care. However, this is not the case. The care of rehabilitation patients can be very complex and highly specialised.

This is evident in the diversity and multiplicity of clinical needs in the rehabilitation patient population. In addition to the need for 'improvement in functioning' (AIHW, 2013, p. 11), rehabilitation patients also commonly need management of the presenting health condition and various additional co-morbid conditions (Pryor & Fisher, 2016).

This comes about as a result of earlier transfer to rehabilitation as a consequence of shortening lengths of stay in acute care and the increasing prevalence of chronic health conditions in the Australian population. In 2016, compared to 2007, patients were admitted to rehabilitation after a shorter acute care length of stay (11.4 compared to 13.6 days), more dependent, older (79 compared to 73 years) and with more co-morbidities impacting on rehabilitation (49.8% compared to 42.4%) (McKechnie et al., 2019). These changes underscore the importance of nurses working in sub-acute rehabilitation services possessing acute care medical and surgical skills as well as rehabilitation-specific skills.

This means that though historically rehabilitation patients have been thought to be 'medically stable', this is no longer the case. It is not uncommon for rehabilitation inpatients to become unwell and require readmission to acute care. International studies report 8–40% of patients require return to acute care from rehabilitation (McKechnie, Pryor, McKechnie & Fisher, 2019). A recent retrospective cohort study identified that 18% of patients admitted to an Australian inpatient brain injury rehabilitation unit over a 7-year period from 2012 to 2018 inclusive were required to return to acute care due to medical deterioration or an adverse event (McKechnie, Fisher, Pryor & McKechnie, 2020).

The increasing complexity of rehabilitation patients impacts upon the care that nurses can provide and the skillset needed to provide that care. In addition to their clinical needs, this complexity relates to learning as well as social and emotional well-being needs. For example, preventing common complications such as falls and urinary tract infections are central to nursing practice in rehabilitation care; however, neither is straightforward. Preventing falls can be complex when promoting skill development and independence, especially when the person is cognitively impaired, has balance impairments or is struggling to cope with an altered functional state. Preventing urinary tract infections is a challenge following spinal cord injury when the person is

---

Box 17.1 - Case study (Vivi)

Vivi had a fall 2 weeks ago while celebrating the birth of her first great grandson. This important occasion involved every member of her extended family living in Australia and Vivi did not want to make a fuss. She waited until the next day to show her daughter the bruising on her hip. After surgery for a fractured neck of femur, Vivi remained in acute care for 10 days during which time she was mostly in bed. She did not routinely monitor her blood glucose levels and inspect her feet as she had done at home as this was conducted by the nurses. Following this she was transferred to rehabilitation for reconditioning, with a pressure injury on one heel.

Reflective questions:
1   What actions could nurses take to prevent deconditioning in acute care?
2   What health promotion opportunities were available to nurses providing care for Vivi throughout her hospitalisation?
3   What rehabilitative actions can you implement to promote Vivi's independence and self-care?

---

learning self-management in readiness for lifelong reliance on catheterisation. Nurses with a wide range of clinical and facilitating-learning skills will optimise rehabilitation patient outcomes.

Meeting the diverse needs of a multicultural patient cohort with a multicultural nursing workforce

As the Australian population becomes more diverse it is imperative for rehabilitation nurses to be able to provide culturally safe care to patients from diverse cultural backgrounds. Ethnic minority groups may experience language barriers, socio-economic and insurance difficulties, impacting on access and participation in rehabilitation. A qualitative study (Taylor & Jones, 2014) of English-speaking therapists' experiences of providing stroke rehabilitation to non-English speaking individuals found that language barriers delayed and limited the assessments and treatments.

Culture can influence the nurse–patient therapeutic relationship. This can negatively impact the patient's engagement and experience of rehabilitation. Preconceived notions about individuals based on their culture, language and appearance or cultural stereotypes hinder the development of therapeutic nurse–patient relationships. For example, the simple use of Australian lingo can be very confusing and sometimes interpreted as being offensive for people from non-Australian backgrounds and when English is not their first language. Whether it is the patient using Australian jargon to a nurse from a different cultural background or a nurse using Australian jargon to a patient from a non-Australian background, the lack of understanding may lead to misinterpretation and feelings of confusion and mistrust. Nurses need to be mindful of the language they use in patient interactions as colloquial language may lead to further misunderstanding.

Nurses need an understanding of the sociocultural context, attitudes and norms of each of their patients, including beliefs about their illness and disability, and the role of family, gender and religion in their life to optimize patient engagement with rehabilitation and rehabilitation patient outcomes (Smith-Wexler, 2014). For example, the role of the family in people's lives can be culturally different. For some cultures, it is normal for patient decision-making to be delegated to other family members whereas others may not want any family involvement in their rehabilitation.

When the nursing workforce is multicultural and the patient population is multicultural, this can be a challenge. However, the solution is simple – be truly person-centred; look beyond cultural stereotypes or differences to find out what really matters to the person who is the patient.

Inequity of access to rehabilitation

Inequity of access to rehabilitation in Australia takes several forms. According to AROC (2019), there is inequity in access to inpatient rehabilitation services for people living in remote and outer regional areas of Australia with 68% of public and 77% of private rehabilitation services in major cities and the remainder in inner regional areas. Individuals from low socio-economic areas are less likely to attend private inpatient services, with almost double the number of private rehabilitation services in high socio-economic areas than low socio-economic areas (AROC, 2019). However, the location of specialist inpatient rehabilitation services, for example, for brain injury or spinal cord injury, in major cities further disadvantages individuals living in regional, rural and remote areas as these services are in major cities.

When defining rehabilitation as a service type, there are economic constraints placed on a patient's journey with a defined start time (admission date) and an expected end date with an expected measurable patient outcome being functional gain. For most patients, the doing of rehabilitation is not confined to their inpatient rehabilitation stay, rather it begins during their acute care admission and continues in the community after inpatient rehabilitation discharge. There is a variability in access to rehabilitative services after discharge and it is somewhat dependent on health and disability funders. Within an impairment group, there is disparity in rehabilitation services that a person receives based on how a person has sustained their injury. For example, in NSW people who sustain a severe injury, such as brain injury, spinal cord injury, amputations, burns and permanent blindness resulting from a motor vehicle accident receive treatment, rehabilitation and care through icare lifetime care (icare, 2017). This means that a person with spinal cord injury sustained in a motor vehicle accident in NSW could be funded for different services than a person who sustained a similar injury following a fall at home.

While inequity such as this can be an everyday reality at the individual patient level in rehabilitation units, nurses have little control over the policies and processes that bring them about. A more far-reaching aspect of inequality of access to rehabilitation stems from the way we think about the nature of rehabilitation. The perception that rehabilitation is provided only by specialist rehabilitation services perpetuates access inequity for a far greater number of patients. Rehabilitation is everybody's business and all clinicians (especially nurses) need to possess rehabilitation skills and know when to use them. For example, nurses are ideally placed to contribute to the prevention of functional decline in hospitalised patients, with a recent review of the literature (Ley, Khaw, Duke & Botti, 2019, p. 3049) reporting that 'walking at least twice a day for approximately 20 mins in total appeared to be associated with less functional decline in older patients of variable physical capabilities, and the overall efficacy of twice-daily exercise to reduce functional decline was supported'.

Opportunities for nursing in relation to rehabilitation

Human functioning as the third health indicator following mortality and morbidity (WHO, 2019) recognises the importance of scaling up rehabilitation services internationally (WHO, 2017) and the development of rehabilitation as a speciality sub-acute type of healthcare in Australia creates many opportunities for nursing. These relate to the positioning of rehabilitation within nursing as a whole and the role of nursing within sub-acute rehabilitation services.

Rehabilitation in nursing

In this chapter you have been encouraged to think about rehabilitation as everybody's business, and the need for nurses to possess and use rehabilitation skills across healthcare settings and diagnostic groups regardless of patient age has been stressed. This thinking is in line with the Australasian Rehabilitation Nurses' Association, which promotes rehabilitation as a philosophy of practice for all nurses regardless of their practice context as follows:

> Rehabilitation is a process, the outcome of which is maximised when rehabilitative nursing care is provided throughout the entire episode of health care or illness trajectory regardless of the diagnosis, prognosis, age or setting. Therefore, all nurses should be adequately prepared to deliver nursing care that is rehabilitative. (Australasian Rehabilitation Nurses' Association, 2002)

Pryor (2002) refers to this as using a rehabilitative approach, a philosophy of care which facilitates rehabilitation through the development of therapeutic interpersonal relationships. It relies on the nurse using a repertoire of interpersonal skills and rehabilitative techniques to assess the patient, taking into consideration their context at that point in time and their goals, and to approach every patient interaction as a potential rehabilitative moment. Though it is argued that the rehabilitative approach should be part of every nurse's practice regardless of their practice contexts, this does not mean the demise of the speciality practice of rehabilitation nursing. It simply means that nurses would be better positioned to meet a wider range of their patients' needs if they understood rehabilitation as a philosophy of care and used this thinking to inform the development of skills that meet their patients' rehabilitation needs. The knowledge and skill base for the speciality practice of rehabilitation nursing builds upon this generic foundation.

Nursing in sub-acute rehabilitation

In the recently conceptualised program logic for rehabilitation in NSW (NSW Agency for Clinical Innovation Rehabilitation Network, 2019), the five core influencing activities listed earlier in the chapter were identified as the key contributors to rehabilitation patient outcomes. For three of these, nursing is well positioned to take a leadership role within the rehabilitation sector: coordinated goal-directed synergistic teamwork, enabling self-management and providing a facilitatory environment.

Rehabilitation teams commonly comprise a wide range of clinical disciplines working closely with the patient. Increasing patient complexity adds another dimension to this with the creation of meta-teams including some members from outside the sub-acute rehabilitation service within health and beyond (Wade, 2016b). As the only discipline with a twenty-four seven presence in sub-acute rehabilitation services across Australia, nursing has a responsibility to oversee and coordinate each patient's rehabilitation and the input of all team members.

Related to this is the challenge of accurately measuring each patient's activity as a genuine and valuable contribution to their own rehabilitation. This is vital as it positions the person who is the patient as a crucial member of their rehabilitation team. Technologies in the form of step counters are useful here.

Regarding enabling self-management, there is a pressing need for measures that demonstrate the value of nursing in rehabilitation services beyond the management of acute and chronic health conditions and complications, as these are aspects of nursing across all settings. Nursing could be a key mechanism for increasing the intensity of rehabilitation which is advocated in recent studies (for example, Scrivener, et al., 2019). This begins with nurses understanding that every interaction with a patient could be a 'rehab moment', an opportunity to address a patient's learning needs and to coach patients to self-care (Australasian Rehabilitation Nurses' Association, 2003; Pryor, 2009).

Interventions focused on enabling self-management are enhanced when the physical, social and attitudinal environment is purposefully and intentionally manipulated to facilitate patient rehabilitation (NSW Agency for Clinical Innovation Rehabilitation Network, 2019). This is an area long-overdue for further development.

Conclusion

This chapter explored a range of issues about the role of nurses in relation to rehabilitation. People requiring specialist rehabilitation services have complex care needs stemming from a range of impairment types as well as their co-morbid health conditions. Nurses are required to have specialist knowledge and clinical skills in addition to interpersonal skills to support and facilitate patients to undertake rehabilitation. Nurses are uniquely positioned to be at the forefront to help prevent functional decline across healthcare settings and to facilitate independence as key contributors to assessment and management of care in rehabilitation services.

Online resources

1 Australasian Rehabilitation Nurses' Association (ARNA): https://www.arna. com.au/
2 Association of Rehabilitation Nurses (ARN): https://rehabnurse.org/
3 NSW Agency for Clinical Innovation (ACI) Rehabilitation Network Principles to Support Rehabilitation Care: https://www.aci.health.nsw.gov.au/__data/assets/pdf_file/0014/500900/rehabilitation-principles.pdf
4 Stroke Foundation Clinical Guidelines for Stroke Management: https://informme.org.au/en/Guidelines/Clinical-Guidelines-for-Stroke-Management

References

Australasian Rehabilitation Nurses' Association. (2002). *Position Statement: Rehabilitation nursing – scope of practice* (2nd Ed.). https://www.arna.com.au/ARNA/Publications/Position_Statements/ARNA/Publications/Position_Statements.aspx?hkey=3db477cc-cbb9-423f-bf5d-4523c08b83c4

Australasian Rehabilitation Nurses' Association. (2003). Rehabilitation nursing competency standards for registered nurses. Melbourne: Australasian Rehabilitation Nurses' Association.

Australasian Rehabilitation Outcomes Centre. (2018). *Length of stay and functional independence measure change benchmarks of completed episodes in Australia, calendar year 2018.* https://ahsri.uow.edu.au/content/groups/public/@web/@chsd/documents/doc/uow256895.pdf

Australasian Rehabilitation Outcomes Centre. (2019). *Equity of access to inpatient Rehabilitation Services in Australia.* AROC Information Series, No. 1 AU. Wollongong, NSW: Australasian Rehabilitation Outcomes Centre.

Australasian Rehabilitation Outcomes Centre. (2018). *LOS and FIM change benchmarks of completed episodes in Australia. Calendar year benchmarks (2018) – Australia.* Wollongong, NSW: Australasian Rehabilitation Outcomes Centre.

Australian Institute of Health and Welfare (AIHW). (2013). *Development of nationally consistent sub-acute and non-acute admitted patient care data definitions and guidelines.* Cat. No. HSE 135. Canberra: AIHW. https://www.aihw.gov.au/getmedia/01d815ba-3d66-48c9-a9ec-aaa5825c19f2/15425.pdf.aspx?inline=true

Australian Institute of Health and Welfare (AIHW). (2018). Australia's hospitals 2016 17 at a glance. Health services series no. 85. Cat. No. HSE 204. Canberra: AIHW. https://www.aihw.gov.au/getmedia/d5f4d211-ace3-48b9-9860-c4489ddf2c35/aihw-hse-204.pdf.aspx?inline=true

Australian Institute of Health and Welfare (AIHW). (2019a). *People with disability in Australia 2019: in brief.* Cat. No. DIS 74. Canberra: AIHW.

Australian Institute of Health and Welfare (AIHW). (2019b). *Admitted patient care 2017–18: Australian hospital statistics.* Health services series no. 90. Cat. No. HSE 225. Canberra: AIHW. https://www.aihw.gov.au/getmedia/df0abd15-5dd8-4a56-94fa-c9ab68690e18/aihw-hse-225.pdf.aspx?inline=true

icare. (2017). What is reasonable and necessary treatment, rehabilitation and care. https://www.icare.nsw.gov.au/injured-or-ill-people/motor-accident-injuries/who-we-care-for/#gref

Ley, l., Khaw, D., Duke, M., & Botti, M. (2019). The dose of physical activity to minimise functional decline in older general medical patients receiving 24-hr acute care: a systematic scoping review. *Journal of Clinical Nursing, 28*(17–18), 3049–3064.

McKechnie, D., Pryor, J., Fisher, M., & Alexander, T. (2019). Examination of the dependency and complexity of patients admitted to in-patient rehabilitation in Australia. *Australian Health Review.* https://doi.org/10.1071/AH18073

McKechnie, D., Pryor, J., McKechnie, R., & Fisher, M. (2019). Predictors of readmission to acute care from inpatient rehabilitation: a systematic review. *PM&R, 11*(12), 1335–1345. https://dx.doi.org/10.1002/pmrj.12179

McKechnie, D., Fisher, M. J., Pryor, J., & McKechnie, R. (2020). Predictors of unplanned readmission to acute care from inpatient brain injury rehabilitation. *Journal of Clinical Nursing, 29*, 593–601. doi: org/10.1111/jocn.15118

National Health Service England. (2016). Commissioning guidance for rehabilitation. https://www.england.nhs.uk/wp-content/uploads/2016/04/rehabilitation-comms-guid-16-17.pdf

New South Wales Agency for Clinical Innovation Rehabilitation Network. (2019). *Principles to support rehabilitation care.* Chatswood, NSW: New South Wales Agency for Clinical Innovation. https://www.aci.health.nsw.gov.au/__data/assets/pdf_file/0014/500900/rehabilitation-principles.pdf

Ozer, M. N. (1999). Patient participation in the management of stroke rehabilitation. *Topics in Stroke Rehabilitation, 6*(1):43–59.

Pryor, J. (2002). Rehabilitative nursing – a core nursing function across all settings. *Collegian*, *9*(2), 10–15.

Pryor, J. (2009). Coaching patients to self-care: a primary responsibility of nursing. *International Journal of Older People Nursing*, *4*, 79–88.

Pryor, J. (2014). Editorial. The principles of rehabilitation. *Journal of the Australasian Rehabilitation Nurses' Association*, *17*(1), 2–3.

Pryor, J., & Dean, S. (2012). The person in context. In S. Dean, R. Seigert, W. Taylor (eds). *Interprofessional rehabilitation: a person centred approach.* (pp. 135–165). Chichester, West Sussex: Wiley-Blackwell.

Pryor, J., & Fisher, M. (2016). Nursing management of illness, injury and complications in rehabilitation. *Journal of the Australasian Rehabilitation Nurses' Association*, *19*(3), 19–30.

Scrivener, K., Pocivi, N., Jones, T., Dean, B., Gallagher, S., Henrisson, W., Dean, C. (2019). Observation of activity levels in a purpose-built, inpatient, rehabilitation facility. *Health Environments Research & Design Journal*, *12*(4), 26–38

Smith-Wexler, L. (2014). Cultural competency in TBI rehabilitation: working together with the ethnic minority population with TBI. *Spotlight on Disability Newsletter*, *6*(2). https://www.apa.org/pi/disability/resources/publications/newsletter/2014/12/rehabilitation

Stroke Foundation. (2019a). Clinical Guidelines for Stroke Management. https://informme.org.au/en/Guidelines/Clinical-Guidelines-for-Stroke-Management

Stroke Foundation. (2019b). National stroke audit: acute services report 2019. https://informme.org.au/stroke-data/Acute-audits

Taylor, E., & Jones, F. (2014). Lost in translation: exploring therapists' experiences of providing stroke rehabilitation across a language barrier. *Disability and Rehabilitation*, *36*(25), 2127–2135.

Wade, D., (2015). Rehabilitation – a new approach. Part Two: the underlying theories. *Clinical Rehabilitation*, *29*(12), 1045–1054.

Wade, D., (2016a). Rehabilitation – a new approach. Part Four: a new paradigm, and its implications. *Clinical Rehabilitation*, *30*(2), 109–118.

Wade, D., (2016b). Rehabilitation – a new approach. Part Three: the implications of the theories. *Clinical Rehabilitation*, *30*(1), 3–10.

World Health Organization. (2001). *International classification of functioning, disability and health.* Geneva: World Health Organization.

World Health Organization. (2017). *Rehabilitation 2030: a call for action. Rehabilitation: key for health in the 21st century.* https://www.who.int/disabilities/care/KeyForHealth21stCentury.pdf

World Health Organization. (2019). *Rehabilitation 2030. Health policy and systems research agenda for rehabilitation 10 and 11 July 2019.* (https://www.who.int/rehabilitation/Global-HSPR-Rehabilitation-Concept-Note.pdf

World Health Organization & World Bank. (2011). *World Report on Disability.* WHO Press, Geneva, Switzerland. https://www.who.int/disabilities/world_report/2011/report.pdf?ua=1

Wynter-Blyth, V., & Moorthy, K. (2017). Prehabilitation: preparing patients for surgery. *British Medical Journal*, *358*, j3702.

18 Nursing in aged care contexts

*Sarah Yeun-Sim Jeong, Sharyn Hunter
and Larissa McIntyre*

Chapter objectives

This chapter will offer the reader:

* An insight into the history and current contexts of nursing older people
* An outline of the key health issues facing older people
* A description of contemporary contexts where the nursing of older people occurs
* An opportunity to build a knowledge base and develop nursing skills specific to older people
* An overview of future challenges to nursing and nurses who practice in this area

Introduction

Australians have one of the longest life expectancies in the world. A 65-year-old man and woman in 2014–16 are expected to live another 20 years and 22 years, respectively. In 2016, 15% of Australians (3.8 million) were aged 65 and over, and this number is expected to grow 22% of population (9 million) by 2057 (AIHW, 2018a).

This ageing of the Australian population presents both challenges and opportunity. It requires a reorientation of our society towards meeting the needs of older people including the provision of appropriate healthcare services. Nurses, who provide care to older Australians, must understand the policy shifts, funding systems and the implications of these to be able to deliver quality care that is evidence-based and consistent with the regulatory requirements of the Australian Government.

This chapter provides an overview of the changing health issues that older Australians face and the necessary health services to meet their needs. The chapter also offer insights on where and how nurses can promote better health for older Australians.

Historical and current contexts of nursing older people

In the 19th century, universal healthcare did not exist and access to healthcare was limited for many older Australians. The common causes of death have shifted from infectious diseases impacting the very young and the very old in the first half of the century (ABS, 2001) to degenerative diseases among older age groups in the latter half of the century (AIHW, 2018b). During the 20th century, the health and welfare of older Australians has continued to improve greatly, nevertheless many older Australians still need to access supports as they age. There are two major components of the

Australian Aged Care System with quality care at the core: long-term residential care and home or community-based care with respite care available within both.

The Australian aged care sector is regulated by the Aged Care Act 1997. The majority of funding for health and aged care services comes from the Federal Government with State, Territory and local governments, insurers and individual Australians provide additional resources. Despite some government subsidises, it is a user-pays system and users are expected to contribute and are charged fees and payments by service providers based on their assets for the provision of services (My Aged Care, 2019).

Key issues related to older people

Cultural diversity

Of the total number of Australians who were aged 65 years and over in 2016, over one-third (37%) were born overseas, the majority in non-English speaking countries (AIHW, 2018a). There are a number of barriers for older Australians with Culturally and Linguistically Diverse (CALD) background to accessing health and aged care services due to socio-economic disadvantage related to language and other cultural barriers, risk of unemployment, and inadequate provision of culturally sensitive services and coordinated support (Principe, 2015).

In 2016, Aboriginal Torres Strait Islander people made up 3% of the total Australian population. At that time, 17% (108,000) of Aboriginal Torres Strait Islander people were aged 50 years and over, and 5% (31,000) were aged 65 years and over and less than 1% were aged 85 years and over. Given that ageing-related conditions affect Aboriginal Torres Strait Islander people at a younger age than non-indigenous Australians, care needs increase for Aboriginal and Torres Strait Islander people who are aged 50 years and over (AIHW, 2018a).

Chronic conditions

In general, chronic disease contributes to more than 70% of the disease burden in Australia (NSW Health, 2013; AIHW, 2018a). The burden of chronic disease is increased with the ageing population with 87% of older Australians living with at least one chronic condition such as cancer, cardiovascular disease and diabetes (AIHW, 2019). Dementia and Alzheimer disease affected 328,000 Australians (9% of 3.8 million people aged 65 and over in 2016) and this number is expected to double by the year 2046 to around 833,000. It is anticipated that the demand that dementia places on health and aged care services will increase in the future (Dementia Australia, 2014; AIHW, 2012). The prevalence and impact of chronic diseases overshadow healthy behaviours that older Australians engage in to maintain physical and mental health. For example, older Australians have lower rates of smoking (AIHW, 2017) and consume more fruits and vegetables than younger cohorts (ABS, 2015) consume.

Key considerations in the delivery of care

Family/informal carers

As they age, many of the needs of Australians aged 65 years and over will be met by informal carers (e.g. family members, friends, neighbours) (ABS, 2016). In 2015, 94%

Box 18.1 - Case study (Lorna)

Lorna was a 61-year-old woman who identified as Aboriginal Torres Strait Islander with end stage renal failure (ESRF) living in a residential aged care (RAC) facility. Lorna was a loner with few external supports. She had no children, and her closest friend lived locally but was without transport and could not afford the taxi charges to visit.

Lorna was undergoing haemodialysis thrice weekly. Other co-morbidities were Parkinson's disease, insulin dependent diabetes mellitus (IDDM), ischemic heart disease (IHD), peripheral vascular disease (PVD) and hypertension (HT).

Lorna made a decision to withdraw from haemodialysis knowing well of the consequences.

Reflective questions:

1　What social determinants of health had impacted upon Lorna during her lifetime?
2　Do you believe it is important to understand someone's cultural identity? Why?

---

older Australians reported that they had someone outside the household who could support them in a time of crisis (ABS, 2016). Informal carers, often the spouse or a female family member, play an essential role throughout the life stage and especially at the later stages of a person's life. Although caregiving can increase family togetherness and satisfaction, it is common that carers experience considerable adverse physical, psychological and financial consequences (Van't Leven et al., 2013).

Social and mental wellbeing, and gerotranscendence

In the world of abundant materials and technologies, old age is often portrayed as a time of dependency and burden. However, older Australians promote and maintain their social and mental wellbeing by engaging in continued learning with around 13% of people aged 65 years and over engaged in employment, education or training in 2016 (AIHW, 2018a). They also actively participate in regular social engagement through community groups, sports, societies and volunteering. In 2016, around 20% of Australians aged 65 and over volunteered their time within the previous 12 months, providing time, service or skills through an organisation or group (AIHW, 2018a).

Older people in the last phase of life turn inwards and reflect on their entire life as a way to reach peace as well as enjoying small things and viewing oneself in the perspective of contribution made to the future. This phenomenon is known as 'gerotranscendence' (Tornstam, 1997; 2011)

The experience of older people with gerotranscendence was reported in various countries including Sweden, Australia and Korea (Jeong, McMillan, & Higgins (2012); Wadensten, 2010; Yoon, 2012). These studies found that older adults undergoing gerotranscendence enjoy low levels of stress and high satisfaction with life despite their reduced physical, mental, financial and social capacity.

Advance care planning (ACP) is a process that involves thinking, in advance, about what medical care one would like should one be unable to make or communicate decisions about their own care or treatment. An Advance Care Directive (ACD) is a written statement by those who can make medical decisions for themselves for the time when one is unable to make decisions (NSW Health, 2017).

End-of-life care and Advance Care Planning

An ACD is an important outcome of ACP and can only be made by an adult with decision-making capacity whilst an Advance Care Plan can be written by the person or on the person's behalf. Another important outcome of ACP includes an appointment of substitute decision-maker who would make medical decisions on behalf of the individuals. ACDs should include what is important to the person such as values, life goals and preferred outcomes (NSW Health, 2017). It is ideal if ACP happens earlier in life, when the person is still well and capable of making decisions. The benefits of ACP are well documented; ACP improves the quality of end-of-life (EOL) care, patient and family satisfaction, increased sense of control, and reduces stress, anxiety and depression in surviving relatives (Jeong, Higgins & McMillan, 2011; 2012).

Despite this, uptake of ACP and documentation of ACDs have been low in Australia (Jeong et al., 2015). Nurses are in the best position to help older people with ACP and should increase their knowledge and confidence in ACP and EOL care. It is important for nurses to initiate and support patients and family caregivers to engage in conversations about future healthcare preferences (Jeong et al., 2015).

Box 18.2 - Case study (Bill)

Bill is a 69 year old, white man with a history of Cirrhosis of the liver, previous IV drug use (maintenance dose Methadone), Type 2 diabetes mellitus, ischaemic heart disease, COPD, peripheral neuropathy, anxiety, and depression.

Bill was transferred to residential aged care home for palliative care due to complications during gluteal operative washout which included, intraoperative large bleed and ICU admission, and a stage 3 pressure injury sacrum and R heel.

Advance Care Directives were completed with Bill, his sister, the GP and a RN.

Reflective questions:

1 What role do you think Bill's previous IV drug use might have played in his illness and care?
2 What factors should be considered when discussing Bill's ACD?
3 What role can the registered nurse (RN) play in the conversation?

Australian practice contexts

Although family and other informal carers play an important role in caring for older people, 80% of people aged 65 and over access some form of government-funded aged care service before death (AIHW, 2015). These include services provided by general practitioners (GPs), specialists, nurse practitioners (NPs), and allied health professionals in hospitals and clinics in the form of respite and support services, transition services and community/home-based and RAC (AIHW, 2018b). However, it is nursing staff who are responsible and accountable for an accurate assessment of care needs and the delivery of care to older Australians in a cost-effective way in various settings.

Practice nurses in general practice

In 2016–17, 29% of the total 130 million claims for un-referred general practice was made by people aged 65 and over (Department of Human Services, 2018). Nurses are key members of multidisciplinary primary healthcare teams in general practice. Their roles vary, but can include organising and coordinating clinical care, promoting patient, family, carer and community wellbeing, and liaising with others to promote continuity of care (ACN, 2015). For example, practice nurses play an integral role in an Australian Government initiative of the '75+ Health Assessment'. Practice nurses conduct a holistic and comprehensive health assessment of people aged 75 years and over, then design interventions to improve the health of the older person who has been assessed (APNA, 2017).

Nurses in hospitals

Older people accounted for 42% of the same-day hospitalisations, 41% overnight hospitalisations and 20% of emergency department presentations in 2016–17 (AIHW, 2018b). These statistics demonstrate that the main client group of hospital services are people aged 65 and over, and nurses are the key healthcare professionals in this context. A comprehensive understanding of older peoples' needs is increasingly being recognised as the critical and special knowledge required by nurses in acute hospital settings. Nurses in acute hospital settings will need to develop expertise in the care of older people with complex and multiple chronic conditions. Working in a multidisciplinary team with older people and their families provide nurses with an exciting opportunity to practise holistic and person-centred care and initiate innovative care that is integrated and coordinated.

Nurses in home and community care

Government-funded home and community care services support older people to live independently in their own homes. The Commonwealth Home Support Program provides basic maintenance and support services (e.g. centre-based day care, domestic assistance and social support) to people in the community whose independence is at risk. In 2016–17, more than 720,000 people aged 65 years and over received home support services (Department of Health, 2017).

The Home Care Package (HCP) Programme aims to assist older people with more complex needs to continue living at home (Department of Health, 2017). In 2017, the Australian Government introduced the consumer directed care (CDC) service model for the HCP Programme. Under this model, older people (>65 years of age) manage their allocated budget and decide what services they wish to purchase and who will deliver these (e.g. showering, cleaning, nursing and allied health-care) (Department of Social Services, 2015). Nurses, as care coordinators in HCP Programmes, provide needs assessments, goal setting and care planning, information about what funding is available and how funds can be spent, and conduct monitoring and reassessment to ensure that the package continues to be appropriate for consumers (Department of Social Services, 2019). CDC is currently only available for HCPs; however, the Government has plans to introduce CDC into RAC in the future (Aged Care Guide, 2019).

Nurses in residential aged care

There were more than 200,000 older adults living in 2,700 RAC homes across Australia in 2016–17 (AIHW, 2018a). This equates to about 6% of people aged 65 and older, and represents one of society's most vulnerable and dependent populations. The capacity of the RAC sector has been gradually expanding reflecting the ageing population who are living longer with chronic diseases.

Nurses are responsible and accountable for an accurate reflection of nursing care needs and the delivery of care to residents in a cost-effective way. When an older person is admitted to a RAC, it is the responsibility of nurses to assess residents for funding purposes and classify them according to the Aged Care Funding Instrument (ACFI). The ACFI is the primary funding tool for RAC. It assesses people across three domains: activities of daily living, behaviours and complex care. It is this funding that is calculated for each resident, which is used to provide care and services in RAC. These assessments are then reviewed randomly by Department of Health Validators to ensure the claims are accurate (Department of Health, 2018).

Aged Care Quality and Safety Commission

The Aged Care Quality and Safety Commission (ACQSC) oversees compliance with care standards and management of complaints across all federally funded aged care services including RAC, home care, and National Aboriginal and Torres Strait Islander Flexible Aged Care Program (NATSIFACP). Accreditation cycles are for three years with at least two visits per year to a RAC by the ACQSC, and at least once every two years for NATSIFACP providers (Department of Health, 2019).

The new Aged Care Quality Standards (Quality Standards) were introduced into all federally funded programs on 1 July 2019. This means that all services are measured against the same standards. In particular, RAC services must comply with the Aged Care Quality Standards (Aged Care Quality Commission, 2019) to be eligible to receive Australian Government subsidy for their care recipients (Department of Health, 2019). Nurses who work in this sector are responsible for the delivery of care in accordance with these standards.

Challenges facing nurses and nursing profession

Frequently, members of the public fail to understand the indispensable role of nurses in aged care until a relative or significant others require care. Nurses make a difference in the lives of older people every day but are often overlooked by policy makers and not recognised as vital components of our healthcare system. Nurses in aged care are also undervalued within the nursing profession and society, particularly when the media focus heavily on negative portrayals of aged care, ignoring more positive stories. The belief also exists that the care older people require does not need to be delivered by qualified nurses. This is reflected in the fact that the bulk of care provided by Australia's 366,000 aged care workers continues to be delivered by Unregulated Health Care Workers with limited training (ACN, 2019; Mavromaras et al., 2017). These workers represent 75% of the aged care workforce in primary, acute and RAC settings and are supervised by a small number (15%) of RNs. Future regulation of the untrained aged care workforce is of particular importance (ACN, 2019; Mavromaras et al., 2017), and the important roles and functions of nurses in aged care services need to be recognised.

International evidence demonstrates the positive relationship between the number of RNs and quality of care (Dellefield, Castle, McGilton, & Spilsbury, 2014). However, 63% of 2,240 aged care services in Australia reported a shortage of RNs (41%) and main reason for skill shortages were lack of suitable applicants (80%), slow recruitment processes (21%) and specialist knowledge required (19%) (Mavromaras et al., 2017). These issues draw attention to educational and structural issues influencing the availability and capacity of RNs to deliver informed, responsive, expert and compassionate healthcare to older Australians. The absence of a coordinated effort to develop the next generation of Australian gerontological nurse leaders in practice, education and research warrants critical discussion and strategic planning. For the preparation of nurses for future, nursing care for older people and associated aspects of care (e.g., psychogeriatrics, palliative care) need to be specialised as gerontological nursing and to be embedded in undergraduate university education.

Advanced training and specialisation at Masters and PhD level in gerontological nursing is required to provide visionary leadership in the quest to ensure nursing excellence for older people. Gerontological Nurse Practitioners (GNPs) have played significant roles in the care of older people in various settings in the USA since the 1970's (Small 1994). Gerontological nursing in Australia has been slow to adopt the GNP role, although NPs have practised in Australia for over 15 years. This innovative role is expected to improve access to primary health services for older people and reduce unplanned hospitalisations, provide cost-effective and timely care to all but especially at-risk populations through various care contexts including outreach services in rural and remote communities. GNPs work in collaboration with other health professionals to assess older patients and establish and implement care plans. They conduct comprehensive geriatric assessments within the NP scope of practice, order and interpret diagnostic tests and treat a variety of conditions. GNPs may also undertake medication reviews and provide case coordination for older patients with complex needs. It is necessary to adopt new models of care that will allow system-wide gerontology trained nurse clinical leadership by GNPs with adequate Pharmaceutical Benefits Scheme and Medical Benefits Schedule items (ACN, 2015).

Box 18.3 - Community Nurse study

I work as a RN in a Community Health Service. My work as a community nurse involves conducting a comprehensive assessment to identify an older person's care needs and goals, and ensuring the care they need are met at home. I develop care plans with the older person and families, and coordinate care which may require consultations with GPs and other allied healthcare professionals such as Physiotherapist and Occupational therapist. I also provide clinical care such as wound care (simple and complex) and medications. What is the most rewarding when caring for older people at home is that I feel privileged to be welcome at their own home and to develop special therapeutic relationship with the older person and families. While I provide care, I am greatly appreciated by them and the conversations I have with them make me feel that I am very important and special.

Reflective questions:
1 How does the role of a nurse in a community health service differ from a nurse working in a surgical unit in a hospital?
2 What aspects of communication would differ between a nurse and an older person in their own home compared to an acute care situation?

Conclusion

Negative images of nursing older people overshadow and undermine the invaluable contribution that nurses make in aged care services. It is by no means easy to fully unpack the interlinked and complicated nature of all the issues related to delivering safe and quality care to our vulnerable older population. Nursing older people provides nurses with an opportunity to master the care of people with chronic and degenerative diseases, to build a speciality pathway in gerontological nursing, dementia care or palliative care, and to work in a speciality that truly understands person-centred and holistic care for older people while developing key relationships with the people you are providing care for, their families and friends.

As nurses we are privileged to be part of an older person's life journey and to recognise the significant skills and knowledge it takes to work with older people in various healthcare settings. It is a speciality that by its nature must be innovative and one of change – ask yourself 'is this a speciality you would like to be part of?'

Online resources

1 AIHW :https://www.aihw.gov.au
2 GEN aged care data: https://www.gen-agedcaredata.gov.au/
3 My Aged Care https://www.myagedcare.gov.au/assessment/prepare-your-assessment
4 Australian College of Nursing (ACN) Policy Chapter (Ageing) https://www.acn.edu.au/policy/policy-chapters

References

Aged Care Act 1997 (Cth) Act No. 87 of 1997 (Austl.). https://www.legislation.gov.au/Details/C2013C00389

Aged Care Guide (2019). Consumer Directed Care: Flexibility and choice in the direction of your future. Retrieved from https://www.agedcareguide.com.au/information/consumer-directed-care

Aged Care Quality Commission. (2019). Aged Care Quality Standards: Introduction. Retrieved from https://www.agedcarequality.gov.au/standards/guidance-introduction

Australian Bureau of Statistics (ABS). (2001). Australian Social Trends. Retrieved from https://www.abs.gov.au/AUSSTATS/abs@.nsf/allprimarymainfeatures/2B10DB7CF54F4A76CA25709F0025EF97?opendocument

Australian Bureau of Statistics (ABS). (2015). *National Health Survey: first results, 2014–15.* ABS cat. no. 4364.0. Canberra: ABS.

Australian Bureau of Statistics (ABS). (2016). *Survey of disability, ageing and carers: summary of findings, Australia, 2015.* ABS cat. No. 4430.0. Canberra: ABS.

Australian College of Nursing (ACN) (2015). *Nursing in general practice: a guide for the general practice team.* Canberra: Australian College of Nursing.

Australian College of Nursing (ACN). (2019). *Regulation of the unregulated health care workforce across the health care system – a White Paper by ACN 2019.* Canberra: ACN.

Australian Institute of Health and Welfare (AIHW) (2012). *Dementia in Australia.* Cat. No. AGE 70. Canberra: AIHW.

Australian Institute of Health and Welfare (AIHW) (2015). *Use of aged care services before death.* Data linkage series no. 19. Cat. No. CSI 21. Canberra: AIHW.

Australian Institute of Health and Welfare (AIHW) (2017). *National Drug Strategy Household Survey 2016: detailed findings.* Cat. No. PHE 214. Canberra: AIHW.

Australian Institute of Health and Welfare (AIHW) (2018a). *Older Australia at a glance.* Cat. No. AGE 87. Canberra: AIHW. Retrieved from https://www.aihw.gov.au/reports/older-people/older-australia-at-a-glance/contents/summary

Australian Institute of Health and Welfare (AIHW) (2018b). *GEN fact sheet 2016–17: Services and places in aged care.* Canberra: AIHW.

Australian Institute of Health and Welfare (AIHW) (2019). Chronic disease. Retrieved from https://www.aihw.gov.au/reports-data/health-conditions-disability-deaths/chronic-disease/overview

Australian Primary Health Care Nurses Association (APNA). (2017). *Improving patient outcomes: primary health care nurses working to the breadth of their scope of practice- Position statement.* Melbourne: APNA.

Dellefield, M. E., Castle, N. G., McGilton, K. S., & Spilsbury, K. (2015). The relationship between registered nurses and nursing home quality: an integrative review (2008-2014). *Nursing Economics, 33*(2), 95–108, 116.

Dementia Australia. (2014). What is it like to live with dementia? Retrieved from https://www.dementia.org.au/wa/about-us/news-and-media/media-releases/2014/what-is-it-like-to-live-with-dementia

Department of Health. (2017). *2016–17 Report on the Operation of the Aged Care Act 1997.* Canberra: DoH.

Department of Health. (2018). Basic subsidy amount (Aged Care Funding Instrument). Retrieved from https://agedcare.health.gov.au/aged-care-funding/residential-care-subsidy/basic-subsidy-amount-aged-care-funding-instrument

Department of Health. (2019). Current quality assessment arrangement including unannounced accreditation audits. Retrieved from https://agedcare.health.gov.au/quality/current-quality-assessment-arrangements-including-unannounced-re-accreditation-audits

Department of Health and Ageing. (2012). *Consumer Directed Care (CDC) in Australian Government packaged care programs 2010–2011.* Canberra: DOHA

Department of Human Services. (2018). Medicare Australia statistics, MBS Group by patient demographics reports. Canberra: DHS. Viewed 05 February 2018.

Department of Social Services. (2015). Home Support Programme. Commonwealth Home Support Programme (CHSP) Guidelines Overview. Canberra: Australian Government DOSS. Retrieved from https://www.dss.gov.au/sites/default/files/documents/06_2015/chsp_programme_guidelines_-_accessible_version_29_june_5pm.pdf

Department of Social Services. (2019). What is consumer directed care? Retrieved from https://agedcare.health.gov.au/sites/g/files/net1426/f/documents/04_2015/what_is_consumer_directed_care_0_0.pdf

Health Workforce Australia (HWA). (2014). Nursing Workforce Sustainability, Improving Nurse Retention and Productivity. Retrieved from https://www.health.gov.au/internet/main/publishing.nsf/Content/29418BA17E67ABC0CA257D9B00757D08/$File/Nursing%20Workforce%20Sustainability%20-%20Improving%20Nurse%20Retention%20and%20Productivity%20report.pdf

Jeong, S., Higgins, I., & McMillan, M. (2011). Experiences with advance care planning: older people and family members' perspective. *International Journal of Older People Nursing, 6,* 176–186. doi:10.1111/j.1748-3743.2009.00201.x

Jeong, Y. S., McMillan, M. A., & Higgins, I. J. (2012). Gerotranscendence: the phenomenon of advance care planning. *Journal of Religion and Spiritual Aging, 24*(1–2), 146–163.

Jeong, S., Ohr, S., Pich, J., Saul, P., & Ho, A. (2015). 'Planning ahead' among community-dwelling older people from culturally and linguistically diverse background: a cross-sectional survey. *Journal of Clinical Nursing, 24*(1–2), 244–255. doi:10.1111/jocn.12649

Mavromaras, K. Knight G, Isherwood L, Crettenden A, Flavel J, Karmel T, Moskos M, Smith L, Walton H & Wei Z. (2017). 2016 National Aged Care Workforce Census and Survey – the aged care workforce, 2016. Department of Health. Publication number 11848. Retrieved from https://agedcare.health.gov.au/sites/g/files/net1426/.../nacwcs_final_report_290317.pdf

My Aged Care (2019). Understanding costs. Retrieved from https://www.myagedcare.gov.au/understanding-costs

New South Wales Health. (2013). NSW chronic disease management program – connecting care in the community: Service model 2013. Retrieved from https://www.aci.health.nsw.gov.au/__data/assets/pdf_file/0016/201832/ACI13-011-CDMP-services-web.pdf

New South Wales Health. (2017). Making an Advance Care Directive. Retrieved from https://www.health.nsw.gov.au/patients/acp/Publications/acd-form-info-book.pdf

Phillips, J., Parker, D., & Woods, M. (2018). We've had 20 aged care reviews in 20 years – will the Royal Commission be any different? *The Conversation,* 20 September 2018 Retrieved from https://theconversation.com/weve-had-20-aged-care-reviews-in-20-years-will-the-royal-commission-be-any-different-103347

Principe, I (2015). Issues in Health Care in South Australia for people from culturally and linguistically diverse backgrounds: a scoping study for the Health Performance Council. file:///C:/Users/sarah/Sarah%20OneDrive%20Business/OneDrive%20for%20Business/Sarah%202017/Aged%20Care/SA%202015%20CALD%20scoping%20study%20final.pdf

Small, N. (1994). The role of gerontological nurse practitioner in nursing homes. *Nursing Homes, 43*(4), 48–50.

Tornstam, L. (1997). Gerotranscendence in a broad cross-sectional perspective. *Journal of Ageing and Identity, 2*(1), 17–36.

Tornstam, L. (2011). Maturing into gerotranscendence. *The Journal of Transpersonal Psychology, 43*(2), 166–180.

Van't Leven, N., Prick, A. E., Groenewoud, J. G., Roelofs, P. D., de Lange, J., & Pot, A. M. (2013). Dyadic interventions for community-dwelling people with dementia and their family caregivers: a systematic review. *International Psychogeriatrics*, *25*(10), 1581–1603. doi:10.1017/s1041610213000860

Wadensten, B. (2010). Changes in nursing home residents during an innovation based on the theory of gerotranscendence. *International Journal of Older People Nursing*, *5*, 108–115.

Yoon, M. (2012). An Exploratory study on the affecting factors of gerotranscendence in Metropolitan area in Korea. *Journal of Welfare for the Aged*, *56*, 7–31.

19 Remote area nursing

Sue Lenthall, Terrie Ivanhoe and Kylie Stothers

Chapter objectives

This chapter will offer the reader:

- An outline of the role of a remote area nurse
- An outline of the key health issues facing people in very remote Australia, in particular Aboriginal and Torres Strait Islander peoples
- An outline of cultural adaptation, cultural safety/responsiveness framework that underlie remote nursing practice

Introduction

Remote area nurses (RANs) have been around for more than one hundred years with the first bush nursing posts established in 1911. RANs, along with Aboriginal and Torres Strait Islander Health Practitioners/Workers are the main health providers in very remote Australia. Remote area nursing is not an accredited role, rather is self-identified by individual registered nurses or identified by employers. Generally, RANs are nurses working in very remote areas of Australia. The most commonly accepted geographical classification is the Accessibility and Remoteness Index of Australia (ARIA+) which classify areas 'major cities', 'inner regional', 'outer regional', 'remote', and 'very remote', a continuous varying index with values ranging from 0 (high accessibility) to 15 (high remoteness), and is based on road distance measurements from over 12,000 populated localities to the nearest service centres in five size categories based on population size (University of Adelaide, 2019-

RANs work in an advanced practice role, often in a cross-cultural situation that operates with separate language, knowledge and cultural systems to that of the health providers (Lenthall et al. 2011). The current RAN workforce is generally ageing, mainly female, and work in a variety of health facilities, predominately nurse led primary health care clinics without inpatients, but also in mines and remote tourist sites (Lenthall et al. 2011, Lenthall et al, 2018). Many nurses find the high workload and type of work, emotionally demanding (Lenthall et al. 2011), and there is a high turnover rate, 148%, in the Northern Territory (Russell, et al, 2017). However, RANs also report moderate to high levels of job satisfaction and work engagement (Opie, et al 2010). There are also have higher levels of resilience among RANs compared to their hospital colleagues (Lenthall, 2015). Most nurses enter the remote workplace with little or no understanding of the remote environment or the context and are unprepared for the complexities and challenges of providing quality health care to a mainly marginalised group of people (Lenthall,2009). This chapter provides an introduction to remote area nursing and an overview of the key issues.

Context of remote area nursing

Although the population in very remote Australia only makes up 3% of the total Australian population, the majority of the land mass in Australia is classified as remote or very remote. A large proportion of people living in remote Australia are Aboriginal and/or Torres Strait Islander peoples and the main industries are pastoral, mining, and fishing. Remote communities tend to be small, dispersed, and highly mobile with most in areas of climatic extremes such as the deserts in Central Australia, Western Australia and the tropical areas in northern Australia (Wakerman 2004; Lenthall et al. 2011, Lenthall & Dade-Smith 2016).

Australians living in remote areas generally experience poorer health than their major city counterparts, likewise mortality rates increase with remoteness. For instance, in 2015, people living in remote and very remote Australia had a mortality rate 1.3 times higher than people living in major cities (655 per 100,000 population compared with 522 per 100,000). Rates of coronary heart disease, diabetes, road transport accidents and suicide are considerably higher compared to those living in major cities (AIHW 2017).

People living in remote and very remote areas generally have poorer access to, and use of, health services and higher rates of avoidable hospital admissions. In 2013–14, the rate for emergency hospital admissions involving surgery was highest for people living in very remote areas (22 per 1,000 population) and fell with decreasing remoteness to be lowest among people living in major cities (12 per 1,000). People living in remote and very remote areas are also disadvantaged with regards to education and employment opportunities and income (AIHW 2017).

Indigenous Australians constitute a large proportion of remote area populations. In 2016, 48% of people living in very remote areas and 18% of people living in remote areas were Indigenous (ABS, 201). The poor health status of Indigenous Australians has been well recognised and accounts for a large portion of the health problems within remote areas. (AIHW, 2015). In 2017, the age-standardised death rate for Aboriginal and Torres Strait Islander people living in New South Wales, Queensland Western Australia, South Australia and the Northern Territory as 9.8 per 1,000, 1.8 times the rate for non-Indigenous people. There have been improvements in life expectancy for Indigenous people, with an increase of 2.5 years for males and 1.9 years for females since 2012. However, the 'gap' between Indigenous and non-Indigenous people in Australia is not closing (Australian Indigenous HealthInfoNet, 2019). There is clear evidence that social and cultural determinants of health, including early life experiences, social and economic position in society, exposure to stress, educational attainment and exclusion from participation in society contribute to the poor health status of Indigenous peoples in Australia (Australian Indigenous HealthInfoNet, 2019). Nevertheless, Indigenous people in remote areas self-report higher levels of wellbeing compared to Indigenous Australians in urban areas (Schultz et al, 2019). This may be due to the stronger connections to country and more opportunities to participate in cultural practices such as art and craft, ceremony, caring for country, and hunting and gathering (Schultz et al, 2019).

Remote area nursing practice

There are far fewer doctors and allied health professionals in remote Australia, compared to urban areas, with around 65% fewer occupational therapists, podiatrists, optometrists and psychologists, 50% less physiotherapists and 40% less pharmacists compared to major cities (NRHA, 2019). Accuracy of the number of medical practitioners in remote Australia is problematic. Nurses are the most evenly distributed health professions, with the highest distribution (unlike other professions) in very remote areas, with similar percentage of nurses to population between the different area classifications. Health care in very remote areas is generally provided through community Primary Health Care Clinics, with many being run by Aboriginal Community Controlled Health Organisations (ACCHO). In most instances, clinics are the first contact for all health care from emergencies to end of life care. RANs manage medical emergencies and trauma, stabilising patients before they are evacuated to definitive care and respond to all acute medical presentations. This work is often done with medical doctors on the end of a phone or video link.

In addition, clinics provide age-appropriate 'wellness' check-ups (e.g. well women's, men's and children's checks), to detect, monitor and assist with self-management of chronic disease; and provide end-of-life care. Their skills include the ability to examine, diagnose, provide and dispense medications as part of routine practice. They also undertake community development and health promotion activities following a Primary Health Care approach and conduct public health programs, including screening and surveillance, early intervention and prevention of illness advice (Aitken et al, 2019).

Cultural adaptation

Many RANs, particularly those who work in remote Aboriginal and Torres Strait Islander communities may experience a process of cultural adaptation. Living and working in another culture can be a positive learning and growth experience. However, many RANs first go through a negative stage which has been referred to as 'culture shock', 'the anxiety that results from losing all our familiar signs and symbols of social intercourse' (Adler, 1975, p 13).

There are five stages of cultural adaptation. The *first stage* is the honeymoon stage, also known as the fascination, stage. This is where the individual feels a sense of euphoria, excitement and enthusiasm. (Oberg 1960)). The **second stage** has been referred to as the rejection or disenchantment stage, and is when the culture 'shock' begins to set in. It is in this stage that language barriers and the misunderstanding of cultural cues begin to cause trouble for the RAN. It is common to reject the 'other' culture and develop a hostile and aggressive attitude. RANs are likely to associate with people from their own culture and avoid interaction with people from the 'other'. This stage can mimic racism and some people will leave at this stage, returning to their home culture with a continuing negative view of the 'other culture'. (Muecke, Lenthall and Lindeman, 2011). The **third stage** has been described as the adjustment or beginning resolution stage. Here, the visitor begins to form a more balanced and open-minded view of the other culture and starts to develop relationships with people from the other culture. The *fourth stage* is the effective functioning stage where the beliefs and beliefs are accepted are legitimate and valid. The RAN feels as if he/she knows what's their doing and that living and working in another culture is a privilege. Some authors have also identified an additional stage which occurs when someone who has been working in a remote community returns to their own culture. This has been called 'reverse culture shock'. Many have found as distressing if not more that the initial shock of moving to another culture, perhaps because reverse culture shock is often unexpected (Muecke, Lenthall and Lindeman, 2011). There are a number of strategies that may assist a nurse to work their way through the cultural adaptation process. Realise that what you are experiencing is normal; be open-minded and curious; find a cultural ally; seek out positive experiences of the 'other' culture; use your observation skills; ask questions; give yourself (and others) permission to make mistakes; take care of your physical health; seek out support from colleagues; try not to appear racist; be patient, the rewards of reaching effective functioning are great.

Foundations of remote area nursing

The key foundations of remote area nursing are cultural safety/responsiveness and Primary Health Care, the later described as an approach or philosophy that permeates the whole healthcare system. It is a way of doing healthcare, not so much in what is done, but rather *how* it is done (Aitken et al, 2019). Indigenous health services and remote area nurses have been leaders in Australia in implementing comprehensive primary health care which is more fully described in Chapter 6.

Culturally safe and responsive practice

Cultural safety

Cultural safety is a phrase originally coined by Maori nurses and nursing students who felt that they and their people were unsafe in the mainstream health system. They defined cultural safety as nursing practice where there is no assault on a person's identity (Papps & Ramsden 1996) and as:

> The effective nursing practice of a person or family from another culture, and is determined by that person or family. …. The nurse delivering the nursing care will have undertaken a process of reflection on their own cultural identity and will recognise the impact their personal culture has on their professional practice. Unsafe cultural practice comprises any action which diminishes, demeans or disempowers the cultural identity and wellbeing of an individual.

Cultural safety involves recognition of power balances and historical, political, social and economic structures. Rather than treating people regardless of their ethnic and social background, cultural safety requires that patients are treated regardful of their backgrounds. The beginning step of cultural safety is described as cultural awareness that leads to cultural sensitivity, through the acceptance and respect for differences, creating environment that is spiritually, socially and emotionally safe (Williams et al, 2016).

The Nursing and Midwifery Board of Australia's code of conduct for nurses (2018) states that *'culturally safe and respectful practice requires having knowledge of how a nurse's own culture, values, attitudes, assumptions and beliefs influence their interactions with people and families, the community and colleagues'* (NMHA, Code of Conduct, p9).

Cultural safety has been endorsed by the Congress of Aboriginal and Torres Strait Islander Nurses and Midwives (CATSINaM), who emphasise that cultural safety is as important to quality care as clinical safety. However, the 'presence or absence of cultural safety is determined by the recipient of care, it is not defined by the caregiver' (CATSINaM, 2014, p. 9).

Cultural responsiveness

Indigenous Allied Health Australia (IAHA), a national not for profit, member-based Aboriginal and Torres Strait Islander allied health organisation has taken cultural safety one step further with the cultural responsiveness framework. IAHA describes working in a culturally responsive way as a strengths-based, action-oriented approach to achieving cultural safety that can facilitate increased access to affordable, available, appropriate and acceptable health care (IAHA, 2019).

As suggested above, cultural safety describes a state in which we (RAN's) should be aiming to reach in their practice. That is safe, accessible, patient-centred and informed care. Action is needed, at the individual, organisational and systems level to enable a change in practice. Cultural responsiveness is the practice (or action) that can enable us to do this. IAHA has developed the Cultural Responsiveness in Action: An IAHA Framework as a tool to support individuals and organisations to embed culturally safe and responsive practices (IAHA, 2019 V2). The IAHA Framework is based on Aboriginal and Torres Strait Islander ways of knowing, being and doing and aims to facilitate and transform practice. The IAHA Framework presents six key capabilities that show the relationship and interconnectedness between each capability, they are not hierarchical or linear in relationship but more of a framework to enable continual self-reflection and action.

Capability 1: Respect for the centrality of cultures: Identifies and values cultures, both group and individual, as central to Aboriginal and Torres Strait Islander health, wellbeing and prosperity.

Capability 2: Self-awareness: Self-awareness in this context refers to continuous development of self-knowledge, including understanding personal beliefs, assumptions, values, perceptions, attitudes and expectations, and how they impact relationships with Aboriginal and Torres Strait Islanders peoples.

Capability 3: Proactivity: The ability to anticipate issues and initiate change that creates the best possible outcomes. It involves acting in advance of a possible situation, rather than reacting or adjusting.

Capability 4: Inclusive engagement: Provides Aboriginal and Torres Strait Islander people with opportunities to participate by reducing barriers and engaging in meaningful and supportive ways.

Capability 5: Leadership: Inspires others and influences change in contributing to the transformation of the health and well-being of Aboriginal and Torres Strait Islander individuals, families and communities.

Capability 6: Responsibility and accountability: The process of owning our role and monitoring progress in addressing inequities between Aboriginal and Torres Strait Islander peoples and other Australians.

In the Australian context, we have many diverse cultures, in order to work in a culturally safe manner, the onus is on the individual, organisation and/or system to reflect on one's own culture and its impact on their clients/patients. The IAHA Framework is a tool, which supports the individual/organisation to embed a lifelong journey of reflection on their own practice when working in a cross-cultural environment, examining dominant cultures, biases, stereotypes and myths.

Safety

The safety of RANs has been a concern for some time. Traditionally RANS have been required to attend call outs afterhours on their own. In 2016, a remote area nurse, Gayle Woodford was raped and murdered while responding to a call out on her own in a remote community in the APY lands in South Australia. Before this it was accepted by many for RANs to attend call outs at night by themselves. This has never been a safe situation was it wasn't until Gayle's murder that RANs and their supporters really lobbied for the use of escorts or second responders. There is now much more attention to the safety of RANS and Aboriginal Health Practitioners/workers. In South Australia, Gayle's law, requiring that health professionals be accompanied on callouts was passed in 2017 (SA Health, 2019). In the Northern Territory it is not a law but the NT Department of Health and most Aboriginal Community Controlled Health Organisations (ACCHO) have made a second responder a requirement. The responses in other areas of the country have been mixed. The basis of remote health workforce safety and security is never working alone when on call or in situations involving risk to your being, (CRANAplus 2017) and nurses are encouraged not to accept contracts without an assurance that they will not work alone.

CRANAplus Safety and Security Guidelines for Remote & Isolated Health (2017), available from https://crana.org.au/resources/safety-security-in-remote-healthcare, include information on hazard identification and risk management as well as a number of safety tools. These include (1) a Safety Audit Tool, Safety Flow Charts on Responding to critical events, escalating events and call outs; and (2) a Rapid Risk Assessment Tool.

Clinical practice

Remote area nurses often move across into remote area work from the acute care setting with no experience of the environment. Whilst the experience that they bring is valuable, it often does not prepare them for the working environment. Emergency nurses are great at the emergency work, midwives are great with the women's health and babies, mental health nurses are at ease with counselling and dealing with mental health issues, however most nurses are not experienced across the broad spectrum required in the remote primary health care setting. Many nurses therefore work using an acute care approach within a PHC setting and attempt to apply models of client consultation designed for acute episodes of care for single-cause diseases. However, illness in remote areas is often chronic, complex, multi-system and multifactorial in origin and management. The RAN is also, in most instances, the first contact person for the person seeking health care in the remote setting. Therefore, the skills needed are varied and require the nurse to have a broad theoretical and clinical understanding of health care needs, how to assess and clinically reason and how to communicate in an effective manner. While RANs treat emergencies, and provide health promotion and public health services, the majority of their work is seeing individual clients waiting in the waiting room.

The RAN model of consultation

The RAN Model of Consultation is a comprehensive, systematic approach to client assessment that manages the risk to the client, the nurse and the organization. It was developed from a combination of expert opinion, literature and trial and feedback from RANs. It represents a systematic comprehensive approach to each client consultation and has seven principles and eight steps (Lenthall et al, 2015). The principles include the following, (1) Culturally safe approach, (2) Holistic and Comprehensive approach, (3) Systematic, comprehensive history, (4) Shares power with the client, (5) Provides coordination and continuity of care, (6) Encourages clinical reasoning and (7) Promotes clinical safety and quality.

The RAN model of consult is a series of steps that enables the health care provider to formulate a working hypothesis and obtain relevant information to establish a diagnosis (final hypothesis). Whilst not every step may be relevant for every consult it is important to have a sequential problem solving approach when consulting with patients to develop your clinical reasoning skills and minimise the risk of a poor outcome. The steps include (1) Open consultation, (2) History, (3) Clinical examination, (4) Assessment and discussion, (5) Negotiate a management plan, (6) Close consultation, (7) Documentation, and (8) Reflection (Lenthall et al, 2015).

Becoming a remote area nurse

Remote area nursing is an advanced practice role and some preparation is necessary for the role. Most employers seek nurses with three to five years' experience before they are employed as RANs. However, there are small but growing number of positions for relatively inexperienced RANs. These are mainly with the state and Territory Health Departments. Experience in emergency care, child health, primary health care and Indigenous health is valuable. A small remote regional hospitals are often useful places to gain the required experiences in a supported environment.

RAN courses

CRANAplus run a number of short courses, including *Remote Emergency Care (REC)* and *CRANAplus Remote Maternity Care (MEC)*. Completion of these is a requirement by the NT Department of Health. More information is available from https://crana.org.au/education/education-information/courses. Employers also encourage RANs to complete the *Pharmacotherapeutics for RANs*, an online short course through the Centre for Remote Health, https://www.crh.org.au/post-graduate-award-courses/ graduate-certificate-in-remote-health-practice. There are also a number of free online courses through the Remote Area Health Corp (RAHC), https://www.rahc.com.au/ elearning.

A longer workshop of two weeks, Transition to Remote Area Nursing is available through the Centre for Remote Health, https://www.crh.org.au/short-courses-and-workshops/transition-to-remote-area-nursing.

There are also some award courses aimed at preparing remote area nurses for practice through Flinders University such as The Graduate Certificate and Graduate Diploma in Remote Health Practice and the Master of Remote and Indigenous Health.

Conclusion

Over the last 20 years, remote area nursing has been recognised as a speciality. In doing so, there has been an emphasis on professional development and the need to improve the preparedness of nurses for the remote setting. Nurses working in the remote setting work across the lifespan from birth to end of life care and provide first line care from emergencies to non-acute presentations. It is essential that nurses move or incorporate their acute care model of practice to a primary health care model based on a preventive approach. A reflective approach to practice will enable the nurse to identify their own learning needs and seek out resources to meet these needs. Whilst RAN's work in isolated areas and often away from direct clinical supervision, their practice should always be open to scrutiny. Providing health care to vulnerable groups of people is serious business and requires skilled, prepared nurses who are prepared to be ongoing learners and reflective practitioners.

References

Adler, P.S. (1975). The transitional experience: an alternative view of culture shock, *Journal of Humanistic Psychology*, *15*(4): 13–23.

Aitken, R. L., Lenthall, S., & Mackay, B. (2019). Rural and remote area nursing. In D. Brown, H. Edwards, T. Buckley, & R. L. Aitken (Eds.), *Lewis's Medical Surgical Nursing: Assessment and Management of Clinical Problems* (5th ANZ). 9-1 – 9-14 Elsevier.

Australian Bureau of Statistics. (2016). *Australian Statistical Geography Standard (ASGS): Volume 5 – Remoteness Structure,* July 2016. https://www.abs.gov.au/ausstats/abs@.nsf/mf/ 1270.0.55.005

Australian Indigenous HealthInfoNet. (2019). Overview of Aboriginal and Torres Strait Islander health status, 2018. Australian Indigenous HealthInfoNet, https://healthinfonet. ecu.edu.au/about/news/6001/,

Australian Institute of Health and Welfare. (2015). *The health and welfare of Australia's Aboriginal and Torres Strait Islander peoples 2015.* Cat. no. IHW 147, https://www.aihw.gov. au/getmedia/584073f7-041e-4818-9419-39f5a060b1aa/18175.pdf.aspx?inline=true

Australian Institute of Health and Welfare (AIHW). (2019). Acute rheumatic fever and rheumatic heart disease in Australia, https://www.aihw.gov.au/reports/indigenous-australians/ acute-rheumatic-fever-rheumatic-heart-disease

Australian Institute of Health and Welfare (AIHW). (2019). *Rural & remote health.* https://www.aihw.gov.au/reports/rural-health/rural-remote-health

Congress of Aboriginal and Torres Strait Islanders Nurses and Midwives (CATSINaM). (2014). Towards a shared understanding of terms and concepts: strengthening nursing and midwifery care of Aboriginal and Torres Strait Islander Peoples, https://www.catsinam.org. au/static/uploads/files/catsinam-cultural-terms-2014-wfwxifyfbvdf.pdf

CATSINaM. (2017). *Position statement: Embedding cultural safety across Australian nursing and midwifery,* https://www.catsinam.org.au/static/uploads/files/embedding-cultural-safety-accross-australian-nursing-and-midwifery-may-2017-wfca.pdf

Council of Remote Area Nurses of Australia plus, CRANAplus) (2017). *Working Safe in Remote and Isolated Health Handbook,* https://crana.org.au/uploads/pdfs/CRA_Safety_ Booklet_online.pdf

Indigenous Allied Health Australia (IAHA). (2019). *Cultural Responsiveness in Action: An IAHA Framework,* 2nd Ed, IAHA.

Lenthall, S., Wakerman, J., & Knight, S. (2009). The frontline and the ivory tower: A case study of service and professional-driven curriculum. *Australian Journal of Rural Health, 17*(3), 129–133. https://doi.org/10.1111/j.1440-1584.2009.01056.x

Lenthall, S. (2015). *Back from the edge, reducing stress among remote area nurses in the Northern Territory.* Flinders University. https://flex.flinders.edu.au/file/d3331394-2e9a-4c13-9718-bc0eef2462aa/1/ThesisLenthall2015.pdf

Lenthall, S., Wakerman, J., Opie, T., Dunn, S., MacLeod, M., Dollard, M., ... Knight, S. (2011). Nursing workforce in very remote Australia, characteristics and key issues. *Australian Journal of Rural Health, 19*(1), 32–37. https://doi.org/10.1111/j.1440-1584.2010.01174.

Lenthall S., Wakerman, J., Dollard, M.F., Dunn, S., Knight, S.M., Opie, T., MacLeaod, M. (2018). Reducing occupational stress among registered nurses in very remote Australia: A participatory action research approach' *Collegian, 25*(2), 181–191, Open Access DOI: https://www.collegianjournal.com/article/S1322-7696(17)30092-6/pdf

Lenthall, S., Knight, S., Foxley, S., Gordon, V., Ivanhoe, T., & Aitken, R. (2015). The remote area nurse model of consultation. *International Journal of Advanced Nursing Studies, 4*(2), 149. https://doi.org/10.14419/ijans.v4i2.4963

Lenthall, S., Dade-Smith, J. (2016). Chapter twelve, remote health practice in Dade-Smith J (ed) *Australia's Rural, Remote and Indigenous Health* 3e, (pp 285–315). Elsevier.

Muecke, A., Lenthall, S., & Lindeman, M. (2011). Culture shock and healthcare workers in remote indigenous communities of Australia: What do we know and how can we measure it. *Rural and Remote Health, 11*(2), 1–13.

National Rural Health Alliance. (2019). Allied health workforce in rural, regional & remote Australia factsheet, https://www.ruralhealth.org.au/sites/default/files/publications/fact-sheet-allied-health.pdf

Oberg K. (1960). Cultural shock: adjustment to new cultural environments. *Practical Anthropology, 7,* 177–182.

Opie, T., Dollard, M., Lenthall, S., Wakerman, J., Dunn, S., et al. (2010). Levels of occupational stress in the remote area nursing workforce. *Australian Journal of Rural Health, 18,* 235–241.

Papps, E. & Ramsden. I. (1996). Cultural safety in nursing: the New Zealand experience, *International Journal for Quality in Health Care, 8*(5), 491–497, https://doi.org/10.1093/ intqhc/8.5.491

Russell, D. J., Zhao, Y., Guthridge, S., Ramjan, M., Jones, M. P., Humphreys, J. S., & Wakerman, J. (2017). Patterns of resident health workforce turnover and retention in remote communities of the Northern Territory of Australia, 2013-2015. *Human Resources for Health, 15*(1), 1–12. https://doi.org/10.1186/s12960-017-0229-9

SA Health. (2019). *Gayle's Law,* SA Health website https://www.sahealth.sa.gov.au/wps/wcm/ connect/public+content/sa+health+internet/about+us/legislation/gayles+law,

Schultz, R., Quinn, S. J., Abbott, T., Cairney, S., & Yamaguchi, J. (2019). Quantification of interplaying relationships between wellbeing priorities of Aboriginal people in remote Australia. *International Indigenous Policy Journal, 10*(3), 1–23. https://doi.org/10.18584/ iipj.2019.10.3.8165

University of Adelaide, Hugo Centre for Migration and Population Research. (2019). *Accessibility/Remoteness Index of Australia (ARIA),* https://www.adelaide.edu.au/hugo-centre/services/aria, accessed 19/12/2019.

Wakerman, J. (2004). Defining remote health. *Australian Journal of Rural Health, 12*(5), 210–214. https://doi.org/10.1111/j.1440-1854.2004.00607.

Williams R., Dade-Smith J., & Sharp, R.J. (2016). Chapter three, cultures and health, in Dade-Smith J (ed), *Australia's Rural, Remote and Indigenous Health* 3e, pp 45–75, Elsevier.

20 Sexuality and sexual health

Professional issues for nurses

Marika Guggisberg

Chapter objectives

This chapter will offer the reader:

- Insight into the concepts of sexuality and sexual health
- An outline of sexual rights and sexual health promotion
- Components including reproductive health and gender dysphoria
- A discussion of sexuality and sexual health and sexual violence using the example of sexual minorities as one vulnerable subpopulation
- An opportunity to build a knowledge base and develop nursing skills specific to sexual health promotion and intervention in relation to sexually transmissible infections
- Practice considerations important to nursing

Introduction

The current literature indicates that health professionals including nursing students require specific knowledge in the area of sexuality and sexual health to be able to provide holistic and effective care (Blakey & Aveyard, 2017). This chapter offers an overview of issues related to sexuality, sexual health and sexual violence along with some practice considerations and strategies to promote sexual health for patients with whom nurses interact using the example of sexual minorities.

Sexuality

Sexuality forms part of a person's daily living and as such is an important component of overall health and wellbeing (Evcili & Demirel, 2018; Gruskin, Yadav, Castellanos-Usigli, Khizanishvili, & Kismödi, 2019; Malta et al., 2018). Nursing care, therefore, includes being responsive to patients' sexual health needs. However, nurses and nursing students often experience embarrassment in relation to sexuality (Ollivier, Aston, & Price, 2019) and fear that addressing sexuality issues will be perceived by patients as offensive (Blakey & Aveyard, 2017). Nurses are also concerned that they lack knowledge and skills to engage patients in a conversation about sexuality, and some believe that sexuality is not a priority in patient care (Bates, 2011). Consequently, there is a need to enhance understanding of sexuality in nursing and nurses' ability to relate well to self and others in relation to sexuality.

Sexuality, sexual health and sexual rights as individual concepts are inextricably interconnected (Gruskin, et al., 2019). Understanding sexuality and interpersonal skills are characteristics of competent nurses who acknowledge that sexual rights are a part of people's human rights (Temmerman, Khosla, & Say, 2014).

Sexual rights

The World Association for Sexual Health that sexual rights are encompassed within human rights and are therefore already recognised in national laws, international human rights conventions and other consensus documents (Gruskin et al., 2019; Guggisberg, 2018). These sexual rights include the right of all persons to achieve the highest standard of health in relation to sexuality and to be free of any form of coercion, discrimination and violence. Everyone has the right to seek, receive and provide information in relation to their sexuality including respect for bodily integrity, choice of partner, the decision to be sexually active or not, consensual sexual relations and reproductive decisions. Consequently, people have the right to pursue a satisfying, safe and pleasurable sexual life without any unwanted short- or long-term consequences. To achieve these goals, it is important that all health professionals including nurses have an understanding about their own and other people's sexuality, sexual rights and sexual health.

Sexual health

Sexual health has been identified by the World Health Organization (2018) as an important component of overall health and wellbeing. It is defined as 'a state of physical, emotional, mental and sexual well-being related to sexuality' (Sadovsky & Nusbaum, 2006, p. 3). According to this definition, sexual health goes beyond identifying and treating sexual problems such as sexually transmitted infections, which is a critical component of sexual health care prevention and intervention.

Practitioners, researchers and policy makers have recognised that despite the acknowledgement that sexual health care forms part of clinical nursing practice, it is often neglected (Ollivier et al., 2019; Ozan, Duman, & Çiçek, 2019). The reasons for lack of engagement of health care professionals in sexual health discussions with patients are complex and manyfold. They include lack of knowledge and skills in relation to sexuality, believing that the issue is too sensitive to address, health practitioners' own insecurity about their sexual identity, and lack of confidence (Evcili & Demirel, 2018). A gap between patient expectations and nursing care can be created in relation to intervention for identified sexual health problems (Ozan, et al., 2019), and also in relation to preventative psychosexual education, which is what Blakey and Aveyard (2017) referred to as 'sexual health promotion' (p. 3906).

Sexual health promotion

Sexual health promotion has been defined as 'the process of enabling people to increase control over their sexual health that should be based on people's needs and abilities' (Khalesi, Simbar, Azin, & Zayeri, 2016, p. 2489). In practice, this includes supporting patients in having enjoyable sexual interactions that are free of fear, guilt and shame as well as communicating trauma-informed understandings to those who have become or are vulnerable to sexual violence (Blakey & Aveyard, 2017; Queensland Health, 2016). Even though nurses and nursing students may feel uncomfortable discussing sexuality issues including risks of sexual violence, research evidence indicates that psychosexual education is a very important part of patient care (see for example Bal & Sahiner, 2015); sexual health promotion has been found to be effective in raising awareness of specific sexuality issues and improving health outcomes of individuals. Furthermore, benefits of discussing sexuality issues with patients include improved knowledge of sexual rights and the ability to challenge misconceptions and stereotypes around vulnerable subpopulations.

For nurses, providing information about sexuality, screening and treatment in a non-judgemental and sensitive way helps patients to make informed decisions about their sexual health and health behaviour. Therefore, sexual health promotion may reduce the burden of disease associated with sexual health. As examples, the following topics will be discussed subsequently: sexually transmissible infections and reproductive health and gender dysphoria.

Sexually transmissible infections

Sexually transmissible infections (STIs) are defined as 'different bacterial, viral and parasitic infections which are transmitted through sexual contact' (Australian Government, 2018, p. 10). STIs pose a significant public health challenge in Australia, with some infections continuing to increase. For example, the prevalence of Syphilis is rising among Aboriginal and Torres Strait Islander peoples and Gonorrhoea in men who have sex with men (MSM). The Australian Government (2018) noted that there is a specific need to increase knowledge about STIs not only in the general community but also among health professionals. Raising awareness on the issue of STIs includes knowledge about the preventative role of condom use and engaging patients in discussions about the long-term consequences and emphasising the importance of STI testing and early treatment if infections are identified. Patients may need to be reminded that even if they have been identified with a notifiable STI, they have the right to sensitive and confidential treatment and that sexual health education is an integral part of preventative strategies to reduce the risk of future infections. STIs, while generally transmitted through sexual contact, can be transmitted orally and through blood contact.

Reproductive health

Women have been recognised to be particularly at risk of notifiable STIs with statistics indicating a continuous rise of infections since 2012, particularly Gonorrhoea and Syphilis. It is well known that women may experience serious reproductive consequences including mother-to-child transmission of STIs during child birth (Australian Government, 2018). Prevention activities may involve pre-exposure prophylaxis (PrEP), which consist of providing psychosexual education and early intervention to those women who have been newly diagnosed with STIs to assist patients navigate available care options.

Psychosexual education may include informing female patients that untreated STIs can lead to complications and health consequences such as pelvic inflammatory disease, infertility, ectopic pregnancy and even foetal and neonatal death. Preventative

health information including screening and testing may contribute to positive reproductive health outcomes. Sexual health education includes promoting contraceptive
measures such as the use of condoms (for females and males), which may act as a
physical barrier against STIs. The use of condoms has been found to be effective in
preventing STIs including HIV (Queensland Health, 2016).

Gender dysphoria

A person may experience discomfort or even distress due to feelings of incongruence
in relation to biological sex and gender identity. Nurses who understand difficulties arising from gender dysphoria may be able to communicate awareness, support
patients sensitively and provide referrals to specialist services without discrimination.
Such approaches to coordinated care indicate understanding of the importance of
working effectively as an interdisciplinary team using a 'sex positive' (Gruskin et al.,
2019, p. 6) understanding of sexual health promotion free of stigma and shame. The
provision of sexual health information and education is understood as an effective way
that reduces any form of overt and covert sexual discrimination.

Specific subpopulations

Sexual health is a right that applies to every person equally. Importantly, it has been
recognised that certain population groups require particular attention to achieve and
maintain highest standards of sexual health and wellbeing (Kismödi, Cottingham,
Gruskin, & Miller, 2015) due to their vulnerability to sexual health-related problems
that impact their overall health and wellbeing, even across generations (Australian
Government, 2018). These include sexual minorities, Aboriginal and Torres Strait
Islander peoples, individuals with disabilities, sex workers and individuals in custodial settings. It is important to note that there is considerable overlap and these groups
are not mutually exclusive. As an example, one subpopulation will be discussed below:
individuals identifying as sexual minorities.

Sexual minorities

The issue of gender identity and sexual orientation is important and needs to be
acknowledged in sexual health care. Not only patients but also nurses may identify
as non-heterosexual. As a nurse, discussing sexual health in relation to sexual minorities requires particular sensitivity and understanding of vulnerability issues (Ollivier
et al., 2019). This section examines individuals identifying as lesbian, gay, bisexual,
transgender, intersex and other sexuality, sex and gender diverse (LGBTI+) as a specifically vulnerable group in relation to primary health care.

   The Australian Institute of Health and Welfare (2018) indicated that an estimated
11% of the Australian population identify as LGBTI+, which acknowledges 'other sexuality'. Sexual orientation is defined by 'an emotional, romantic, sexual or affectionate
attraction' (Australian Psychological Society, 2010, p. 1) that is felt towards other individuals and whether or not this attraction is to those of the same sex, a different sex,
or both sexes. Importantly, sexual orientation is not fixed and firmly determined. It is
more accurately described as variable in same-sex and other-sex attraction and involvement at different times and situations throughout a person's life (Crooks & Baur, 2017).

Sexual fluidity. Importantly, sexual orientation is not fixed and stably determined. It is more accurately described as variable in same-sex and other-sex attraction and involvement at different times and situations throughout a person's life (Crooks & Baur, 2017). The preference of sexual partners can vary over time. For example, Diamond (2008) followed 89 young women over a 10-year period. Her study found that many women changed their sexual identity, sometimes numerous times, over the duration of the 10 years. Diamond concluded that female sexual responsiveness was flexible and dependent on the situation the women found themselves in.

Sexual identity. Sexual identity goes beyond what sex someone has been assigned at birth and to whom the person is attracted to (Crooks & Baur, 2017). For example, a person who is attracted to individuals of the same sex can be lesbian, gay, bisexual or transgender. Some individuals define their sexual identity in terms of asexuality, celibacy, or engaging in particular sexual practices such as BDSM (bondage, dominance, sadism and/or masochism). In this regard, the National LGBTI Health Alliance (2014) stated that 'gender identity and expression is best seen as a flexible socially-constructed spectrum rather than as a fixed binary classification' (p. 22). This means that cultural norms of acceptance are shifting to allow sexual identity formation to occur more openly. It is generally considered to begin in adolescence in the context of the adolescent life, which includes family, school, peer and neighbourhood and workplace influences (Rosenthal, 2013).

Minority stress. LGBTI+ individuals experience stressors related to their sexual orientation. Minority stress includes internal stressors such as anticipated rejection or internalised homophobia, and external stressors such as experiencing homophobia and heterosexism (Walters, Chen, & Breiding, 2013). Not only are many LGBTI+ individuals subject to the direct prejudice and discrimination associated with homophobia, but they may also experience pervasive heterosexism. Consequently, fear of being stigmatised in the workplace or educational setting can be a particular acute issue and can deter LGBTI+ individuals from gaining further education or entering careers.

While marginalised status has been associated with shame, not only mental health problems but also increased health risk behaviours have been noted in the literature. Minority stress is closely associated with physical and mental health problems (Walters, et al., 2013). This is due to social withdrawal and feelings of loneliness LGBTI+ individuals feel isolated from their community. Mental health problems, which may be related to a sense of helplessness, exacerbate health risk behaviours such as alcohol/other drug use issues as a coping mechanism, all of which may be related to a complex interaction with homophobia/heterosexism (Australian Institute of Health and Welfare, 2018).

Sexually transmissible infections. The prevalence of STIs among LGBTIQ+ individuals has been found to be greater when compared to the general population (Australian Government, 2018). Men who identify as gay and MSM have been found to be disproportionately affected by STIs when compared to the general population. The rate of notifiable infections is particularly high among HIV-positive men who usually live in urban areas (Australian Government, 2018). The reason for this vulnerability has been associated with unprotected anal intercourse with casual encounters. Prevention education emphasising the importance of condom use along with regular STI testing and PrEP as a HIV prevention measure was emphasised by the Australian Government (2018). A concerning trend has been observed among gay and MSM in that casual sex partners omit consistent condom use (Australian Government, 2018).

Rolle and colleagues (2018) indicated an increased vulnerability to STIs, including the risk to contract HIV/AIDS through impaired negotiation powers for safe sex and forced unprotected intercourse. The inability to negotiate safe sex is related to unequal power in the relationship, fear of violence and inability to control sexuality (Walters et al., 2013).

Sexual violence. There are important differences when considering sexual violence among LGBTI+ women and men in comparison to heterosexual couples. For example, concerns about inclusivity and an increasing gender-neutral stance have been identified as 'de-gendering' (Frazier & Falmagne, 2014, p. 481) when discussing the issue of sexual violence among LGBTI+ individuals. It is not always recommended to use inclusive language when addressing sexual violence as this fails to recognise the high levels of sexual violence among sexual minorities (Gruskin et al., 2019). Achieving justice for LGBTI+ women and men requires acknowledgement of the dynamics of sexual violence among LGBTI+ individuals, which highlights the gendered dimension beyond the traditional heterosexual paradigm.

Importantly, sexual violence occurs in intimate relationships of all sexual orientations. However, sexual victimisation also relates to heteronormativity and marginalisation of individuals identifying as Aboriginal and Torres Strait Islander (Guggisberg, 2019; Northern Territory Government, 2019) or culturally and linguistically diverse (Australian Government, 2018), which adds an additional dimension to those patients who identify as not exclusively heterosexual.

Research among non-heterosexual individuals is still underdeveloped. Current insight suggests that the prevalence of Same-Sex Intimate Partner Violence (SSIPV) is even higher when compared to IPV among heterosexual people (Blondeel et al., 2018; Gehring & Vaske, 2017). However, it is commonly acknowledged that prevalence rates are unreliable for several reasons including different participant groups, and methods used along with reluctance to report sexual victimisation similar to heterosexual individuals (Blondeel et al., 2018).

Some data suggest that approximately one in three males and one in two females identifying as a sexual minority have experienced physical and/or sexual forms of SSIPV in their life time. However, variations exist among sexual minorities with bisexual women experiencing the highest rate with 61% followed by lesbian women with 44%, 37% of bisexual men and gay men experiencing the lowest rates with 26% (Rolle et al., 2018). Messinger (2011) argued that minority stress likely contributed to the higher prevalence of SSIPV. Individuals with nonexclusive heterosexual attraction experience their sexual orientation as a risk factor for sexual and other forms of IPV because of sexual stigma (Blondeel et al., 2018).

In relation to sexual violence, in a systematic review of 76 studies, transgender women have been identified as the most victimised group with prevalence rates ranging from 11.8% to 68.2% (Blondeel et al., 2018). Blondeel and colleagues (2018) stated that the high prevalence of sexual victimisation among transgender women is likely to be explained through victim/survivors' engagement in sex work rather than same-sex or opposite-sex IPV.

Practice considerations

The role of nurses across all practice settings encompasses discussing sexual health (including sexual health promotion) with the patient, the partner, the carer and other health professionals. Nurses may be involved in sexual health promotion and assertiveness training to address sexual rights as human rights and inform about specific vulnerabilities being recognised in certain subpopulations.

Raising awareness and developing knowledge about STIs and their consequences, particularly among identified vulnerable population groups is critically important. Nurses should provide psychosexual education to their patients about reducing sexual risk behaviours (e.g., promoting condom use) on a regular basis. Consistent condom use has been found to be one of the most effective protection strategies (Australian Government, 2018). Routine care should involve sexual health promotion strategies including STI education, testing and early intervention.

When working with sexual minorities, interventions should be tailored to the specific needs of LGBTI+ clients rather than using protocols for heterosexual individuals. This includes awareness of the complexities of belonging to a marginalised community group and using appropriate terminology, communicating acceptance and considering confidentiality issues. Importantly, supervision and professional development should form part of professional practice when working with LGBTI+ patients.

Communicating acceptance. Nurses should be aware of the stressors that patients can face as a result of their sexual orientation and ensure that they convey acceptance of their sexuality. All health professionals are encouraged to enquire about patients' sexual orientation in an open but sensitive way, without fear of being intrusive. Furthermore, it is important to be aware of inclusive language. It may be advisable to negotiate the language used with each patient (Australian Psychological Society, 2010).

Confidentiality. It is important for nurses to exercise care with confidentiality in terms of their patients' sexuality and disclosures of sexual orientation. It is advisable to include a written policy that ensures that information about patients' sexual health issues is kept secure and that their sexuality issues are discussed and addressed professionally. If a patient identifies as LGBTI+, nurses should be alert to signs that the patient may have concerns about 'coming out' (disclosing their sexual identity). Demonstrating awareness of sexuality includes communicating that this is a process rather than an event, given that heterosexuality is commonly assumed and that patients are reassured that all information is kept strictly confidential. Even when LGBTI+ patients are open about their sexual identity, they can still find themselves monitoring their surroundings and trying to gauge nurses' attitudes towards them. In this regard, it is important to note that nurses should avoid assuming that the 'correct' position is that the patient reveals their sexual orientation, as this may not be the best outcome for them in their specific situation.

Empowerment. The concept of empowerment in nursing has become important in relation to patients' health care outcomes and job satisfaction. There are different forms of empowerment relevant to clinical nursing (Connolly, Jacobs, & Scott, 2018). These include workplace empowerment and psychological empowerment. Workplace empowerment encompasses nursing managers and teaching staff being supportive, exhibiting a positive attitude towards student nurses and understanding the importance of a supportive and nurturing environment, as this promotes personal empowerment. Nurses who have sufficient resources (competency and support) perceive themselves as confident within themselves. They tend to have a positive attitude towards promoting their patients' health and wellbeing, which results in patients' empowerment (Connolly et al., 2018). In relation to sexuality and sexual health, there is an interconnectedness between nurses' and patients' sense of empowerment to openly and freely discussing intimate issues in a supportive and confidential environment. Nurses have the opportunity to create and maintain an environment that promotes a 'sex positive' stance, enabling patients to learn about sexuality, sexual health promotion and to discuss issues that allow health professionals to help optimise their patients' health and wellbeing in the long term. Patient empowerment is, therefore, dependent on nurses experiencing a sense of competency in relation to addressing sexuality and sexual health with their patients on a routine basis.

Conclusion

This chapter examined a range of issues on sexuality, sexual health and prevention and intervention measures with focus on STIs. STIs disproportionately impact specific subpopulations and, therefore they may benefit from targeted prevention approaches. It was suggested that nurses are uniquely positioned to be at the forefront of improving sexuality issues and promote sexual health for individuals across Australia. Sexual health promotion includes preventative screening along with raising awareness and providing information about infections that can be transmitted through sexual contacts. By adopting a sexual health promotion focus, using a patient-centred and empowerment approach to nursing care with the understanding that patients are experts of their own life who deserve professional and unbiased psychosexual education and support, positive outcomes will likely result.

Online resources

1 Sexual minority support services: https://au.reachout.com/articles/lgbtqi-support-services
2 Indigenous health and welfare services: https://www.aihw.gov.au/indigenous-health-welfare-services/about
3 Australian Institute of Health and Welfare. (2019). Family, domestic and sexual violence in Australia: Continuing the national story. Canberra, ACT: https://www.aihw.gov.au/getmedia/b0037b2d-a651-4abf-9f7b-00a85e3de528/aihw-fdv3-FDSV-in-Australia-2019.pdf.aspx?inline=true
4 Australian Institute of Family Studies. (2019). Australian child protection legislation. Sydney, NSW: https://www.aihw.gov.au/reports-data/health-welfare-services/child-protection/child-protection-legislation-by-jurisdiction
5 Australian Institute of Health and Welfare. (2019). The health of Australia's prisoners 2018. Canberra, ACT: https://www.aihw.gov.au/getmedia/2e92f007-453d-48a1-9c6b-4c9531cf0371/aihw-phe-246.pdf.aspx?inline=true
6 RACGP. Guidelines for preventive activities in general practice, the red book. Sexually transmissible infections: https://www.racgp.org.au/clinical-resources/clinical-guidelines/key-racgp-guidelines/view-all-racgp-guidelines/red-book/communicable-diseases/sexually-transmissible-infections

References

Australian Government. (2018). *Fourth National Sexually Transmissible Infections Strategy 2018-2022*. Canberra, ACT: Department of Health, Commonwealth of Australia.

Australian Institute of Health and Welfare. (2018). *Australia's health 2018:* In brief. Canberra, ACT: Author. Retrieved from: https://www.aihw.gov.au/getmedia/fe037cf1-0cd0-4663-a8c0-67cd09b1f30c/aihw-aus-222.pdf.aspx?inline=true

Australian Psychological Society. (2010). *Guidelines for psychological practice with lesbian, gay, and bisexual clients.* Melbourne, VIC: Author.

Bal, M., & Sahiner, N. C. (2015). Turkish nursing students' attitudes and beliefs regarding sexual health. *Sexuality and Disability, 33,* 223–231.

Bates, J. (2011). Broaching sexual health issues with patients. *Nursing Times, 107,* 20–22. Retrieved from: https://www.nursingtimes.net/clinical-archive/sexual-health/broaching-sexual-health-issues-with-patients-02-12-2011/

Blakey, E. P., & Aveyard, H. (2017). Student nurses' competence in sexual health care: A literature review. *Journal of Clinical Nursing, 26,* 3906–3916. https://doi.org/10.1111/jocn.13810

Blondeel, K., de Vasconcelos, S., Garcia-Moreno, C., Stephenson, R., Temmerman, M., & Toskin, I. (2018). Violence motivated by perception of sexual orientation and gender identity: a systematic review. *Bulletin of the World Health Organization, 96,* 29–41. Retrieved from: https://www.who.int/bulletin/volumes/96/1/17-197251/en/

Connolly, M., Jacobs, S., & Scott, K. (2018). Clinical leadership, structural empowerment and psychological empowerment of registered nurses working in an emergency department. *Journal of Nursing Management, 26,* 881–887. https://doi:10.1111/jonm.12619.

Crooks, R. T., & Baur, K. (2017). *Our sexuality* (13th edition). Boston, MA: Cengage Learning.

Diamond, L. (2008). *Sexual fluidity: Understanding women's love and desire.* Cambridge, MA: Harvard University Press.

Evcili, F., & Demirel, G. (2018). Patient's sexual health and nursing: a neglected area. *International Journal of Caring Sciences, 11,* 1282–1288. Retrieved from: http://www.internationaljournalofcaringsciences.org/docs/72_evcili_original_10_2.pdf

Frazier, K. E., & Falmagne, R. J. (2014). Empowered victims? Women's contradictory positions in the discourse of violence prevention. *Feminism & Psychology, 24,* 479–499. https://doi.org/10.1177/0959353514552036

Gehring, K. S., & Vaske, J. C. (2017). Out in the open: the consequences of intimate partner violence for victims in same-sex and opposite-sex relationships. *Journal of Interpersonal Violence, 32,* 3669–3692. https://doi.org/10.1177/0886260515600877

Gruskin, S., Yadav, V., Castellanos-Usigli, A., Khizanishvili, G., & Kismödi, E. (2019). Sexual health, sexual rights and sexual pleasure: meaningfully engaging the perfect triangle. *Sexual and Reproductive Health Matters, 27,* 1–12. https://doi:10.1080/26410397.2019.1593787

Guggisberg, M. (2019). Aboriginal women's experiences with intimate partner sexual violence and the dangerous lives they live as a result of victimization. *Journal of Aggression, Maltreatment & Trauma, 28,* 186–204. https://doi.org/10.1080/109266771.2018.1508106

Guggisberg, M. (2018). The impact of violence against women and girls: a life span analysis. In M. Guggisberg, & J. Henricksen (eds.). *Violence against women in the 21st century: Challenges and future directions* (pp. 3–27). New York, NY: Nova Science Publishers.

Khalesi, Z. B., Simbar, M., Azin, S. A., & Zayeri, F. (2016). Public sexual health promotion interventions and strategies: a qualitative study. *Electronic Physician, 8,* 2489–2496. Retrieved from: https://www.ncbi.nlm.nih.gov/pmc/articles/PMC4965198/pdf/epj-08-2489.pdf

Kismödi, E., Cottingham, J., Gruskin, S., & Miller, A. M. (2015). Advancing sexual health through human rights: the role of the law. *Global Public Health, 10,* 252–267. Retrieved from: https://www.ncbi.nlm.nih.gov/pmc/articles/PMC4318115/

Malta, S., Hocking, J., Lyne, J., McGavin, D., Hunter, J., Bickerstaffe, A., & Temple-Smith, M. (2018). Do you talk to your older patients about sexual health? Health practitioners' knowledge of, and attitudes towards, management of sexual health among older Australians. *Australian Journal of General Practice, 47.* https://doi:10.31128/AJGP-04-18-4556

Messinger, A. M. (2011). Invisible victims: same-sex IPV in the national violence against women survey. *Journal of Interpersonal Violence, 26,* 2228–2243. https://doi:10.1177/0886260510383023.

National LGBTI Health Alliance. (2014). *Working therapeutically with LGBTI clients: A practice wisdom resource.* Newton, NSW: Author. Retrieved from: https://www.beyondblue.org.au/docs/default-source/default-document-library/bw0256-practice-wisdom-guide-online.pdf

Northern Territory Government. (2019). *The Northern Territory's Domestic, Family & Sexual Violence Reduction Framework 2018–2018.* Winnellie, NT: Author. Retrieved from: https://territoryfamilies.nt.gov.au/domestic-violence/domestic-and-family-violence-reduction-strategy

Ollivier, R., Aston, M., & Price, S. (2019). Let's talk about sex: a feminist poststructural approach to addressing sexual health in the healthcare setting. *Journal of Clinical Nursing, 28*, 695–702. https://doi.org/10.1111/jocn.14685

Ozan, Y. D., Duman, M., & Çiçek, Ö. (2019). Nursing students' experiences on assessing the sexuality of patents: mixed method study. *Sexuality and Disability.* https://doi.org/10.1007/s11195-019-09567-6

Queensland Health. (2016). *Queensland Sexual Health Strategy 2016–2021.* Brisbane, QLD: Department of Health. Retrieved from: health.qld.gov.au/qh-sexual-health-strategy.pdf

Rolle, L, Giardina, G, Caldarera, A. M., Gerino, E., & Brustia, P. (2018). When intimate partner violence meets same sex couples: a review of same sex intimate partner violence. *Frontiers in Psychology, 1506,* 1–13. https://doi.org/10.3389/fpsyg.2018.01506

Rosenthal, M. S. (2013). *Human sexuality: From cells to society.* Belmont, CA: Wadsworth Cengage Learning.

Sadovsky, R., & Nusbaum, M. (2006). Sexual health inquiry and support is a primary care priority. *Journal of Sexual Medicine, 3,* 3–11. https://doi:10.1111/j.1743-6109.2005.00193.x

Temmerman, M., Khosla, R., & Say, L. (2014). Sexual and reproductive health and rights: a global development, health, and human rights priority. *The Lancet, 384,* e30–e31. https://doi:10.1016/S0140-6736(14)61190-9.

Walters, M. L., Chen, J., & Breiding, M. J. (2013). *The national intimate partner and sexual violence survey (NISVS): 2010 findings on victimization by sexual orientation.* Atlanta, GA: National Center for Injury Prevention and Control, Centers for Disease Control and Prevention. Retrieved from: https://www.cdc.gov/violenceprevention/pdf/nisvs_sofindings.pdf

World Health Organization. (2018). *Sexual and reproductive health: Defining sexual health.* Geneva, Switzerland. Retrieved from: http://www.who.int/reproductivehealth/topics/sexual_health/sh_definitions/en

Part III

Diverse and distinctive practice areas

21 Nursing and people with cosmetic and related concerns

Elissa J O'Keefe and Robin Curran

Chapter objectives

This chapter will offer the reader:

- Insight into the history and current contexts of nursing and people with cosmetic and related concerns.
- An outline of the key health issues facing people with cosmetic and related concerns.
- A description of contemporary contexts of the nursing of people with cosmetic and related concerns occurs.
- An opportunity to build a knowledge base and develop nursing skills specific to people with cosmetic and aesthetic concerns.
- An overview of future challenges to nursing and nurses who practice in this area which is both cosmetic and medical in nature.

Introduction

One of the largest trends globally is the seeking of wellness solutions and the health and beauty industry is booming (CB Insights, 2019). Consumers are driving the provision of cosmetic and aesthetic treatments and procedures and actively seek Registered Nurses out as a provider of choice. Cosmetic medical and surgical procedures are defined as 'operations and other procedures that revise or change the appearance, colour, texture, structure or position of normal bodily features with the sole intention of achieving what the patient perceives to be a more desirable appearance or boosting the patient's self-esteem'. (Australian Health Ministers' Advisory Committee, 2011, p2) The most common procedures are the administration of muscle relaxants into the face and/or dermal filler for volume loss of the face, reduction of unwanted body or facial hair, non-invasive facial rejuvenation, chemical peels, and skin resurfacing (International Society of American Society for Aesthetic Plastic Surgery, 2017). All these treatments are within the scope of practice for appropriately educated and trained nurses.

Data released by the American Society of Aesthetic Plastic Surgeons (ASAPS, 2017) shows nearly a quarter of a million more cosmetic procedures were performed in the USA in 2018 compared to 2017. In Australia, consumer spending on non- and minimally invasive treatments increased by 15% (2011–12) with a total estimated annual expenditure of $644.7 million (Cosmetic Physicians Society of Australia, 2012).

According to recent statistics, Australians spend over $1 billion on cosmetic proce-
dures (Latouff, 2017) and approximately $350 million on one specific brand of botuli-
num toxin injections alone (Duncan, 2018). Annual growth of the sector is estimated
at 10% globally with Australians spending more per capita than any other country
globally (Cosmetic Physicians College of Australia, 2016). This increase is driven
by consumer demand for antiaging products, non-surgical procedures and minimally invasive procedures.

Cosmetic nursing has as its genesis the two separately recognised specialty areas
of dermatology nursing and plastic surgery nursing. This is because nurses originally involved in the provision of cosmetic and medical aesthetic treatments were
typically based in dermatology and plastic surgery clinics. There has been a shift in
context of practice, and it is not unusual for Registered Nurses to work in a variety of
settings beyond this including owning and operating their own businesses. The cosmetic nursing skill sets developed and honed in the dermatology and plastic surgery
settings were transferable and cosmetic nursing is now being developed as unique
specialty distinct from them.

A diverse range of healthcare professionals work in the field of cosmetic medicine
including plastic surgeons, dermatologists, neurologists, dentists, general physicians
and practitioners, as well as nurses (O'Keefe & Hoitink, 2013). Despite the growth of
the sector, the Australian evidence-base for cosmetic nursing is limited related to a lack
of research and published papers. Nevertheless, O'Keefe and Kushelew (2016) have discussed nursing credibility and practice standards and described how cosmetic nursing
already fits into the legislative and clinical governance frameworks in the Australian
health care system. Furthermore, the breadth of the scope of practice of cosmetic
nurses including the provision of skin care advice and referral, skin cancer checks,
management of common skin disorders, prescription of medical grade skin care products, laser and other light based therapies, skin resurfacing, removal of benign lesions,
dermal fillers, administration of muscle relaxants, skin tightening and mesotherapy is
made explicit.

Mesotherapy is a non-surgical, minimally invasive method of drug delivery that
consists of multiple intradermal or subcutaneous injections of a mixture of com-
pounds 'melange' in minute doses (Konda et al., 2013). Plant extracts, homeopathic
agents, pharmaceuticals, vitamins and other bioactive substances can be used, but
alcohol- or oil-based substances should not be used for mesotherapy because of the
risk of cutaneous necrosis.

The term 'mesotherapy' is derived from the Greek words 'mesos' meaning 'middle0'
or 'mean' and 'therapeia' meaning 'to treat medically,' i.e. injecting into the middle layer
of skin or 'intradermothera'. The depth of penetration of the needle should not exceed 4
mm for it to be effective.

Throughout Australia, nurses are the cornerstone of many practices within the private hospital and community cosmetic medicine setting as they perform a majority
of the non-surgical cosmetic procedures. Neither the Australian Institute of Health
and Welfare nor the Nursing and Midwifery Board of Australia maintain statistics
on the number of nurses working in cosmetic practice, but conservative estimates are
that there are approximately two thousand full time equivalent registered nurses and

between twenty and thirty nurse practitioners (Australian College of Nursing, 2020). However, as this area of nursing not yet recognised as a discrete specialty area, the exact number is difficult to quantify and requires further research.

Specialty recognition

The challenge for cosmetic nurses in Australia is professional recognition; unlike their British (British Association of Cosmetic Nurses, 2013), Canadian (**Canadian** Society of Aesthetics Specialty Nurses, 2019) and United States (Plastic Surgical Nursing Certification Board, 2020) counterparts, cosmetic nursing in Australia doesn't currently meet the criteria for being recognised as a specialty primarily because there is no cosmetic specialty nursing group in Australia that has developed processes for recognition (NMBA, 2019). Furthermore, there is no process for licensure, endorsement, credentialing, validation or certification as developed overseas nor is there a robust body of research unique to the Australian context to support this emerging scope of practice.

The Australian College of Nursing (ACN) have recently launched a Graduate Certificate in Cosmetic Nursing (ACN, 2019a) with the first student intake commencing in 2020. The ACN have also started a Cosmetic Nursing Community of Interest which already has just over one hundred and thirty members (ACN, 2020). The gathering of a critical mass of interested nurses, a new educational and career pathway and increasing professional commitment is building. These new pioneers will be charged to conduct research, build the evidence base and document their place in the Australian healthcare context.

Key issues facing people requesting cosmetic procedures

People requesting cosmetic and related care are generally well, female and aged 18–55 (ASAPS, 2017) and have an income that allows discretionary spending on appearance medicine (Goh, 2009). Treatments sought are generally to enhance appearance or correct a perceived defect. An example of an enhancement may include the administration of botulinum toxin A to the muscles of the forehead, crow's feet (lateral canthal lines) and frown (glabellar complex) and lip augmentation. An example of a correction of a defect may include the correction of asymmetry caused by Bell's Palsy, cerebrovascular accident or motor vehicle accident; or control of adult acne using medical grade skin care, chemical skin peels and photobiomodulation technology and then skin resurfacing to correct scarring or tone skin.

> Photobiomodulation (PBM) is a treatment method based on research findings showing that irradiation with certain wavelengths of red or near-infrared light has been shown to produce a range of physiological effects in cells, tissues, animals and humans (Heiskanen & Hamblin, 2019).

In today's society the importance of physical appearance shaped by the media is arguably more persuasive than ever, especially among younger generations and through newer forms of media such as Social Networking Sites (SNS) (Fardouly & Vartanian, 2016). Utilising social media to promote cosmetic treatments is governed by the Therapeutic Goods Advisory code developed by the Therapeutic Goods Advisory (TGA, 2018). The TGA recognises that social media provides a valuable platform for sharing views about products, but there are important considerations around therapeutic goods. The code provides a social media policy that sets out acceptable guidelines on photography, endorsements, testimonials and product promotion and it is expected that nurses and other health practitioners adhere to these.

Key considerations in the delivery of care

Unlike most other areas of nursing practice, cosmetic nursing is a potentially lucrative market that is at risk of being driven by sales and profit rather than the best interest of the patient. This can cause pressure on the delivery of services especially when the demands and expectations of patients are not in alignment with the reality of the planned treatment. It is also an area where incentives from major pharmaceutical companies or skincare companies may be provided to the nurse in the form of additional income, personal treatments or skincare product and this must be disclosed to the patient (Parliament of NSW, 2019). It is vital that advertising guidelines issued by the Therapeutic Goods Administration are followed to prevent misleading promotions and advertising (TGA, 2019a, TGA, 2019b).

It is important that nurses also recognise inappropriate treatment seeking behaviours such as people with Body Dysmorphic Disorder (BDD).

> Body Dysmorphic Disorder (BDD) is a type of mental illness where the individual perceives a serious defect in something about themselves that does not exist.

It is thought that this cohort is overly represented in the cosmetic medicine industry and one study (Conrado, 2009) estimated the prevalence rate of patients with BDD in a dermatology clinic to be up to 15%. Individuals with BDD seek out cosmetic treatments in order to reduce body dissatisfaction related to their appearance concerns and believe that changing their appearance with these treatments will resolve these appearance concerns (Verhoef & Mulkins, 2012). However, these treatments do not usually resolve their concerns and a high level of distress and concern remains or becomes heightened (Crerand et al., 2005; Wilhelm et al, 2014). It is imperative for cosmetic nurses to be aware of, screen for and refer people with BDD for appropriate assessment and treatment. Validated screening tools to assess for BDD are available (Danesh et al, 2015).

Australian practice contexts

As the uptake of products such as dermal fillers, botulinum toxin and energy-based treatments like laser, fat reduction and skin tightening have continued to grow, so opportunities for nurses to pursue career opportunities in this area have increased. The context of care for cosmetic nurses is variable. Nurses practice in collaboration with medical colleagues such as with cosmetic physicians, plastic surgeons or dermatologists in private or public healthcare settings. They can also work in nurse-led clinics or independently in private practice. Common domains within which they work include but are not limited to the provision of skin care advice and referral, skin cancer checks, management of common skin disorders, prescription of medical grade skin care products, laser and other light based therapies, skin resurfacing, removal of benign lesions, administration of dermal fillers, muscle relaxants and deoxycholic acid, skin tightening and mesotherapy.

It is of interest to note here that there is a discrete sub-specialty of cosmetic nurses self-identifying as 'nurse injectors' with a significantly reduced scope of practice compared to that described by O'Keefe and Kushelew (2016) where their role is primarily to exclusively administer dermal filler and muscle relaxants. Nurse injectors who have based their career and livelihood on this restricted scope of practice may be vulnerable if poison legislation, standards, policies or product change occur and they find themselves with eroded skills and limited opportunity.

High powered Class 4 lasers are used in cosmetic nursing for a number of different patient presentations including but not limited to the reduction of benign lesions, vascular abnormalities, pigmentation and tattoos and the resurfacing of skin for scars or rhytids. The legislation regarding the use of Class 4 lasers is variable across states and territories in Australia (ARPANSA, 2019). In Queensland, Tasmania and Western Australia nurses are required to comply with relevant legislation. The minimum national requirement according to the current *Safe use of lasers and intense light sources in health care* (SAI, 2018) is a laser/IPL safety certificate which should be renewed every two years to remain clinically relevant. In Queensland and Western Australia, a logbook of supervised hours is required by a full licence holder before signing off the competency for any clinician to independently practice, including nurses. A validated tool to assess a nurse's competency (or indeed any provider's competence) in laser and other energy-based therapies is not available and further research into this is warranted.

Professional exemplars from overseas

The United Kingdom (UK) (British Association of Cosmetic Nurses, 2013) and the United States of America (American Nurses Association, 2013, American Society of Plastic Surgical Nurses Inc, 2015, Plastic Surgical Nursing Certification Board, 2020) recognise that nurses working in a cosmetic medicine or aesthetic context are a specific cohort of the nursing profession. In the UK they are referred to as 'nurses in aesthetic medicine' while in the USA 'non-surgical aesthetic nursing' is recognised as being part of plastic surgical nursing. In the UK the British Association of Cosmetic Nurses has been established since 2010. BACN have in excess of 600 members and have developed educational frameworks, competencies and training. Their *Integrated Career and Competency Framework for Nurses in Aesthetic Medicine* builds on a previous 2007 Royal College of Nursing (RCN) document and continues to be accredited by RCN (British Association of Cosmetic Nurses, 2013). The American Society of Plastic Surgery Nurses (ASPSN) has been established since 1975 and has in excess of one thousand members. The mission of ASPSN is to employ education and research to promote practice excellence, nursing leadership, optimal patient safety, and outcomes by using evidence-based practice as a foundation of care. They hosted their first aesthetic symposium in 2004 and aesthetic nursing was affirmed as a significant part in their strategic direction at their 2014 conference and board meeting. (American Society of Plastic Surgical Nurses Inc, 2015). In the future, Australian cosmetic nurses will be charged with developing and validating their scope of practice and place in the health care landscape (NMBA, 2019; NMBA, 2015) and would do well to learn from their international counterparts.

Conclusion

The evidence indicates a role for nurses in the provision of cosmetic and related concerns, but the future is unclear. Cosmetic nursing in Australia is likely to evolve into a recognised specialty. To achieve this, cosmetic nurses will be charged with validating and further defining what their scope of practice is and how it is differentiated from dermatology nursing and plastic surgical nursing. The paucity of rigorous research reported in the peer reviewed literature is a concern as it essentially renders the work of this group invisible. Cosmetic nurses should be encouraged to conduct research and publish consistently as part of their post graduate education and daily work. A professional peer support network is essential to guide the development of the area and processes for licensure, endorsement, credentialing, validation or certification. The authors look forward to being involved in the evolution of this emerging context of practice.

Online resources

1 Allergan Australia (2016). *Medical Aesthetics Face Value Survey:* http://www.allerganmedicalinstitute.com.au/
2 Australian College of Nursing Cosmetic Nurses Graduate Certificate (2020): https://www.acn.edu.au/education/postgraduate-course/cosmetic-nursing
3 Australian College of Nursing Cosmetic Nurses Community of Interest (2020): https://www.acn.edu.au/membership/coi/coi-leads#cosmetic-nurses
4 International Society of Plastic and Aesthetic Nurses (ISPAN): http://ispan.org/

References

American Society for Aesthetic Plastic Surgery. (2017). Procedural Statistics. Retrieved August, 2019, from https://www.surgery.org/media/statistics.

American Nurses Association. (2013). Plastic Surgery Nursing: Scope and standards of practice. https://www.fishpond.com.au/Books/Plastic-Surgery-Nursing/9781558104822?utm_source=googleps&utm_medium=ps&utm_campaign=AU&gclid=CjwKCAiA-vLyBRBWEiwAzOkGVA1yzvEiJ6y7oiwxXyIzINmhwCWBxJggp52P1e6xuB4jHNi1EVssNRoCGV8QAvD_BwE

American Society of Plastic Surgical Nurses Inc. (2015). *Core Curriculum for Plastic Surgical Nurses.*

Australian Radiation Protection and Nuclear Safety Agency (ARPANSA). (2019). *Do I need a licence?* Retrieved February 17, 2020, from https://www.arpansa.gov.au/regulation-and-licensing/licensing/information-for-licence-applicants/do-i-need-a-licence.

Australian College of Nursing (2020). Personal communication with members of the Cosmetic Nurses Community of Interest.

Australian Health Ministers' Advisory Committee. (2011). *Cosmetic Medical and Surgical Procedures: A National Framework (Final Report).* Commonwealth of Australia. https://www.coaghealthcouncil.gov.au/Projects/Independent-Review-of-NRAS-finalised/ArtMID/524/ArticleID/82/Cosmetic-Medical-and-Surgical-Procedures-A-National-Framework

British Association of Cosmetic Nurses. (2013). *An integrated career and competency framework for nurses in aesthetic medicine.* British Association of Cosmetic Nurses. Cancer Council (2019). *Skin Cancer.* Retrieved September 26, 2019, from https://www.cancer.org.au/about-cancer/types-of-cancer/skin-cancer.html

Canadian Society of Aesthetics Specialty Nurses. (2019). Retrieved August 22, 2019, from https://csasn.org/

CB Insights. (2019). *Wellness Trends*. Retrieved September 26, 2019, from https://www.cbinsights. com/reports/CB-Insights_Wellness-Trends-2019.pdf?utm_campaign=wellness-trends_2019

Conrado, L. A. (2009). Body dysmorphic disorder in dermatology: Diagnosis, epidemiology and clinical aspects. *Anais Brasilieros de Dermatologia, 84*(6), 569–581. https://doi. org/10.1590/S0365-05962009000600002

Cosmetic Physicians College of Australia. (2016). *Australia's Spend On Cosmetic Treatments Tops $1 Billion: Non-surgical cosmetic treatments in Australia continue to soar* https://cpca.net. au/wp-content/uploads/2016/05/31-05-2016_AUSTRALIAS_SPEND_ON_COSMETIC_ TREATMENTS_TOPS_1_BILLION.pdf

Crerand, C. E., Phillips, K. A., Menard, W., & Fay, C. (2005). Nonpsychiatric medical treatment of body dysmorphic disorder. *Psychosomatics, 46*(6), 549–555. https://doi.org/10.1176/ appi.psy.46.6.549.

Danesh, M., Beroukhim, K., Nguyen, C., Levin, E., & Koo, J. (2015). Body dysmorphic disorder screening tools for the dermatologist: A systematic review. *Practical Dermatology* (February 2015). https://practicaldermatology.com/articles/2015-feb/body-dysmorphic-disorder-screening-tools-for-the-dermatologist-a-systematic-review-s?c4src=issue:feed

Duncan, A. (2018). *Aussies get more procedures per capita than America, spending over a billion dollars last year alone.* https://www.sbs.com.au/news/the-feed/australia-is-outdoing-the-us-in-cosmetic-surgery

Fardouly, J., & Vartanian, L. R. (2016). Social media and body image concerns: Current research and future directions. *Current Opinion in Psychology, 9*, 1–5. https://doi.org/10.1016/j. copsyc.2015.09.005

Ferencak, K. (2019, August 10). *Tempted to tweak? Here's our guide.* Body+Soul. https:// www.bodyandsoul.com.au/beauty/how-to/tempted-to-tweak-heres-our-guide/news-story/ f1b15eb26b7668225ac097e3bd578a5d

Goh, C. L. (2009). The Need for Evidence-Based Aesthetic Dermatology Practice. *Journal of Cutaneous and Aesthetic Surgery, 2*(2), 65–71. https://doi.org/10.4103/0974-2077.58518

Heiskanen, V., & Hamblin, M. (2018). Photobiomodulation: Lasers *vs.* light emitting diodes?' *Photochemical and Photobiological Science, 17*, 1003–1017. https://doi.org/10.1039/ C8PP90049C

Latouff, A. (2017). *Call for tighter regulation at beauty salons offering cosmetic injections.* https://www.abc.net.au/news/2017-08-31/injections-by-beauty-salons-unacceptable,-surgeons-say/8861120

Konda, D., & Thappa, D. M. (2013). Mesotherapy: What is new?. *Indian Journal of Dermatology, Venereology and Leprology, 79*, 127–34. http://doi.org/10.4103/0378-6323.104689

Nursing and Midwifery Board of Australia. (2019). *Fact sheet: Advanced nursing practice and specialty areas within nursing.* Retrieved February 17, 2020, from https://www.nursingmidwiferyboard.gov.au/Codes-Guidelines-Statements/FAQ/fact-sheet-advanced-nursing-practice-and-specialty-areas.aspx

Nursing and Midwifery Board of Australia. (2015). *Position statement on specialist recognition and the nursing profession.* Retrieved February 17, 2020, from https://www.nursingmidwiferyboard.gov.au/News/2015-02-18-position-statement.aspx

O'Keefe, E. J., & Hoitink, S. (2013). Pioneering a cosmetic, skin rejuvenation and aesthetic nursing model of practice. *Australian Nursing Journal, 21*(2), 36–37.

O'Keefe, E. J., & Kushelew, I. (2016). Asserting credibility and capability: Professional practice standards in Australia. *Journal of Aesthetic Nursing, 5*(2).

Parliament of NSW. (2019). *Cosmetic Health Service Complaints in New South Wales.* Retrieved September 26, 2019, from https://www.parliament.nsw.gov.au/ladocs/inquiries/ 2476/Final%20Report%20-%20Cosmetic%20Health%20Service%20Complaints%20in% 20New%20South%20Wales.PDF

Plastic Surgical Nursing Certification Board. (2020). Get Certified: CANS from https://psncb. org/CANS/

SAI. (2018). *Safe use of lasers and intense light sources in health care 4173: 2018*. SAI Global. https://infostore.saiglobal.com/en-us/Standards/AS-NZS-4173-2018-99065_SAIG_AS_AS_208306/

Therapeutic Goods Advisory (TGAa). (2019). *Advertising: Sample social media acceptable use policy*. Retrieved September 26, 2019, from https://www.tga.gov.au/advertising-sample-social-media-acceptable-use-policy

Therapeutic Goods Advisory (TGAb). (2019). *Cosmetic injections*. Retrieved February 18, 2019, from https://www.tga.gov.au/cosmetic-injections

Verhoef, M. J., & Mulkins, A. (2012). The healing experience-how can we capture it? *Explore (NY), 8*(4), 231–236. https://doi.org/10.1016/j.explore.2012.04.005

Wilhelm, S., Phillips, K. A., Didie, E., Buhlmann, U., Greenberg, J. L., Fama, J. M., et al. (2014). Modular cognitive-behavioral therapy for body dysmorphic disorder: A randomized controlled trial. *Behavior Therapy, 45*(3), 314–327. https://doi.org/10.1016/j.beth.2013.12.007

22 Nursing in the Australian correctional system

Linda Starr and Claire Newman

Chapter objectives

This chapter will offer the reader:

- An overview of the key characteristics of the Australian prison population.
- Insight into the complexity of health issues experienced by incarcerated individuals.
- A description of what nursing in the prison environment involves.
- An overview of the challenges faced by nurses working in the prison environment.

Introduction

There are more than one hundred public and private correctional centres across Australia providing minimum, medium and maximum security facilities for men and women. In addition to correctional centres, there are remand centres, pre-release centres, forensic mental health facilities and juvenile detention centres.

> Individuals charged with a criminal offense may be ordered by a court to be held in a remand centre until their trial or sentencing. Pre-release centres have programs that support incarcerated persons to be gradually released from custody to the community. Forensic mental health facilities provide care to patients with a mental illness who have been in contact with the criminal justice system. Juvenile detention centres detain young offenders who have been remanded in, or sentence to, custody.

Nurses are the largest health work force in the correctional system. Nurses attend to incarcerated individuals for assessment upon reception into the prison through to their transfer back into the community. Although there are no specific practice standards developed, nurses are bound by their code of ethics, conduct and professional standards to deliver high quality evidence-based nursing care to those seeking health care in prison.

Key characteristics of the Australian prison population

As of June 2018 there were just over 40,000 adults incarcerated in Australia (Australian Bureau of Statistics, 2018b). New South Wales (NSW) has the largest prisoner population (32%), followed by Queensland (21%), Victoria (18%), Western

Australia (16%), South Australia (7%), Northern Territory (4%), Australian Capital Territory (1%) and Tasmania (1%) (Australian Bureau of Statistics, 2018b). Males account for more than 90% of the Australian adult prison population (Australian Bureau of Statistics, 2018b).

Aboriginality

More than a quarter (approximately 11,000) of incarcerated adults, and more than half (approximately 500) of incarcerated young people in Australia, are Aboriginal (Australian Bureau of Statistics, 2018b; Australian Institute of Health and Welfare, 2018). This is a vast overrepresentation of Aboriginal people in custody compared to 2% found in the non-Aboriginal population (Australian Bureau of Statistics, 2018a). Incarcerated Aboriginal people have higher rates of mental health problems and chronic health conditions compared to non-Aboriginal Australians (Indig, McEntyre, Page & Ross, 2009). Aboriginal people in custody are likely to be affected by inter-generational trauma (Sivak & Cantley, 2017). Aboriginal persons in prison require culturally appropriate nursing care; see Chapter 6 for more information on providing culturally appropriate nursing care.

Aboriginal people in Australia have experienced trauma as a result of historical events. Trauma associated with the colonisation of Indigenous land includes exposure to violence, forced removal of children, displacement from Country and institutionalisation. Trauma may be passed down from those who experienced it directly to future generations through destructive behaviours, parenting practices, family disintegration, and mental health issues. This is known as intergenerational trauma.

Social disadvantage

Socially disadvantaged minority groups are also overrepresented in the prison population (Binswanger, Redmond, Steiner, and Hicks, 2012). This includes people with intellectual and developmental disabilities. Incarcerated individuals are more likely than persons in the general community to have: been placed in care as a child, had a parent incarcerated during their childhood; left school without qualifications; and been incarcerated previously (Justice Health and Forensic Mental Health Network, 2017). They are also likely to have been homeless and/ or had limited utilisation of health services prior to incarceration. Social disadvantage is associated with poorer physical and mental health outcomes and has been attributed to the escalation of age-related illnesses in incarcerated adults (Baidawi et al., 2011).

Complex health issues of incarcerated individuals

Incarcerated individuals, as a population, generally have complex health issues. Co-morbidity of health conditions further adds to the complexity of health issues of incarcerated individuals; having physical, mental and substance misuse disorders is a frequent occurrence. Prison nurses need to understand the implications of co-morbidity of disorders with regards to the management of patient care.

Chronic health conditions

Chronic health conditions are more prevalent in incarcerated individuals compared to the general population and include hepatitis C, hypertension, asthma, diabetes and arthritis (Justice Health and Forensic Mental Health Network, 2017).

Mental health conditions

Mental health conditions are more prevalent in the prison population than in the community. Depression and anxiety are the most common mental health disorders reported by incarcerated individuals. For example, in NSW 38% of incarcerated individuals participating in a health survey reported having been diagnosed with depression, 25% with anxiety, 17% with psychosis, and 10% with Post-Traumatic Stress Disorder (Justice Health and Forensic Mental Health Network, 2017). There is also a high prevalence of suicide and self-harm behaviours amongst incarcerated individuals.

Substance misuse disorders

Substance withdrawal is a common health concern for persons entering the prison system. In NSW, more than 85% of incarcerated individuals participating in a health survey reported having misused drugs other than alcohol, 20% reported drug abuse or dependence, and 13% reported alcohol abuse or dependence (Justice Health and Forensic Mental Health Network, 2017). Drug use, including injecting drugs, in prison is also common (Kinner, Jenkinson, Gouillou and Milloy, 2012). Incarcerated individuals have access to drug and alcohol health services in prison. In NSW, it is estimated that one in 10 prisoners will be participating in a prison-based methadone program (Justice Health and Forensic Mental Health Network, 2017).

Ageing prison population

There are a rising number of elderly individuals incarcerated in the prison system. Older incarcerated adults are five times more likely to have chronic health conditions such as hypertension, heart disease and diabetes (Field & Archer, 2019). The management of dementia, impaired cognitive-function and physical disability in older prisoners have also been recognised as key challenges for prison-based health services (Field & Archer, 2019; Patterson, Newman & Doona, 2016).

What does nursing in the prison system involve?

Nurses in the prison system are responsible for providing routine heath care to incarcerated individuals. Providing routine health care includes: administering medications, providing counselling and health promotion, conducting physical exams, providing first aid and completing referrals to specialist services. Nursing management of individuals in the prison system also forms part of the nursing role in prison. This includes: undertaking comprehensive health assessments; and planning, implementing and evaluating care. Nurses are also responsible for undertaking health screening for individuals entering the prison system. Components of the prison nursing role are outlined below:

- **Drug and alcohol:** Prison nurses are responsible for the assessment and management of drug and/or alcohol intoxication and withdrawal. Nurses also undertake the assessment and review of individuals receiving Opioid Substitution Treatment.
- **Primary care:** Prison nurses are responsible for the management of acute and chronic health conditions. Sub-specialities of primary care nursing in the prison system include women's health, older person's health, and end-of-life care.
- **Population health:** Prison nurses undertake the screening and management of blood-borne viruses and sexually transmissible infections. Prison nurses also provide public health services including disease prevention (immunisation, surveillance and infection control), communicable diseases outbreak management, environmental health, and health promotion and education.
- **Adolescent health:** Nursing care of young people in juvenile detention centres involves the management of acute health conditions, sexual health care and pregnancy-related care. There is a focus on collaborative working with a range of agencies (including education and health-based programs) provided to incarcerated young people.
- **Mental health:** Prison nurses with postgraduate mental health qualifications may have a specialist role in providing case management based nursing care to incarcerated individuals with severe mental disorders who have complex mental health needs. Care is provided to individuals housed in specialist mental health units within the prison system and to individuals located in the mainstream prison population.
- **Forensic mental health:** Nurses with postgraduate mental health qualifications, or nurses undertaking a Transition to Practice Program, may specialise in forensic mental health. Nurses working in forensic mental health provide care to mentally disordered offenders; otherwise known as forensic patients. Forensic mental health patients may be cared for within specialist prison-based units or in secure hospital environments. Forensic mental health nursing involves working with a multidisciplinary team to provide mental health assessment and intensive treatment.

Challenges faced by nurses working in the prison environment

Delivering high quality health care in the prison environment can be challenging (Pont et al., 2018). The culture of correctional services is focused on security and risk management. The physical nature of the setting is characterised by high walls securing the perimeters of the buildings, surveillance technology and internal bars, locked doors, segregation, and limited freedom of movement. The environment created as a result is embedded in control, security, discipline and order (Walsh, Freshwater, and Fisher 2012). Outside of emergencies, nursing access to prisoners is governed by custodial priorities and prison policy. Activities related to security and order, such as the transfers of incarcerated individuals between prisons and prisoner-behaviour management, take precedence over the delivery of planned nursing care. This can frustrate the efforts of nursing staff in delivering health education and primary health care to a mobile population.

Box 22.1 - Case study (Max)

Max is a 67-year-old prisoner who according to the correctional officers has become increasingly agitated over the past few weeks and his behaviour is disturbing other prisoners. The correctional officers are asking the nurse for Max's medical notes and for the nurse to give Max something to make him sleep and be more manageable. Max tells the nurse he is fine but worried that the correctional officers are going to make him take medication that will reduce his control and awareness of his surroundings. Max also tells the nurse that he is worried about his wife who is unwell and asks the nurse to take a note he has written and personally deliver this to her.

Reflective questions:

1 What steps should the nurse take in addressing the correctional officers' concerns?
2 Does Max have the right to refuse treatment?
3 Should the nurse take the letter to Max's wife in the hope this will help Max become more settled?
4 Do the correctional officers have a right to Max's case notes?
5 How should the nurse respond to the correctional officers' requests?

The conflict between care and custody

The tension between the philosophical ideologies underpinning health and security is often referred to as a conflict between care and custody (Dhaliwal and Hirst, 2016: Hörberg, 2015; Hernandez-Sherwood, 2012; Walsh, Freshwater, and Fisher 2012). It is vital that nurses working in the prison environment recognise the potential impact of this tension on developing and maintaining a therapeutic relationship with their patients. Nurses also need to ensure that they continue to work from a nursing perspective and not a custodial one; avoiding becoming institutionalised in a system where security is prioritised over health care. For instance, nurses should not be involved in security issues such as body cavity searches, use of restraint/force, or decisions on punishment. Nevertheless, it is important that the nurse understands and adheres to the policies and practices regarding safety and security that are enforced in the prison setting in order to contribute to maintaining a safe environment. This includes forming respectful and collaborative professional relationships with correctional officers.

Ethical considerations

Nurses working in correctional settings need to be cognisant of the ethical issues that present in this forum and the challenges that may impact on ethical decision making. It is important in adhering to the principle of justice that nurses fairly and equally distribute nursing care and resources to patients without discrimination. This requires a non-judgemental approach with a focus on the health needs of the patient and not the crime for which they have been incarcerated for (Jacob, 2014; Dhaliwal and Hirst, 2016). Despite their incarceration, individuals still have a right to consent and refuse treatment and the nurse has a duty to ensure that this is upheld. Due to the nature of the setting, and the need for security, there is little privacy in correctional settings.

Prison nurses, however, have an obligation to preserve patients' confidentiality regarding their health care.

Professional boundaries

Maintaining professional boundaries is crucial in prison-based nursing in the development and maintenance of the therapeutic relationship (Dhaliwal & Hirst 2016). This will also help ensure the nurse approaches the delivery of care objectively and will help them avoid manipulation tactics of individuals who may use such strategies to access health care.

Vicarious trauma

Nurses working in the prison environment are at risk of experiencing vicarious trauma in response to repeated exposure to traumatic material in their professional role (Newman, Eason & Kinghorn, 2019). Traumatic material may be in the form of listening to the personal trauma histories of incarcerated individuals, reading about violent crimes committed, or being exposed to the details of violent incidents that have occurred in the workplace. A nurse with vicarious trauma may experience psychological distress, similar to the symptoms of Post-Traumatic Stress Disorder. Prison-based nurses should be aware of the effects of vicarious trauma, employ strategies to minimise the impact of vicarious trauma and actively promote self-wellbeing.

> Vicarious traumatisation occurs as the result of repeated or extreme indirect exposure to aversive details of traumatic events. Professionals working with traumatised clients are at risk of vicarious trauma.

Conclusion

This chapter discussed the role of prison-based nursing and explored a range of issues faced by nurses working in the Australian prison system. Incarcerated individuals have complex health needs; chronic health conditions, mental health conditions and substance misuse disorders are highly prevalent. The diverse and complex nature of the prison population highlights the need for compassionate high-quality accessible health care for those incarcerated. Balancing the caring role of the nurse with the need to contribute to the security priorities of the institution is what makes correctional nursing a unique and dynamic role in health care.

Online resources

1 Educational resources for correctional nurses (American): https://correctional-nurse.net/
2 Essentials of Correctional Nursing Blog (American): https://essentialsofcorrectionalnursing.com/
3 Forensic mental health nursing resources: https://www.apna.org/i4a/pages/index.cfm?pageid=4653

References

Australian Bureau of Statistics. (2018a). *Australian Demographic Statistics, Sep 2018*. Canberra: Australian Bureau of Statistics.

Australian Bureau of Statistics. (2018b). *Prisoners in Australia, 2018*. Canberra: Australian Bureau of Statistics.

Australian Institute of Health and Welfare. (2018). *Youth detention population in Australia 2018*. Canberra: AIHW.

Baidawi, S., Turner, S., Trotter, C., Browning, C., Collier, P., O'Connor, D., & Sheehan, R. (2011). Older prisoners - a challenge for Australian corrections [online]. Trends and Issues in Crime and Criminal Justice. Retrieved 18 Jun 19 https://search.informit.com.au/documentSummary;dn=711433717814344;res=IELAPA

Binswanger, I., Redmond, N., Steiner, J., and L Hicks, (2012) Health Disparities and the Criminal Justice System: An Agenda for Further Research and Action. Journal of Urban Health: Bulletin of the New York Academy of Medicine, Vol. 89, No. 1

Dhaliwal, K., & Hirst S. (2016). Caring in Correctional Nursing: A Systematic Search and Narrative Synthesis. *Journal of Forensic Nursing, 12*(1), 5–12.

Field, C., & Archer, V. (2019). Comparing health status, disability, and access to care in older and younger inmates in the New South Wales corrections system. *International Journal of Prisoner Health, 15*(2), 153–161. doi: 10.1108/IJPH-04-2018-0017

Hernandez-Sherwood, C. (2012). Correctional facility nursing. *Minority Nurse*, 15–19.

Hörberg, U. (2015). Caring science and the development of forensic psychiatric caring. *Perspectives in Psychiatric Care, 51*(4), 277–284. doi:10.1111/ppc.12092.

Indig, D., McEntyre, E., Page, J., & Ross, B. (2009). *2009 NSW Inmate Health Survey: Aboriginal Health Report*. Sydney: Justice Health.

Jacob, J. D. (2014). Understanding the domestic rupture in forensic psychiatric nursing practice. *Journal of Correctional Health Care, 20*(1), 45–58. doi: 10.1177/1078345813505444.

Justice Health and Forensic Mental Health Network. (2017). *2015 Network Patient Health Survey Report*. Sydney, Australia.

Justice Health and Forensic Mental Health Network, & Juvenile Justice NSW. (2017). *2015 Young People in Custody Health Survey: Full Report*. Sydney: Justice Health and Forensic Mental Health Network.

Kinner, S., Jenkinson, R.,Gouillou, M., and Milloy, M. (2012). High-risk drug-use practices among a large sample of Australian prisoners Drug and Alcohol Dependence. Volume 126, Issues 1–2, 1 November 2012, Pages 156–160

Newman, C., Eason, M., & Kinghorn, G. (2019). Incidence of Vicarious Trauma in Correctional Health and Forensic Mental Health Staff in New South Wales, Australia. *Journal of Forensic Nursing, 15*(3), 183–192. doi: 10.1097/jfn.0000000000000245

Patterson, K., Newman, C., & Doona, K. (2016). Improving the care of older persons in Australian prisons using the Policy Delphi method. *Dementia, 15*(5), 1219–1233. doi: 10.1177/1471301214557531

Pont, J., Enggist, S., Stover, H., Willimas, B., Greifinder, R., & Wolff H. (2018). Prison Health Care Governance: Guaranteeing Clinical Independence. *American Journal of Public Health, 108*(4), 472–476.

Sivak, L., & Cantley, L. (2017). *Model of Care for Aboriginal Prisoner Health and Well-being for South Australia*. South Australia: South Australian Prison Health Service.

Walsh, E., Freshwater, D., & Fisher, P. (2012). Caring for prisoners: Towards mindful practice. *Journal of Research in Nursing, 18*, 158–168. doi.org/10.1177/1744987112466086.

23 Women's health nursing

Charrlotte Seib and Debra Anderson

Chapter objectives

This chapter provides the reader with:

- An outline of the influence of sex and gender on health
- Insight into the health issues facing women and girls across the lifespan
- A description of how nurses contribute to the advancement of women's health
- An overview of the challenges for nurses working in this area

Introduction

Men and women differ in the ways they experience and respond to health and illness. Understanding how these differences translate into healthcare is important for nurses seeking to provide patient-centred care. This chapter explores the health of women, both biologically and psychosocially, with the goal of informing optimal care.

> Historically, the terms 'sex' and 'gender' and been used interchangeably but there is some important difference should be noted. Sex refers to the biological characteristics that define females and males whereas gender refers to the socially constructed norms that define the roles, expectations and behaviours of men, women, boys and girls

Women's health in Australia

In the past century, women's health has been transformed through medical advancements and improved living standards. However, while women are generally living longer, they are not necessarily healthier (United Nations [UN], 2015). Among Australian women, mental health concerns (anxiety, depressive and drug use disorders) account for half of all disease burden during the middle years, while in women aged 50 years and over, cancer, heart disease and Alzheimer's disease (70 years and older) are significant contributors to health loss (Australian Institute of Health and Welfare [AIHW], 2019a, 2019b; Department of Health, 2018). Furthermore, around half (49%) of Australian women are living with one or more common chronic health condition and the proportion increases in women aged 65 and older (83%) and in some population groups (AIHW, 2019a). For example, women from Aboriginal and Torres Strait Islander backgrounds, culturally or linguistically diverse backgrounds, who are socially or geographically isolated or impoverished, report more risk factors for chronic disease, have less access to quality health care and experience greater relative disease burden (AIHW, 2019a, 2019b; Department of Health, 2018).

According to the National Women's Health Strategy 2020–2030 Australian priority populations include: Aboriginal and Torres Strait Islander women; Pregnant women and their children; Culturally and linguistically diverse women and girls; Members of the lesbian, gay, bisexual, transgender, intersex and queer community; Women and girls from low socioeconomic backgrounds; Women and girls from rural and remote areas; Women and girls living with disability and their carers;and Women and girls affected by the criminal justice system.

Priority areas for Australian women's health

In 2018, the Australian government released the National Women's Health Strategy 2020-2030 (Department of Health, 2018). To drive change and optimise the health of women and girls, five priority areas are being targeted:

Sexual and reproductive health

Maternal, sexual and reproductive health continues to be a determinant of health for Australian females. Since 2015, sexually transmissible infections (STIs) like chlamydia and gonorrhoea have risen in women aged 20–29 years, those living outside major metropolitan centres, and Aboriginal and Torres Strait Islander women (Kirby Institute, 2018). Sexual health literacy can be improved through the availability of appropriate health information and access to clinical services (Department of Health, 2018).

Healthy ageing

The Australia healthcare system is under increasing pressure due to the increasing complexity of older women's health and the prevalence of multiple morbidities. Healthy aging requires acknowledgement of the factors that impact health-related quality of life as they age and better management of the needs of women across the life course (Department of Health, 2018).

Chronic disease and preventive health

More than one-third of chronic disease could be prevented by eliminating key modifiable risk factors (World Health Organisation [WHO], 2005). Among Australian women, tobacco smoking and alcohol consumption remains low, although physical activity and overweight and obesity are increasing (Department of Health, 2018). Investment in awareness and prevention of key risk factors to prevent chronic disease are needed (Department of Health, 2018).

Mental health and wellbeing

Australian women experience a higher proportion of some mental health conditions like anxiety, depression, post-traumatic stress and eating disorders than men

(AIHW, 2019b). Women are also disproportionately affected by a range of life events (pregnancy, motherhood, menopause, caring for others, violence, perinatal loss and socioeconomic disadvantage) which contribute to poor mental health outcomes (AIHW, 2019a, 2019b; Department of Health, 2018).

Conditions where women are overrepresented

Around one in six women have experienced physical and/or sexual violence by an intimate partner, and for many, violence is recurring (Australian Bureau of Statistics [ABS], 2017). Domestic and interpersonal violence against women is a pervasive problem for many Australian women linked with reduced mental health, physical function and general health (Department of Health, 2018).

Women's health nursing beyond childbearing

Women's Health Nurses (WHNs) play an essential role in providing affordable, equitable and accessible healthcare for women across the life course (Australian Women's Health Nurse Association [AWHNA], 2015). The roles of WHNs can include both health promotion, education and direct clinical care and the support of women through community development, advocacy, policy and research in a variety of service contexts (AWHNA, 2019).

Changes in oestrogen levels during menopausal transition can cause the vaginal mucosa to become thinner, drier and less elastic or flexible and change vaginal discharge (North American Menopause Society [NAMS], 2019). Given Alice's age, an age-related reduction in oestrogen comes to mind as a potential cause however, other explanations include

- infection (fungal, bacterial or viral)
- vaginismus (involuntary spasms of the vaginal muscles)
- urinary tract infections or irritation
- cancer
- dermatological conditions

Box 23.1 - Case study (Alice)

Alice is a 50-year-old woman living in a small town around 1 hour from Adelaide. As the nurse on duty, you introduce yourself and invite Alice into a private consulting room. You begin by asking Alice 'What brings you to the clinic today?'. She stares at you and then looks down. You notice that she is rubbing her hands together and you suspect that she might be nervous or embarrassed. Alice explains that her vaginal discharge has recently changed, and she has been experiencing irritation and itchiness for several months. She has no pain, no urinary symptoms and no fever. You explain to Alice that you need to examine her and potentially do some tests. Her pelvic examination is unremarkable, and her abdomen is benign, with no lumps or pain.

Reflective questions:
1 What other questions would you ask Alice about her presenting health concern?
2 What other information would you gather before you examine her?
3 Are there any tests you would recommend?

Box 23.2 - Case study (Alice II)

Reflecting on Alice's symptoms, you decide to ask some more questions not only about her reason for presentation but also about her sexual and reproductive history. You ascertain that the discharge is thin, slightly yellow in colour and has a slightly unpleasant odour; it started about three months ago, shortly after she started having sex with a man she met through a dating site. He is 58 years of age, and they did not use a condom because 'at his age, what are the chances he has a disease. After all, he is newly divorced, too'.

Reflective questions:

1 With the additional information you have just received, does this change your clinical judgement about the possible causes of the discharge?
2 Does this change the tests you would recommend?
3 What additional education/information would you provide Alice?

As rates of separation and divorce have risen, so too have the numbers of midlife and older adults re-partnering and engaging in casual sex. However, condom use remains low (Schick et al., 2010), and rates of sexually transmissible infections (STIs) have doubled in recent years (Lyons et al., 2017). Research has also suggested that older women often feel ill-equipped to negotiate safer sex and condom use (Morison & Cook, 2015) and lack knowledge about and the importance of safer sex (Lyons et al., 2017).

At the same time, older women often experience ageism regarding their sexual health, despite many women wanting the opportunity to discuss their sexual health needs and concerns (Fileborn et al., 2017). Thus, one of the priority actions for the National Women's Health Strategy 2020-2030 is to 'Recognise and equip health care practitioners to support women's sexual wellbeing as they age' to better provide information to midlife and older women on sexual wellbeing (including STIs) (Department of Health, 2018).

Midlife women can also experience menopause-related weight gain (Nejat, Polotsky, & Pal, 2010) and are less likely to comply with lifestyle recommendations (Mishra, Cooper, & Kuh, 2010). However, positive changes in lifestyle behaviours at this time are also likely to maximise opportunities for successful aging (Avis, Colvin, Bromberger, & Hess, 2018). Because of the complexities associated with aging, women's health nursing has evolved into a range of diverse roles not only the provision of

---

Box 23.3 - Case study (Alice III)

From your history, it appears that Alice's knowledge of sexual health is limited, and you believe that she would benefit from information and support. You discuss the tests that you have performed, including a full sexual health screen and cervical screening test, and you provide her with written information to compliment the information you have already provided. You ask Alice to return in one week for the test results.

Reflective questions:

1 Given Alice's age and personal circumstances, is there any additional information you would gather?
2 What other health information do you think would be of benefit to Alice?

direct clinical care, health education and promotion, but also community development, advocacy and evaluation activities across woman's lifespan.

Summary

Women's health nurses provide comprehensive and holistic care for women across
the life course. For many disadvantaged women, women's health nurses provide
effective women-centred care that facilitates assess and participation in health education and promotion activities and clinical care. The National Women's Health
Strategy 2020–2030 (Department of Health, 2018), provides an opportunity for
nurses to expand and improve their practice in relation to the provision of effective
and essential care for women. The five priority areas provide a blueprint for nurses
to effectively target their nursing practice to drive change and improve health for
women and girls.

References

Australian Bureau of Statistics. (2017). *Personal safety survey 2016*. Canberra, Australia:
   Australian Bureau of Statistics.
Australian Institute of Health and Welfare. (2019a). *The health of Australia's females*. Canberra,
   Australia: Australian Institute of Health and Welfare.
Australian Institute of Health and Welfare. (2019b). *Australian burden of disease study: Impact
   and causes of illness and death in Australia 2015*. Canberra, Australia: Australian Institute of
   Health and Welfare.
Australian Women's Health Nurse Association [AWHNA]. (2015). Essentials of Care. Retrieved
   from https://www.womenshealthnurses.asn.au/download/essentials-of-care-2/.
Avis, N. E., Colvin, A., Bromberger, J. T., & Hess, R. (2018). Midlife predictors of health-related
   quality of life in older women. *J Gerontol A*, 73(11), 1574–1580. doi:10.1093/gerona/gly062
Department of Health. (2018). *National women's health strategy 2020–2030*. Canberra,
   Australia: Department of Health.
Fileborn, B., Lyons, A., Heywood, W., Hinchliff, S., Malta, S., Dow, B., Minichiello, V. (2017).
   Talking to healthcare providers about sex in later life: findings from a qualitative study
   with older Australian men and women. *Australasian Journal of Ageing*, 36(4), E50–e56.
   doi:10.1111/ajag.12450
Kirby Institute. (2018). *HIV, viral hepatitis and sexually transmissible infections in Australia:
   Annual surveillance report 2018*. Sydney: Kirby Institute, UNSW Sydney.
Lyons, A., Heywood, W., Fileborn, B., Minichiello, V., Barrett, C., Brown, G., Crameri, P.
   (2017). Sexually active older Australian's knowledge of sexually transmitted infections and
   safer sexual practices. *Australian and New Zealand Journal of Public Health*, 41(3), 259–261.
   doi:10.1111/1753-6405.12655
Mishra, G. D., Cooper, R., & Kuh, D. (2010). A life course approach to reproductive health:
   theory and methods. *Maturitas*, 65(2), 92–97.
Morison, T., & Cook, C. (2015). Midlife safer sex challenges for heterosexual New Zealand
   women re-partnering or in casual relationships. *Journal of Primary Health Care*, 7(2),
   137–144.
Nejat, E. J., Polotsky, A. J., & Pal, L. (2010). Predictors of chronic disease at midlife and
   beyond-the health risks of obesity. *Maturitas*, 65(2), 106–111.
North American Menopause Society. (2019). Sexual Health & Menopause. Retrieved from
   https://www.menopause.org/for-women/sexual-health-menopause-online

Schick, V., Herbenick, D., Reece, M., Sanders, S. A., Dodge, B., Middlestadt, S. E., & Fortenberry, J. D. (2010). Sexual behaviors, condom use, and sexual health of Americans over 50: implications for sexual health promotion for older adults. *The Journal of Sexual Medicine,* 7(s5), 315–329. doi:10.1111/j.1743-6109.2010.02013.x

United Nations, Department of Economic and Social Affairs, Population Division. (2015). *World population ageing 2015.* New York, USA: United Nations.

World Health Organization. (2005). *Preventing chronic diseases: A vital investment.* Geneva, Switzerland: World Health Organization.

24 Nursing men

Andrew Smith, Blake Peck and Daniel Terry

Chapter objectives

This chapter will offer the reader:

- What does it mean to be male?
- Key influences on the health of men today
- Insights into men and their health needs and priorities
- An insight into nursing men in the society irrespective of context
- Challenges for nurses caring for men
- Future challenges to nursing men

Males represent 49.6% of the population; however, they experience a greater burden of disease and are more likely to die younger from preventable causes than females (AIHW, 2019). While males experience a greater burden of health and illness, there are some broader principles that inform the nursing of men. *Men* are not a homogenous group that behave, work or experience the world in the same way; differences exist that impact how men experience health and engage health services (AIHW, 2019). This chapter offers nurses an overview of the points of difference among men, the health issues they experience and key insights into how to better engage and promote the health and wellbeing of men.

> Gender defines characteristics of men and women that are socially constructed, whereas sex refers to characteristics that are biologically determined and impact health. People are born male or female but learn to be men and women. This learned behaviour makes up gender identity and determines gender roles, which also impacts health (WHO, 2001).

The iconoclast of Aussie men has deep roots from colonial days shaped by the gold rush miner, bushranger rebel, Gallipoli digger and the struggling shearer (Webb, 2013). Contemporary imagery of the Aussie male embodies the idealised working-class, beer-swilling, stoic larrikin, which has led to a normalised, yet powerfully entrenched concept of the Australian 'bloke' (Gottschall, 2014).

Until now, the health of the stereotypical toughened Australian man has been long ignored. The Australian Government has developed the nation's first National Male Health Policy (NMHP) (2010), recently updated in 2019, that places the health challenges encountered by men at the forefront of the national health agenda. The policy outlines six priority areas for action which include developing optimal health outcomes, ensuring health equity between different groups of men and different life stages, increasing preventive health, building a strong evidence base and improving access to healthcare. The NMHP offers vital contemporary insights that inform the way nurses can better care for this population group, while highlighting key health issues, contexts and consideration that need to be considered among nurses now and in the future (Commonwealth of Australia, 2010).

What are the influences on men's health?

Expectations of gender

In early life, men are exposed to traditional, local and global expectations that are associated with *hegemonic masculinity*. Hegemonic identities are often underpinned by a tendency toward dominant social positions even in instances where the man does not feel powerful, or does not dominate anyone (Blum et al., 2017). Hegemonic ideas form in early to adolescent years through the portrayal of gendered roles where boys are strong, powerful and independent, and all that is not hegemonic is not male nor valued (Blum et al., 2017). Importantly, this view of masculinity is not fixed, yet represents the masculinity which occupies the dominant position and speaks largely to societal and patriarchal influences that are so often portrayed by men in authority and exert an influence across the society (Connell, 2005). While these expectations of men often afford greater opportunity and perceived power, in comparison to females, hegemonic ideas have been shown to impact the health of men into adult life.

> Hegemony as a singular term relates to the concept of dominance, power and authority within a culture. Hegemonic masculinity is characterised by attributes such as strength, independence and lack of vulnerability (Connell, 2005).

Men and risk

Hegemonic ideas operate to define what it means to be a man in society and place pressure on younger men to conform to the dominant ideology often with developmental consequences (Blum et al., 2017). Amin et al. (2018) suggest that men aged 15–24 years are exposed to distinct risks and vulnerabilities that tend to be gendered such as higher rates of road-traffic accidents as well as suicide, alcohol and drug use, with alcohol and drug use featuring highly as a related risk behaviour. Ultimately, behaviours learned in early adulthood will often contribute to risk in later life (Amin et al., 2018).

Cancers and risk

Cancer in Australian men, particularly, bowel, lung and prostate rank highly and pose a considerable burden in terms of mortality and morbidity. Prostate cancer is the most commonly diagnosed male cancer with rates of incidence and mortality increasing with age (AIHW, 2019). Australia has one of the highest global incidences of prostate cancer with 18,000 men diagnosed and 3,500 deaths in 2018 (AIHW, 2019;

Kannan et al., 2018). Despite initiatives focused on improved screening and treatment, traditional views of masculinity, perceptions of sexual function, attitudes to health-care, and health seeking behaviours of men seem to impede diagnosis and treatment (Kannan et al., 2018). In fact, men may often delay seeking initial medical advice and symptom knowledge about cancer. Ultimately, men have a tendency to delay further investigation until symptoms worsen or are prolonged (Fish et al., 2019). This presents a unique risk in this area for men, but also an opportunity for nurses. Currently there are no men's health centres or men's health nurse specific roles; however, the ground is shifting and nurses have adapted to the needs of men in many ways. For example, community mental health nurses may regularly engage men in various non-traditional health context to facilitate mental health support. It is in these contemporary contexts where the role of nurses needs to be considered when nursing men.

Nursing men in society irrespective of the context

Irrespective of the clinical context, it is likely that men play important roles in the lives of the people you are caring for. For example, as a husband, son, father and grandfa-ther each of whom may exert important roles in influencing the life of the person in your direct care. If genuinely providing family-centred care, it is imperative that male members of that family are considered. Nurses therefore have an obligation to involve men in discussions, in decision-making and to recognise that the roles and responsi-bilities of men vary within each family. Genuinely hearing and seeking to understand men is central to sound nursing practice.

Addressing men's health in community settings

Although men access the health system less frequently than women, recent data from the National Men's Health Strategy 2020–2030 shows that the trend of men accessing healthcare is increasing (Commonwealth of Australia, 2019). However, fewer interac-tions with the healthcare system leads to fewer opportunities for health professionals to ask the right questions, assess risk and engage in health promotion that is spe-cific to men and boys. There is a growing evidence to suggest that when a gendered approach is applied by health services, men will change the way they respond to their own health needs (WHO, 2018). Some men and boys have a hegemonic tendency to view the healthcare system as 'feminised', impacting on both the perceived value and accessing the system (Galdas et al., 2015). In this way, healthcare may be perceived by men as having a stronger relationship with the feminised body, ill or weak less-masculine bodies, where seeking healthcare violates the idealised embodiment of the stoic male. In recognition of this, the National Men's Health Strategy 2020–2030 makes several key recommendations to strengthen the capacity of health systems to deliver *appropriate* quality care for men and boys, including the provision of male-focused community health services (Commonwealth of Australia, 2019).

Men's Sheds

Men's Sheds were established in order to provide predominately older men with a com-munity location to participate in a range of activities, in a supportive male-friendly environment to socialise (Wilson et al., 2015). In addition, some sheds participate in mentoring programs between older and younger, at risk, men (Wilson et al., 2013), which have been shown to develop stronger psychosocial support for men by improving their sense of belonging and overall sense of life satisfaction (Taylor et al., 2018). They also create 'safe' male spaces where nurses, such as community nurses, can enact health promotion and health screening, while providing health roadshow, mental health support and comprehensive primary care. Men's Sheds are not there to provide a traditional health service; however, they do offer a supportive health-promoting environment.

Connecting with men in the workplace

Men can often to be hard to engage in health and personal care. The National Men's Health Strategy 2020–2030 suggests outreach programs to connect with men in the workplace. Nurses in workplaces play a key role in the early identification and ongoing surveillance of health issues for men while providing an avenue for structured and opportunistic health promotion programs. For example, Rio Tinto employs Occupational Health Nurses to provide physical healthcare, screening and cessation program, and also focuses on mental health among fly in, fly out workers at their various remote worksites across Australia. This signals an opportunity for nurses in the future to engage with men where they work.

Challenges for nurses caring for men

Men and boys are obligated to adopt a myriad of roles that have widespread implications for wider society. Typically, men in society progress through a continuum of roles from son, partner/husband, father and grandfather, having different health needs and expectations at each stage. While we are only now starting to see the men's health movement catch up to this traditional male trajectory, it is

---

Box 24.1 - Case study (Kevin)

Kevin Jones is a 75-year-old farmer, living and working on the same regional property for all of his life. He has been widowed for 13 years and lives alone. He has three grown up children, two children live outside the State and his middle son lives nearby but leads a busy working life. He was a Vietnam Veteran, an accomplished football player, competing in a number of premierships for his local football club. He is fiercely independent and during his presentation for an episode of atrial fibrillation and subsequent transient ischaemic attack (TIA) to the local hospital, he has verbalised his wish to return home and manage on his own, against the wishes of his family.

Reflective questions:

1 What are the challenges for rural men and being male in a rural location impact heath trajectories and health seeking behaviour?
2 What 'gendered' influences in Kevin's life may have impacted on his health?
3 What do health services need to do differently to capture the needs of males like Kevin?
4 What can nurses learn by considering the impact of gender on Kevin's health in providing effective care?

less representative of the nuances of the roles that the modern man might identify with: single fathers, ex-husband/partner, stepsons or stepfathers or step grandfather, and also employer/employee, community or religious leader, professional or voluntary public servant. Although these roles come with a level of complexity, it is important that men's health strategies and nurses engaging with men promote inclusivity of marginalised male roles and develop health promotion initiatives that focus on developing a positive image of boys and men to promote more equitable gender roles.

Future challenges to nursing men

Given men do not live as long and have poorer health outcomes compared to women, there remains a health inequality within the health system (AIHW, 2019). The Australian Government, through the NMHP, has sought to remind health services, professional and community members that gender is a determinant of health and good health means more than simply addressing biological differences. The NMHP seeks to address a number of current inequalities experienced by males, while providing a framework to realise good health. Nevertheless, there remain future challenges, some of which are known and other that remain unknown (Commonwealth of Australia, 2010).

As society progresses, the stereotype of the misogynistic male has shifted. Society is now a place where men are perpetually portrayed in the media and popular culture as inept and bumbling fools, where microaggression or 'hidden' misandry is accepted, and where men who are nurses continue to encounter negative stereotypes (Synnott, 2016). It is also a society where social media movements such as #MeeToo, #NotOkay and #HowIWillChange call out and seek to address sexual harassment and other gender-based violence against women (PettyJohn et al., 2018). These fundamental shifts can and have had a positive public health opportunity for women and should be embraced by all (O'Neil et al., 2018). Nevertheless, it has been suggested that this shift in society has given rise to a phenomenon where being a man is considered pathological, where all men are considered 'broken' (Synnott, 2016). This emerging popular culture, where positive social media movements and poor stereotypes of men coexist, is a new and unrealised challenge for men's health and healthcare needs in the future. However, nurses of both sexes, who understand and appreciate that men hail from all walks of life and how and where they are situated in society, will have the necessary foundations to recognise differences and respond in gendered ways that make it easier for men to receive the healthcare they require (Commonwealth of Australia, 2010).

Conclusion

This chapter explored a range of issues about the role of nurses in supporting the health of men taking into consideration the impact of gender stereotypes and the risks that contribute to their vulnerability and complexity. In providing nursing care to men, this chapter highlights the following:

- A health inequity exists in men when compared to women, on average they die younger from health issues, are diagnosed later and engage differently with health services and professionals.

- The context of health and help seeking for men may be impacted by societal influences related to gender and they should not be compared to women or in fact other men.
- The care and education of men needs to be individualised and implemented with an understanding of their own life experiences, role and exposure to risk.

Online resources

1 Australian Men's Health Forum: https://www.amhf.org.au/nurses_give_tips_on_working_with_men
2 National Male Health Policy: http://www.health.gov.au/malehealthpolicy
3 Australian Men's Sheds Association: https://mensshed.org/

References

AIHW. (2019). *The health of Australia's males.* Retrieved from http://www.health.gov.au

Amin, A., Kagesten, A., Adebayo, E, & Chandra-Mouli, V. (2018. Addressing gender socialization and masculinity norms among adolescent boys: policy and programmatic implications. *Journal of Adolescent Health. (62) 3.* S3-S5. doi: 10.1016/j.jadohealth.2017.06.022

Australian Government Department of Health and Ageing. (2013). *National Mental Health Report 2013: Tracking progress of mental health reform in Australia 1993–2011.* Retrieved from http://www.health.gov.au

Blank, L., Baxter, S., Buckley Woods, H., Goyder, E. Lee, E. Payne, N., & Rimmer, M. (2015). What is the evidence on interventions to manage referral from primary to specialist non-emergency care? A systematic review and logic model synthesis. *Health Services and Delivery Research*, 3(24), 1–429.

Blum, R.W., Mmari, M.A., & Moreau, C. (2017). It begins at 10: How gender expectations shape early adolescence around the world. *Journal of Adolescent Health*, 61(4), S3–S4. doi:10.1016/j.jadohealth.2017.07.009

Commonwealth of Australia. (2010). *National male health policy: Building on the strengths of Australian males.* Canberra: Commonwealth of Australia. Retrieved from https://consultations.health.gov.au.

Commonwealth of Australia. (2019). *National Men's Health Strategy 2020–2030.* Canberra: Commonwealth of Australia.

Connell, R. W. (2005). *Masculinities (2nd edn).*Crows Nest, NSW: Allen and Unwin.

Fish, J. A., Prichard, I., Ettridge, K., Grunfeld, E. A., & Wilson, C. (2019). Understanding variation in men's help-seeking for cancer symptoms: A semistructured interview study. *Psychology of Men & Masculinities*, 20(1), 61–70. https://doi.apa.org/doi/10.1037/men0000152

Galdas, P., Darwin, Z.J., Fell, J., Kidd, L., Blickem, C., McPherson, K., Richardson, G. (2015). A systematic review and metaethnography to identify how effective, cost-effective, accessible and acceptable self-management support interventions are for men with long-term conditions (SELF-MAN). *Health Services and Delivery Research*, 3(34), 1–301.

Gottschall, K. (2014). Always the larrikin: Ben Mendelsohn and young Aussie manhood in Australian cinema. *Continuum*, 28(6), 862–875.

Kannan, A., Kirkman, M., Ruseckaite, R., & Evans, S. M. (2019). Prostate care and prostate cancer from the perspectives of undiagnosed men: A systematic review of qualitative research. *British Medical Journal Open*, 9(1), e022842. doi:10.1136/bmjopen-2018-022842

O'Neil, A., Sojo, V., Fileborn, B., Scovelle, A., & Milner, A. (2018). The #MeToo movement: An opportunity in public health?. *Lancet*, 391(10140), 2587–2589.

PettyJohn, M. E., Muzzey, F. K., Maas, M. K., & McCauley, H. L. (2018). # HowIWillChange: Engaging men and boys in the #MeToo movement. *Psychology of Men & Masculinity. 20(4)* 612–622. Advance online publication. doi:10.1037/men0000186

Synnott, A. (2016). *Re-thinking men: Heroes, villains and victims*. London: Routledge.

Taylor, J., Cole, R., Kynn, M., & Lowe, J. (2018). Home away from home: health benefits of men's sheds. *Health Promotion Journal of Australia. 29(3)*. 236–242. https://doi.org/10.1002/hpja.15

Webb, J. (2013). Aussie rules: Writing and social practice in a regional community. *Journal of the Association for the Study of Australian Literature*. 243–251.

WHO. (2001). *Madrid statement: Mainstreaming gender equity in health: The need to move forward*. Retrieved from http://www.euro.who.int/__data/assets/pdf_file/0008/76508/A75328.pdf

Wilson, N. J., Cordier, R., & Wilson Whatley, L. (2013). Older male mentors' perceptions of a Men's Shed intergenerational mentoring program. *Australian Occupational Therapy Journal*, 60, 416–426. doi:10.1111/1440-1630.12090

Wilson, N. J., Cordier, R., Doma, K., Misan, G., & Vaz, S. (2015). Men's Sheds function and philosophy: Towards a framework for future research and men's health promotion. *Health Promotion Journal of Australia*, 26(2), 133–141. doi:10.1071/HE14052

25 Global nursing

Deborah Kirk and Stephanie Wheeler

Chapter objectives

This chapter will offer the reader:

- An outline of skills and preparation needed to work in a global context.
- A description of various opportunities to collaborate abroad and use nursing skills in a global context.
- An overview of the impact of working abroad may have on a long-term nursing career.
- A list of online resources to assist with opportunities and preparation before working abroad.

Introduction

Global health is an area that offers the nurse the opportunity to expand clinical knowledge and skill set, enhance communication skills, develop confidence, experience new cultures and build lifelong collaborative networks. Concurrently, the nurse can partner with international colleagues to support developing health systems and strengthen local health workforce capacity. This chapter will provide an overview for the nurse interested in working internationally with insight into skills needed to work in a global context, appropriate preparation, types of opportunities to collaborate abroad, and the long-term impact it may have on a nursing career. Online resources will be provided to help guide with opportunities and preparation for international experience.

Skills to work globally

Nurses venturing into the global health space require the same excellent clinical nursing skills and core 'soft skills' that all nurses require for best practice, such as communication, professionalism, collaboration, leadership and critical thinking (Liu & Aungsuroch, 2018). To thrive and be effective in international health, nurses are additionally required to be adaptable, creative with limited resource, confident to work with minimal supervision and able to translate complex scientific evidence into culturally accessible information. Importantly, global health nurses must engage in developing cultural competency and self-awareness.

Cultural competency is not a check-box exercise before deployment; it is a deep-learning process led by respectful, humble and genuine curiosity. This positioning best occurs through the development of self-awareness, and an examination of one's own culture and privilege (Borell, Gregory, McCreanor, Jensen, & Barnes, 2009; Hobbs, 2018). In understanding our own cultural assumptions and biases, we are able to encounter others' culture more with a gracious and accepting perspective, rather than orienting – and, often, prejudicing – it in relation to our own (Sharifi, Adib-Haibaghery, Najafi, 2019). White Western people must be sensitively attuned to the history of cultural violence perpetrated against many cultures and nations under colonisation and beyond (MacDonald & Steenbeek, 2015; Richardson, McGinnis, & Frankfurter, 2019). In these contexts, where whiteness has been threatening and destabilising, it is particularly important for the white nurse to actively work to give up privilege in order to centre the local perspective, culture and leadership (Waite & Nardi, 2019).

Developing cultural competency should involve general training on skills, principles and attributes required for cross-cultural work, as well as context-specific training. The latter should extend beyond teaching polite behaviours and the purely visible aspects of culture; it must include an exploration of historical and cultural belief systems and structures that influence health and health behaviours. Without this foundational understanding, it is impossible to work with local colleagues to craft culturally appropriate and acceptable solutions.

While there has long been understanding of the need to centre communities and ensure the cultural appropriateness of health strategies, we continue to see Western approaches be unsuccessfully transplanted into non-Western contexts. For example, during the 2014–2016 Ebola outbreak in West Africa, response teams responded quickly to initiate case isolation and safe burials to minimise disease transmission. However, many processes did not fulfil the cultural and religious obligations of the communities and consequently, many people concealed their sickness or performed secret funerals in order to conduct cultural rites for their loved ones (Pellecchia, Crestani, Decroo, Van, & Al-Kourdi, 2015). The engagement of anthropologists with local community was critical in managing the outbreak; promoting adherence by working together to co-design and implement culturally appropriate and evidence-based practices for use within the community (Fairhead, 2016). Whether in complex emergencies or in longer-term development planning, local expertise must be centred to lead in the development of local solutions to local problems.

We must all enter global health work in a position of humility with a genuine respect for the host country and its people, a spirit of partnership, a strengths-based approach and a willingness to be unseen so that your local colleagues may be championed. Table 25.1 provides a sample of online learning and development resources to prepare for global work.

Table 25.1 Online resources

Resources	Contact	Details
ReliefWeb	https://reliefweb.int/	Online source for reliable and timely humanitarian information on global crises and disasters, and job listings
Devex	https://www.devex.com/	Media platform for the global development community
OpenWHO	https://openwho.org/	WHO's learning and development website for public health issues in emergencies
Coursera	https://www.coursera.org/	Free online learning and development online courses
RedR	https://redr.org.au	Training programs for humanitarian workers

Table 25.2 Considerations before you work globally

- Ensure required travel documents including visas and passport with appropriate expiration period – be aware of legal requirements for each country including allowed length of stay and conditions specific for working in-country, including work permits and insurances
- Professional qualifications and registration process varies for each country. Relevant websites for the registration process should be reviewed for appropriate process. Scope of practice can be different in different countries; ensure your trained scope of practice is communicated clearly, and practice within this.
- Health – Travel insurance (including emergency evacuation coverage), indicated vaccinations, organisation and accessibility of the health sector, personal medication availability. Some countries require proof of certain vaccinations.
- Safety – Consider the political situation of the country and monitor frequently. Undertake security briefings in-country to understand local issues and available emergency services. Consider taking security items, such as personal alarms, door alarms and smoke alarms, which may be difficult to source locally. Be aware of internet and phone connectivity.
- Language – considerations if local language is different than yours, and investing time and finances into learning language, and/or hiring an interpreter
- Cultural awareness – learning local history and culture to understand the current situation and how this impacts on the working environment and population
- Mental health – Ensure a strong support system with the country of origin, as well as developing relationships in-country. Research availability of leisure and exercise activities, as well as formal mental health supports, such as counselling.
- If being deployed through a providing agency, ensure expectations and benefits are clearly articulated and agreed upon prior to departure.
- Financial implications

  - Length of stay has impact on cost, including rent, utilities and day-to-day living costs, which may also require security personnel
  - Ongoing home of origin expenses and tax obligations
  - Travel costs to country, and additional in-country travel costs
  - Consider a financial contingency to account for unforeseen fluctuations in exchange rates

---

As you consider your skills and what it means to work as a nurse globally, there are also a number of practicalities to consider before engaging in another country that must be researched and planned. Being prepared before you go is key to success of the experience. Research into the location, opportunities and financial implications are important first steps in the process. Table 25.2 outlines a number of considerations in choosing the right location, opportunity and the financial considerations.

Types of opportunities

There are many types of global opportunities for nurses from short-term to long-term, volunteer or paid, and clinical or non-clinical. It is important to select an organisation, either government or non-government, that prioritises responsible and sustainable work by ensuring that you will work alongside national counterparts to develop local capacity that remains long after your mission is complete.

Clinical

The level of engagement while working in a clinical setting abroad will be based on regulations surrounding nursing registration in the particular country, followed by

---

Box 25.1 - RN story

I am an RN working in sub-Saharan Africa in a private hospital and community set-ting focusing on children and adults who have acute healthcare needs. I work along-side the local hospital staff and community members to identify the most urgent needs, which include malaria screening and healthcare treatment to remote villages. I have raised funds to support two mobile clinics that now operate 5 days a week. These clinics promote community health programs that truly improve the health of the community through education and improved healthcare practices that the local residents take ownership of. I have been here for 2 years and do not have plans to leave anytime soon.

---

skill level, individual comfort and community needs. Once those parameters are established, there are a variety of opportunities for nursing professionals ranging from home visits in remote communities, primary care in local community health cen-tres or intensive care in the larger urban hospitals. Depending on the setting, clinical activities may include day-to-day readiness for clinics, community health education, health histories and vital signs or medication administration.

Capacity building

In limited resource contexts, the role of the international nurse is to support the develop-ment of capacity in the local health workforce. Although nurses and midwives account for almost half of the 43.5 million health workers worldwide (WHO, 2016), approximately 25% of countries have less than 10 nursing and midwifery personnel per 10,000 popu-lation, compared to 127 per 10,000 in Australia (WHO, 2019). These nurses are often practising across multiple disciplines to service their communities, a feat that is becom-ing more and more complex with the epidemiological shift towards non-communicable diseases and ageing populations in many countries (Gail, Birch, Mackenzie, Bradish, & Annette, 2016). In such situations, nurses can provide technical assistance in the develop-ment of nursing curriculums that best address the needs of the population.

Research

Many health systems are relatively young or are recovering from crises which rendered them fragile. The health workforce in such states may have a greater proportion of junior

---

Box 25.2 - RN story II

I am a nurse practitioner with a passion for oncology nursing. During a short-term mis-sion trip, I met nurses who were employed at a local university in the country. We dis-cussed the need for oncology content to be taught in the nursing program. Through several short-term visits, we were able to collaborate and map oncology throughout the curricula, develop content and conduct workshops to build confidence for the local staff to deliver the material.

Box 25.3 - RN story III

I am an early career nurse researcher interested in chronic disease nursing management. I became involved in global work as a clinician in a developing country early in my career. It was during this time I recognized the need for population-specific evidence to be identified and put into practice. I collaborated with local researchers, academics and clinicians to identify areas of unmet needs for this population and develop a list of priorities for protocol development and areas for future research.

---

nursing professionals who benefit highly from the provision of clinical supervision, training and mentorship. As health systems stabilise and mature, health workers are more able to explore emerging opportunities to contribute to their country's body of evidence (Dalmar et al., 2017; Woodward, Sheahan, Martineau & Sondorp, 2017). Nurse researchers can provide key research support to emerging researchers, ensuring that quality evidence is being generated for their own population and health priorities, in their own language and interpreted for contextualised decision-making (Abdalla, Bortolussi & MacDonald, 2018).

Public health

Nurses who are particularly passionate about health inequities and systemic ways to promote health and prevent disease at a population level may consider exploring the public health space and the requisite postgraduate training in public health (Marmot, 2005). Whilst roles in the public health field are often non-clinical, clinical knowledge and skills are applied in many areas of public health, such as infection prevention and control and case management in an infectious disease outbreak. Nurses also bring a uniquely holistic, whole-of-person, whole-of-society approach to the science of public health – crucial in addressing the complexity of social determinants impacting population health and the appropriate public health response (Donovan & Warriner, 2017).

Impact on career

Working abroad has many benefits that may impact a nursing career and develop a nurse personally and professionally. It can build a resume and demonstrate to an employer adaptability, flexibility and ability to accept the challenge of working in

---

Box 25.4 - RN story IV

I loved clinical work, but always felt drawn to the broader health system issues beyond the hospital environment. I completed a Master of International Public Health and took a role in a World Health Organisation (WHO) country office in the Western-Pacific region. I spent the following years working alongside government counterparts to develop national capacity to detect and respond to public health emergencies. Through the provision of trainings, facilitation of exercise simulations, and the development of processes and structures, we were able to work together to strengthen the country's preparedness for health security threats.

---

an unfamiliar environment. It allows for cultural immersion that will deepen your understanding of another place, its people and the healthcare system. It increases your professional (and personal) network, establishing lifelong colleagues and friends. Additionally, a global network can expand opportunities for jobs or collaborations for research, not just at home, but in other countries.

Conclusion

Global nursing is an emerging career opportunity that should not be overlooked. When considering work of this nature, nurses should spend time identifying their skill set in a global context and in self-awareness of one's own culture to better prepare relating to others. This chapter described several different types of career paths in global nursing to consider. Nurses may choose to work clinically and build on skills developed during undergraduate study, they may choose to function in a supportive role to capacity build others who are in the country or nurses may address the social determinants of health through public health initiatives and research opportunities. Whatever path is chosen, a global nursing experience has the potential to make a life-long impact on your career.

References

Abdalla, S. M., Bortolussi, R., & MacDonald, N.E. (2018). MicorResearch: An effective approach to local research capacity development. *The Lancet Global Health*, 6(4), e377–e378. doi:10/1016/S2214-109X(18)30069-X

Borell, B., Gregory, A., McCreanor, T., Jensen, V., & Barnes, H. (2009). "It's hard at the top but it's a whole lot easier than being at the bottom": The role of privilege in understanding disparities in Aotearoa/New Zealand. *Race/Ethnicity: Multidisciplinary Global Contexts*, 3(1), 29–50. Retrieved from www.jstor.org/stable/25595023

Dalmar, A. A., Hussein, A. S., Walhad, S. A., Ibrahim, A. O., Abdi, A. A., Ali, M. K., Wall, S. (2017). Rebuilding research capacity in fragile states: The case of a Somali-Swedish global health initiative. *Global health action*, 10(1), 1348693. doi:10.1080/16549716.2017.1348693

Donovan, H., & Warriner, J. (2017). Nurses' role in public health and integration of health and social care. *Primary Health Care (2014+)*, 27(8), 20. doi:http://dx.doi.org.virtual.anu.edu.au/10.7748/phc.2017.e1294

Fairhead, J. (2016). Understanding social resistance to the Ebola response in the forest region of the republic of guinea: An anthropological perspective. *African Studies Review*, 59(3), 7–31. doi:http://dx.doi.org.virtual.anu.edu.au/10.1017/asr.2016.87

Gail, T. M., Birch, S., MacKenzie, A., Bradish, S., & Annette, E. R. (2016). A synthesis of recent analyses of human resources for health requirements and labour market dynamics in high-income OECD countries. *Human Resources for Health*, 14, 59. doi:http://dx.doi.org.virtual.anu.edu.au/10.1186/s12960-016-0155-2

Hobbs J. (2018). White privilege in health care: Following recognition with action. *Annals of Family Medicine*, 16(3), 197–198. doi:10.1370/afm.2243

Liu, Y., & Aungsuroch, Y. (2018). Current literature review of registered nurses' competency in the global community. *Journal of Nursing Scholarship*, 50: 191–199. doi:10.1111/jnu.12361

MacDonald, C., & Steenbeek, A. (2015). The impact of colonization and Western assimilation on health and wellbeing of Canadian Aboriginal people. *International Journal of Regional and Local History*, 10:1, 32–46. doi: 10.1179/2051453015Z.00000000023

Marmot, M. (2005). Social determinants of health inequalities. *The Lancet*, 365(9464), 1099–1104. doi:http://dx.doi.org.virtual.anu.edu.au/10.1016/S0140-6736(05)71146-6

Pellecchia, U., Crestani, R., Decroo, T., Van, d. B., & Al-Kourdi, Y. (2015). Social consequences of Ebola containment measures in Liberia. *PLoS One, 10*(12), e0143036. doi:http://dx.doi.org.virtual.anu.edu.au/10.1371/journal.pone.0143036

Richardson, E.T., McGinnis, T., & Frankfurter, R. (2019). Ebola and the narrative of mistrust. *BMJ Global Health*, 4:e001932.

Sharifi, N., Adib-Hajbaghery, M., & Najafi, M. (2019). Cultural competence in nursing: A concept analysis. *International Journal of Nursing Studies, 99*, 103386. doi.org/10.1016/j.ijnurstu.2019.103386

Waite, R., & Nardi, D. (2019). Nursing colonialism in America: Implications for nursing leadership, *Journal of Professional Nursing, 35*(1), 18–25. doi.org/10.1016/j.profnurs.2017.12.013

Woodward, A., Sheahan, K., Martineau, T., & Sondorp, E. (2017). Health systems research in fragile and conflict affected states: A qualitative study of associated challenges. *Health Research Policy and Systems, 15*(1), 44. doi:10.1186/s12961-017-0204-x

World Health Organization (WHO). (2016). Global strategic directions for strengthening nursing and midwifery 2016–2020. Retrieved from https://www.who.int/hrh/nursing_midwifery/global-strategic-midwifery2016-2020.pdf

World Health Organization (WHO). (2019). Global Health Observatory data repository: Nursing and midwifery personnel. Retrieved from http://apps.who.int/gho/data/node.main.HWFGRP_0040?lang=en

26 Nursing and the military

Andrew Ormsby

Chapter objectives

This chapter will offer the reader:

- An insight into the history and context of nursing in the Australian military.
- An outline of the key health issues facing people in the Australian military.
- A description of the contemporary contexts in which military nursing occurs.
- An opportunity to build a knowledge base and develop nursing skills specific to nursing in the military.

Introduction

The primary role of the Australian Defence Force is to defend Australia and its national interests (Davies, 2018). To meet this goal, the Australian Defence Force employs more than 80,000 people across its three service arms (Navy, Army and Air Force) in either a full-time or a part-time capacity (DoD, 2018). The health services that support Australian Defence Force employees comprise both military and civilian health professionals. However, health support on deployed operations (e.g. warlike, peacekeeping, humanitarian assistance, disaster relief and evacuation operations), whether overseas or in Australia, are almost exclusively the domain of uniformed health professionals drawn from the three service arms.

Nurses are an integral part of the Australian Defence Force health services, providing care to the men and women of the Australian Defence Force across a variety of roles and settings. A number of settings in which Australian military nurses work are largely unique to individual service arms (e.g. Navy nurses providing care in a health facility aboard a ship, Army nurses providing care in a field hospital or Air Force nurses providing care in an airplane during an aeromedical retrieval). However, many joint roles exist in which military nurses may work that harness the common skills and experiences of the 'military nurse' across a broad spectrum of operational, health centre, staff or leadership roles as part of a multidisciplinary healthcare team.

Historical context of nursing in the Australian military

An association between nursing and the military has existed since the time of the crusades during the 11th to 13th centuries (Bradley, 2018). However, the work of Florence Nightingale and her nurses during the Crimean War, between 1853 and 1856, arguably remains the best-known global example of military nursing and its positive impact on the care and recovery of soldiers in the time of war (Beck, 2010). Many advances in nursing care emerged during this period that had a positive impact on the mortality and morbidity of the soldiers under the care of Nightingale's nurses.

Nurses have also deployed with Australian military forces to every conflict and major deployment since the Boer War in 1899 (WAM, 2015). The most prominent example of an Australian military nurse is Vivian Bullwinkle, who survived the sinking of the Vyner Brooke, a subsequent massacre at the hands of Japanese soldiers on Bangka Island and three and half years of captivity during the Second World War (Angell, 2011). The conditions in which Australian military nurses have and continue to work are often hazardous, uncomfortable and challenging in their circumstances (Ormsby et al, 2016). Indeed, that nearly 100 Australian military nurses have died in the service of their country underscores the risks associated with military nursing (DVA, 2019).

Key health issues facing people in the Australian military

The Australian military demographic largely comprises a young, fit and healthy workforce who maintain an occupational requirement to be fit for service in Australia and overseas on deployed operations (AIHW, 2018). Nurses are integral to the occupational surveillance, treatment and maintenance of military personnel to meet their primary war-fighting role and in the treatment of wounded, injured or ill personnel (McGinty, 2019). The military nurse needs to be adaptable enough to work across a number of practice domains as both clinical and military leaders. They should possess good clinical assessment and treatment skills, a solid understanding of the Defence occupational workplace, an ability to analyse and distil complex ideas and have strong communication and leadership skills.

Battlefield trauma provides unique challenges for all military healthcare professionals. Nurses work within multidisciplinary teams to treat injuries that may result from such trauma mechanisms as gunshots, mine blasts, burns and motor vehicle crashes. While exposure to battlefield trauma does not occur often, care for the trauma patient remains a key skill for military nurses (Harding, 2010).

Military nurses also need to understand the unique occupational environment in which military personnel work (Westphalen, 2017). The military workplace can be as diverse as a mechanical workshop, an infantry unit, the engine room of a ship, a fuel farm or the cockpit of an aircraft. A sound knowledge of the workplace and a good professional relationship with the people who work in those environments and with whom military nurses often deploy on operations is important to the provision of well-targeted primary and occupational healthcare.

The locations into which military personnel, including nurses, deploy also bring significant challenges to the nursing and healthcare context (Scannell-Desch & Doherty, 2012). Endemic diseases, austere working environments, extremes of weather, local population demographics, and the relative safety and security of deployment locations significantly affect the level and type of care provision. Military nurses not only care for military personnel but also care for local civilian populations and in doing so often need to provide targeted and culturally sensitive care in less than ideal conditions (e.g. care for civilian populations in Indonesia following the 2004 South-East Asian tsunami (DoD, 2005)).

Box 26.1 - Case study (Belinda)

Belinda is an Australian Army nurse deployed to a disaster relief operation in the South Pacific following a cyclone. She is on a task to travel by helicopter to a remote part of the country to provide an assessment of the healthcare needs of the affected civilian population. As part of this task, she will also assess the local environment and community.

Reflective questions:
 1   What should Belinda consider in her assessment?
 2   What is the value of this assessment?

Mental health remains a major challenge to the provision of health services to a population potentially exposed to death, dying and inhumanity on a large scale (Van Hoof et al, 2018). The war-fighting role also exposes individuals to moral conflict when actively engaged in the application of violence on a battlefield (Heath & Beattie, 2019). The military nurse works closely with other health professionals to provide appropriate mental healthcare to affected military personnel.

Contemporary context in which military nurses work

The day-to-day work of a military nurse largely centres on the provision of healthcare to military personnel at defence establishments in Australia. This work incorporates normal civilian clinical nursing roles such as general ward nursing, health promotions and primary healthcare in an outpatients department, particularly early in a career. Nurses that are more senior tend to move into management and command-related roles within the home-based context (AWM, 2017). Where the differences become apparent is in the other roles that military nurses perform, which are as diverse as they are challenging.

Navy nurses may post as part of a ship's complement, providing care to sailors and other personnel while at sea (Grosser, 2018). Typically, Navy nurses provide clinically focussed care in general (primary healthcare and medical/surgical nursing) and speciality areas of nursing (intensive care, emergency and operating theatre) aboard a sea going healthcare facility. A good example of this work environment is the healthcare facility on HMAS Canberra, which contains resuscitation bays, operating theatres and inpatient beds comprising low, medium and high dependency, in conjunction with other ancillary health services such as pharmacy, pathology and radiography (Westphalen, 2018).

Army nurses primarily work within small to large field healthcare facilities when not at their home-based location. Field healthcare facilities form part of land-based trauma system that supports military, domestic and deployed manoeuvre exercises and operations. These nurses may work in primary healthcare teams, trauma teams, general and specialist nursing roles, or in support of forward and tactical aeromedical and land-based retrieval activities. A recent example is the work of Army nurses in a medium-sized field health facility near Baghdad in the Middle East (Kennaway et al., 2017). This facility was similar in capability to the one HMAS Canberra discussed above, but smaller in scale. Existing buildings housed a large part of the facility; however, purposely built tents containing the operating theatre and intensive care beds were also established (SBS, 2016).

Air Force nurses primarily work on airbases in Australia and overseas, supporting Air Force flying operations and activities that enable flying operations. Roles vary

---

Box 26.2 - Case study (Belinda II)

Belinda is carrying a basic field medical kit with limited diagnostic and treatment options, when she has a clearly unwell 6-year-old child brought to her. She conducts an assessment on the child and notes malaise, headaches, myalgia, nausea and vomiting and a sudden onset of high fevers, chills and sweats. Belinda is aware that the region is endemic for Plasmodium Falciparum Malaria, and the potential lethality of the condition if left untreated.

Reflective questions:

1 What can Belinda do immediately to stabilise the child?
2 What treatment options are available for Belinda to consider in her location and elsewhere?
3 Belinda evacuates the child with their mother back to an AUSAID health facility. The health facility confirms the child's condition and she is successfully treated. What other considerations emerge, noting displacement of the child and mother from their home?

---

between occupational aviation nursing duties, nursing within small to large field-based healthcare facilities and in operating within an aeromedical evacuation context (Bown, 2016). Air Force nurses operate independently or in aeromedical evacuation teams primarily caring for military personnel on a variety of aircraft, both military and civilian, across the globe. An example of aeromedical evacuation duties is the retrieval of Australian citizens and approved foreign nationals to Australia following the 2002 and 2005 Bali bombings (Air Force, 2019). These multidisciplinary teams typically comprised generalist and specialist nurses from both the permanent and the reserve (part-time) forces.

Australian military nurses still deploy with, and provide care to, Australian military personnel during times of war (e.g.in current operations in the Middle East), on peace-keeping missions (e.g. United Nations missions) and during humanitarian assistance or disaster relief activities. Military nurses generally deploy jointly (e.g. Australian nurses from the Navy, Army and Air Force deployed to Rwanda between 1994 and 1995), often work alongside Australian civilian nurses, host nation health workers, foreign military healthcare providers and health workers from non-government organizations (e.g. following the Boxing Day tsunami in Indonesia in 2004) (Bullock, 2017). The context within which these nurses work remains challenging and varied.

Nurses provide care to war-fighters (combatants) but maintain a non-combatant status consistent with the protections afforded to them under the Geneva Conventions (ICRC, 2019). These conventions allow nurses, and other healthcare professionals, to carry weapons for personal protection and the protection of their patients (Biedermann, 2017). However, though nurses do not engage in direct action with enemy forces, they are still military officers who discharge professional military responsibilities in addition to those of their professional nursing role.

Conclusion

Military nursing provides a range of challenges to those who pursue this career path whether in a full-time or part-time capacity. While nursing care principles remain consistent with those experienced across the span of the Australian nursing workforce, the military occupational and environmental context is unique. Opportunities to work in sea, land and aviation nursing contexts across the span of operations from warlike, to peacekeeping, to humanitarian assistance and disaster relief have the potential to provide a dynamic, challenging and rewarding career.

The Australian Defence Force offers select nurses the opportunity to develop their nursing skills, broaden their personal and professional horizons, and learn new skills as professional military officers. Nurses are an integral part of the military health team that helps maintain the physical and mental health of military personnel, enabling them to perform the often complex, dangerous and confronting tasks that they undertake in the defence of Australia and its national interests.

Online resources

1 Defending Australia and Its National Interests: https://www.defence.gov.au
2 Defence Jobs Australia – Find Jobs in the ADF: https://www.defencejobs.gov.au/
3 Military Nursing Today: https://www.awm.gov.au/visit/exhibitions/nurses/today/

References

Air Force. (2019). Recent History of Air Force Humanitarian Assistance. Retrieved from https://www.airforce.gov.au/operations/humanitarian-support/recent-history-air-force-humanitarian-assistance

Angell, D. (2011). Vivian Bullwinkle Survivor of the Bangka Island Massacre. *Angellpro*. Retrieved from https://www.ausmed.com/cpd/articles/vivian-bullwinkel

Australian Institute of Health and Welfare (AIHW). (2018). A Profile of Australia's Veterans 2018. Australian Institute of Welfare. Cat.no. PHE 235. Canberra: AIHW

Australian War Memorial (AWM). (2017). Military Nursing Today. Retrieved from https://www.awm.gov.au/visit/exhibitions/nurses/today/

Beck, D. M. (2010). Remembering Florence Nightingale's Panorama: 21st-century nursing – At a critical crossroads. *Journal of Holistic Nursing, 28*(4), 291–301.

Biedermann, N. (2017). Australian military nursing from ANZAC to now: Embracing the ghosts of out nursing ancestors. *Advances in Historical Studies, 6,* 65–77.

Bown, S. (2016). *One woman's war and peace: A nurse's journey through the Royal Australian Air Force*. Wollombi, NSW: Exisle Publishing.

Bradley, M. (2018). War and health care. *Journal of Perioperative Practice, 28*(11), 288.

Bullock, D. (2017). Increasing interoperability through preparedness. Conference Abstract. *Journal of Military and Veterans' Health, 25*(4), 45–46.

Department of Defence (DoD). (2015). *Defence Annual Report 2014-15. Commonwealth of Australia*. Retrieved from https://www.defence.gov.au/AnnualReports/04-05

Department of Defence (DoD). (2018). *Defence Annual Report 2017-18*. Commonwealth of Australia. Retrieved from https://www.defence.gov.au/annualreports/17-18

Davies, G.N. (2018). *Opening address. Air power in a disruptive world: Proceedings of the 2018 Air Power Conference*. Canberra, Australia: Air Power Development Centre.

Department of Veterans' Affairs (DVA). (2019). Wartime Snapshots No.25: Australian Service Nursing. Retrieved from https://anzacportal.dva.gov.au/resources/australian-service-nursing-wartime-snapshots-no25

Grosser, S., White, T., & Cotton, B. (2018). MOHU – Navy MR2E. *ADF Nursing Magazine 2018.* 74–75.

Harding, J. (2010). In the service of peace. In C. McCullagh (Ed.), *Willingly into the Fray: One hundred years of Australian Army nursing* (pp. 323–329). Newport: Big Sky Publishing.

Heath, R., & Beattie, J. (2019). Case report of a former soldier using TRE (Tension/Trauma Releasing Exercises) for post-traumatic stress disorder self-care. *Journal of Military and Veterans' Health, 27*(3), 35–40.

International Committee of the Red Cross (ICRC). (2019). *Practice Relating to Rule 24. Medical Personnel.* Retrieved from https://ihl-databases.icrc.org/customary-ihl/eng/docs/v2_rul_rule25

Kennaway, S., Bottcher, E., & Jone, R. (2017). ANZAC R2E TAJI – Commander's memoirs, April 2015 to December 2016. Conference Abstract. *Journal of Military and Veterans' Health, 25*(4), 14–15.

Lieutenant Colonel Vivian Bullwinkle. Australian War Memorial. Retrieved from https://www.awm.gov.au/collection/P10676383

McGinty, P. (2019). Military and civilian nurses – Nursing is nursing. *ADF Nursing Magazine 2019.* 88–89.

Ormsby, A., Harrington, A. & Borbasi, S. (2016). 'You never come back the same': The challenge of spiritual care in a deployed military nursing context. *Journal of Clinical Nursing, 26*, 1351–1362.

SBS. (2016). Aussie Iraq hospital not like back home. Retrieved from https://www.sbs.com.au/news/aussie-iraq-hospital-not-like-back-home

Scannell-Desch, E., & Doherty, M.E. (2012). *Nurses in war: Voices from Iraq and Afghanistan.* New York, NY: Springer Publishing Company.

Van Hoof, M., Lawrence-Wood, E., Hodson, S., Sadler, N., Benassi, H., Hansen, C., McFarlane, A. (2018). *Mental health prevalence, mental health and wellbeing transition study.* Canberra: The Department of Defence and the Department of Veterans' Affairs.

Western Australian Museum. (WAM). (2015). Australian Nurses at War. Retrieved from https://www.museum.wa.gov.au/whats-on/australian-nurses-war

Westphalen, N. (2017). Occupational and environmental health in the ADF. *Journal of Military and Veterans' Health, 25*(1), 44–52.

Westphalen, N. (2018). Operational test and evaluation, HMAS Canberra: Assessing the ADF's new maritime role 2 enhanced capability. *Journal of Military and Veterans' Health, 26*(1), 35–41.

27 General practice nursing

Elizabeth J Halcomb

Chapter objectives

This chapter will offer the reader:

- An insight into the environment of general practice and an understanding of how this might impact on nurses.
- An outline of the general practice nurses' role.
- An overview of preparation for working in general practice and considerations for seeking employment in this setting.

Introduction

Nurses have worked outside hospital settings for many years both in Australia and internationally. As people living in the community setting experience increasingly complex health issues, multimorbidity and chronic conditions, there is a higher demand for health services in primary care. As the frontline of the health system, primary care plays an important role in preventative care, management of chronic conditions and acute episodic care. Since the mid-2000s, the Australian Government has provided financial incentives and health policy to facilitate building the Australian general practice nursing workforce. This has led to an exponential increase in the number of general practice nurses across Australia. Today there are over 13,000 nurses employed within general practices across Australia (Heywood et al., 2018), with over 63% of general practices employing a nurse (Australian Medicare Local Alliance, 2012). This increase has created challenges for both nurses and general practitioners (GPs), as a primarily medical model of care shifts to a more inclusive multidisciplinary approach to service delivery (McInnes et al., 2017). Understanding these challenges and the unique practice environment of general practice is important for nurses working in this setting to inform their practice.

> PRIMARY CARE = The first point of contact with the health system. In Australia, this is usually a general practice.

> GENERAL PRACTICE NURSE = A registered or enrolled nurse employed to provide nursing care, within their scope of practice, in a general practice.

General practice in Australia

One of the biggest challenges experienced by general practice nurses is understanding and navigating the complexity of the general practice environment (Halcomb et al., 2017). Even clinically experienced nurses who transition from acute to primary healthcare employment experience challenges in adapting to the primary care work environment (Ashley et al., 2018). In the acute care sector, nurses are employed by large organisations, such as the state/territory or private health services. These large organisations have significant infrastructure and professional support, including dedicated nurse educators and structured professional training and development programmes. However, general practice nurses are largely employed by small businesses or corporate chains. These smaller organisations often don't have the same degree of workforce infrastructure. Additionally, many of these small businesses are owned by GPs, creating a complex relationship whereby the GP is both the nurses' employer and clinical colleague (McInnes et al., 2017).

General practices are supported to deliver primary care by Australian government-funded primary healthcare organisations. In Australia these organisations have been restructured several times in recent years, moving from Divisions of General Practice to Medicare Locals and, in July 2015, to 31 Primary Health Networks (Lane et al., 2017). Although the scope and services of these organisations has been slightly different, each iteration has been charged with supporting the delivery of primary healthcare to enhance efficiency and access to healthcare in their region.

General practice funding

Since 1984, Australian general practices have been funded by a blended payment system. The Australian government, via Medicare, provides rebates for specific items of service delivered by particular health professionals (Fisher et al., 2017). While some practices 'bulk bill' patients for consultations and accept the Medicare rebate as the full fee, many others charge patients an additional 'out-of-pocket' co-payment for services (Fisher et al., 2017). Various incentive payments are also offered to general practices from time to time to enhance practice uptake of specific strategies for people with certain health inequities/health needs or to promote employment of nurses and allied health professionals. For example, additional payments have been available for vaccinating children who are more than two months late with their vaccinations, undertaking cervical screening and engaging in quality improvement initiatives within a practice.

Previously, the Medicare schedule included several item numbers to reimburse services delivered by general practice nurses. However, this presented a challenge as it constrained nurses' roles to these specific tasks (Halcomb et al., 2008). This was replaced, in 2012, by the Practice Nurse Incentive Program that gives a block grant to accredited general practices for the delivery of nursing services (Australian Government, 2017). Under this programme, the general practice receives the same reimbursement for nursing services regardless of the activities that the nurse performs. This allows nursing services to be tailored specifically to individual practice needs. However, the nature of Medicare's activity-based funding means that general practices need to consciously manage their workload and models of care to optimise reimbursement. This has significant impact on the collaboration and the roles of individual health professionals (McInnes et al., 2017). It also requires general practice nurses to be much more aware than nurses working in other contexts of the financial aspects of service delivery, including the costs of equipment and consumables (Halcomb et al., 2017).

> BULK BILL = The cost of the consultation or item of service is completely covered by the Medicare rebate and no additional fee is charged to the patient.

General practice nurse's role

The rapid and exponential growth of nursing in Australian general practice created a number of challenges as both nurses and GPs sought to understand how best to incorporate nursing into service delivery within general practice. While in the early years nursing roles were constrained by funding models (Halcomb et al., 2008; McInnes et al., 2017), more recently there has been a shift towards nurses extending their practice to deliver more advanced care (Lane et al., 2017).

All nurses are educated and skilled to deliver nursing care within their scope of practice as described by regulatory frameworks (Nursing and Midwifery Board of Australia, 2019). Therefore, though enrolled nurses, registered nurses and nurse practitioners may all be employed in general practice, the role that they can undertake is distinctly different (Halcomb et al., 2017). Each individual nurse needs to consider the clinical tasks encountered and determine whether they are within their individual scope of practice. This is potentially challenging in general practice, where the nurse is working in relative isolation from other nurses in collaboration with a GP who is perhaps both their employer and colleague and may not fully appreciate their scope of practice.

> SCOPE OF PRACTICE = 'the full spectrum of roles, functions, responsibilities, activities and decision-making capacity that individuals within that profession are educated, competent and authorised to perform'. (Nursing and Midwifery Board of Australia, 2013, p. 1)

Box 27.1 - Case study (Joanne)

Joanne is a recently graduated registered nurse who worked in an aged care facility before being employed by her local general practice. On her first day, the principal GP brings a patient to the nurses' room and tells Joanne that they need their ears syringed as they are having more difficulty hearing than normal. They also need their toenails trimmed as they are rubbing when they wear shoes and as they have diabetes they don't want to develop an ulcer. Joanne tells the GP that she hasn't performed either of these tasks before and is not confident in doing them. The GP responds by saying: 'What do you think I'm paying you for?'

Reflective questions:

1 How can a nurse decide if they are able to undertake a specific clinical task?
2 How could Joanne respond to the GP?
3 Where could Joanne look to seek professional development or support to build her clinical skills?

Box 27.2 - Case study (Sarah)

Sarah is an experienced registered nurse who has worked at Sunnyvale General Practice for over five years. Her first appointment for the day is with Mrs Baker and her 4-year-old daughter Krystal. They have come to the clinic as Krystal is due for her immunisations. During the conversation with Mrs Baker, Sarah notices that she seems flat and looks tired. When Sarah asks Mrs Baker how things are going for her she says she is finding it hard to manage at home. Mrs Baker says that she has put on 15 kilograms since Krystal was born and no longer gets time to go to the gym like she used to. Sarah looks at Mrs Baker's medical record and sees that she has not had a breast check or pap smear since before her pregnancy with Krystal.

Reflective questions:

1 What are Krystal and Mrs Baker's health needs?
2 What could Sarah do to address these issues today?
3 What strategies could be put in place to address these health issues in the medium to longer term?

General practice nurses provide a diverse range of clinical services, depending on their interests, experience and the needs of the individual practice, based on local needs, the practice business orientation and GP interests (Halcomb et al., 2017). For example, a nurse with clinical expertise in cardiovascular disease may develop a role focussed around cardiovascular health screening, assessment and self-management support, whereas a practice with a high proportion of young families may employ a nurse specifically to provide services around child development and parenting issues.

It is common for general practice nurses to be involved in a range of routine health assessments, recalls and reminders for health screening, care planning, immunisation (childhood and influenza), patient education and chronic disease management (Halcomb et al., 2014; Halcomb et al., 2017). Experienced general practice nurses may deliver nurse-directed disease specific clinics, for example, in wound care, women's health or chronic disease. There is growing evidence that interventions provided by general practice nurses can improve health outcomes in a range of conditions.

Professional Practice Standards

To help define and communicate the general practice nurses potential role, the Australian Nursing and Midwifery Federation (2014) developed Professional Practice Standards for nurses practicing in Australian general practice. These Standards build on the regulatory framework for registered and enrolled nurses (Nursing and Midwifery Board of Australia, 2019) to explicitly identify aspects of the nursing role specific to general practice nursing that are dissimilar to other practice settings (Halcomb et al., 2017). The 22 standards are grouped into the four domains of practice, namely, professional practice, nursing care, general practice environment and collaborative care (Australian Nursing and Midwifery Federation, 2014; Halcomb et al., 2017). The performance indicators that underpin each standard provide an opportunity for general practice nurses to critically review their performance and plan ongoing professional development.

Preparation for general practice

Undergraduate nursing education has historically had an emphasis on preparing students for employment in acute care (Calma et al., 2019). However, as a growing number of new graduate nurses are seeking employment outside of the acute hospital (McInnes et al., in press), there is a need to ensure that they are prepared to practice in a range of primary healthcare and community-based settings.

The small business nature of general practice makes it complex to provide large numbers of clinical placements to undergraduate nursing students. Additionally, some students are reluctant to engage in placement experiences in general practice as they have limited understanding of the general practice nurses' role and perceive that this setting has limited learning opportunities (Byfield et al., 2019). However, students who do experience general practice in a clinical placement are often pleasantly surprised by the level of autonomy of the nurse and the complexity of their role (Byfield et al., 2019; McInnes et al., 2019). This experience can shift their perceptions of the viability of primary care as a career option following graduation.

Some nurses believe that gaining clinical experience in acute care is important prior to nurses seeking employment in general practice (Thomas et al., 2018). While acute care settings may provide different opportunities to build confidence and competence in clinical and professional skills, acute care experience is not a prerequisite for general practice employment. However, the general practice environment is quite different to that of acute care. New graduate nurses need to consider these differences and ensure that they are well supported in the workplace. Aspects to consider about employment opportunities include the availability of other registered nurses to provide mentorship and support, the practice's willingness to facilitate professional development, remuneration and working conditions (Calma et al., 2019). Unlike nurses in acute and aged care sectors, nurses working in general practice are not necessarily covered under an Industrial Award. Therefore, new graduate nurses would be well advised to carefully evaluate the individual general practice before considering an offer of employment, especially because nurses are not necessarily prepared for or experienced in negotiation of working conditions (Halcomb et al., 2018).

Conclusion

This chapter explored a range of issues about nursing in general practice. As our population ages and the burden of chronic and complex disease grows, the provision of preventative healthcare and the support for people in the community to live well with their chronic conditions will become increasingly important. Nurses working in general practice are well positioned to improve the health of the practice population through proactive health screening, early intervention and ongoing chronic disease management support. As momentum within the growing nursing workforce of nurses in general practice grows, it is an exciting time to help to shape the role of nurses in this setting and implement models of care that have a real impact on the health and well-being of the community.

Online resources

1 Australian Primary Health Care Nurses Association (APNA): https://www.apna.asn.au/
2 Australian Nursing and Midwifery Federation. (2014). *National practice standards for nurses in general practice*. Melbourne, Victoria: http://www.anmf.org.au/documents/National_Practice_Standards_for_Nurses_in_General_Practice.pdf
3 Nursing in General Practice: A guide for the general practice team: https://acn.edu.au/wp-content/uploads/2017/11/Nursing_in_General_Practice_C20.pdf

References

Ashley, C., Halcomb, E., Brown, A., & Peters, K. (2018). Experiences of registered nurses transitioning from employment in acute care to primary health care – Quantitative findings from a mixed methods study. *Journal of Clinical Nursing, 27*(1–2), 355–362.

Australian Government. (2017). Practice Nurse Incentive Program Guidelines. Retrieved from https://www.humanservices.gov.au/organisations/health-professionals/services/medicare/practice-nurse-incentive-program

Australian Medicare Local Alliance. (2012). *2012 General Practice Nurse National Survey Report*. ACT. http://www.apna.asn.au/lib/pdf/Resources/AMLA2012-General-Practice-Nurse-National-Survey-Report[1].pdf

Australian Nursing and Midwifery Federation. (2014). *National practice standards for nurses in general practice*. Melbourne, Victoria. Retrieved from http://www.anmf.org.au/documents/National_Practice_Standards_for_Nurses_in_General_Practice.pdf

Byfield, Z., East, L., & Conway, J. (2019). An integrative literature review of pre-registration nursing students' attitudes and perceptions towards primary healthcare. *Collegian, 26*(5), 583–593.

Calma, K., Stephens, M., & Halcomb, E. J. (2019). The impact of curriculum on nursing students' attitudes, perceptions and preparedness to work in primary health care: An integrative review. *Nurse Education Today, 39*, 1–10.

Fisher, M., Baum, F., Kay, A., & Friel, S. (2017). Are changes in Australian national primary healthcare policy likely to promote or impede equity of access? A narrative review. *Australian Journal of Primary Health, 23*(3), 209–215.

Halcomb, E., Ashley, C., James, S., & Smythe, E. (2018). Employment conditions of Australian PHC nurses. *Collegian, 25*(1), 65–71.

Halcomb, E. J., Davidson, P. M., Salamonson, Y., & Ollerton, R. (2008). Nurses in Australian general practice: Implications for chronic disease management. *Journal of Clinical Nursing, 17*(5A), 6–15.

Halcomb, E. J., Salamonson, Y., Davidson, P. M., Kaur, R., & Young, S. A. M. (2014). The evolution of nursing in Australian general practice: A comparative analysis of workforce surveys ten years on. *BMC Family Practice, 15*(52). Retrieved from http://www.biomedcentral.com/1471-2296/1415/1452

Halcomb, E. J., Stephens, M., Bryce, J., Foley, E., & Ashley, C. (2017). The development of national professional practice standards for nurses working in Australian general practice. *Journal of Advanced Nursing, 73*(8), 1958–1969.

Heywood, T., & Laurence, C. (2018). An overview of the general practice nurse workforce in Australia, 2012-15. *Australian Journal of Primary Health, 24*(3), 227–232.

Lane, R., Halcomb, E., McKenna, L., Zwar, N., Naccarella, L., Powell Davies, P. G., et al. (2017). Advancing general practice nursing in Australia: Roles and responsibilities of primary health care organisations. *Australian Health Review, 41*(2), 127–132.

McInnes, S., Halcomb, E., Huckel, K., & Ashley, C. (2019). The experiences of new graduate registered nurses in a general practice based graduate program: a qualitative study. *Australian Journal of Primary Health*, 25(4), 366–373.

McInnes, S., Peters, K., Bonney, A., & Halcomb, E. J. (2017). A qualitative study of collaboration in general practice: Understanding the general practice nurse's role. *Journal of Clinical Nursing*, *26*(13–14), 1960–1968.

Nursing and Midwifery Board of Australia. (2019). Professional standards. Retrieved from https://www.nursingmidwiferyboard.gov.au/Codes-Guidelines-Statements/Professional-standards.aspx

Thomas, T. H., Bloomfield, J. G., Gordon, C. J., & Aggar, C. (2018). Australia's first transition to professional practice in primary care program: Qualitative findings from a mixed-method evaluation. *Collegian*, *25*(2), 201–208.

28 Occupational health nursing

Kim Oliver and Bernadette Cameron

Chapter objectives

This chapter will offer the reader:

- An overview of the role of an Occupational Health Nurse (OHN)
- An outline of the key health, mental health and health management issues in nursing the fly-in, fly-out (FIFO) workforce
- Recognising proactive and reactive occupational health management in the work environment
- The importance of health monitoring

Introduction

OHNs have been practicing within the Australian workforce for over 100 years (Mellor & McVeigh 2006). As far back as 1975, the role of the OHN started to evolve from the more generalist nursing style to a consultative role, whereby interpretation and application of current legislation, hazard management and education morphed into their sphere of understanding and practice (Davey 1995). The main focus of working as an OHN is to help keep a workforce safe and healthy, respond to accidents and emergencies, and monitor the wellbeing of a workforce that face unique stressors. The role of the OHN is dynamic and multidisciplinary with a plethora of challenges faced each day through such role complexity. According to the World Health Organisation (WHO, 2001), the OHN can be described as a 'Clinician, Specialist, Manager, Coordinator, Advisor, Health Educator, Counsellor and Researcher' (p. 26).

The role of the occupational health nurse

The role of the OHN has expanded to include the tasks previously undertaken by other members of a healthcare team, such as an occupational hygienist, counsellors, ergonomists and health promotion officers. The role may also encompass facilities management as outlined in the Department of Mines, Industry Regulation and Safety (DMIRS) and communications, where the amalgamation of these duties were previously undertaken by the operations and senior management teams. As outlined by the WHO (2001, p. 32) 'The specialist occupational health nurse may be involved, with senior management in the enterprise, in developing the workplace health policy and strategy including aspects of occupational health, workplace health promotion and environmental health management'.

The OHN may practice autonomously as an individual or as part of a multidisciplinary team dependent upon the size of the workforce or area in which they are located. Usually the larger the company, the more likely they will employ more occupational and allied healthcare workers. Very rarely is a doctor physically located at one facility but may be accessible via satellite phone, covering many different work sites to enable a wider coverage of support. Having extensive acute care nursing knowledge (in either the emergency department, operating theatre or intensive care) along with excellent critical thinking and problem-solving skills coupled with a good grounding in computer programs (such as word processing, data bases and spread sheets) is vital for them. As the OHN often works autonomously and possibly in remote areas of the country, having other OHNs to assist and liaise with is often considered a luxury.

The role of an OHN can be within a construction industry, a surface or underground mine, in the oil and gas industry (on- or off-shore) or domestically in general industries such as large supply chains and transport companies. Work sites in remote locations typically have workers that do not live there, rather their workers are called FIFO workers and this also applies to the OHN. The FIFO role can vary and is dependent on a roster or the 'swing' and there are numerous variations to the swings. For example, it can vary to working one week on, then a week off, or nine days on and five days off, or three weeks on and one week off. The OHN working a FIFO role is typically located within a mine site, in an offshore rig or platform within oil and gas, or a floating production storage and offloading facility. The OHN can also work in a residential posting or a drive-in/drive-out site such as a mine close to country town. All are high-risk environments because they involve working with specialised and often highly dangerous machinery, exposed to dangerous chemicals and work in confined areas that are difficult to access freely. Therefore, they are covered by various legislations, for example, the Work Health and Safety (Mines and Petroleum Sites) Act 2013, the Health and Safety (Mines and Petroleum Sites) Regulation 2014, the National Offshore Petroleum Safety and Environmental Management Authority (NOPSEMA) and DMIRS.

It is recognised by the WHO (2001, p. 45) that '…the complex, highly dynamic processes used by occupational health nurses to deliver health care interventions to working populations in diverse organisations cannot be described simply in a list of core competencies'.

Some of the general duties that OHNs cover can include but are not limited to:

* Initiation and follow-up of first-aid exercises and training
* Participation in emergency response training and exercises
* Identification of health trends within the workforce and measures of health
* Organisation of external providers to deliver education and training on health topics or health initiatives as part of a scheduled health promotion programme, or following health trends analysis or delivery of these programmes by the OHN if external providers are unavailable or budgetary constraints do not allow
* Audits of health management areas within the organisation
* Identification and application of budgetary requirements for workplace health needs
* Development of policies and procedures to ensure health-screening procedures meet legislative organisational and professional requirements

- Conduct risk assessments for both health and safety of the workforce
- Manage injuries and return to work programmes
- Develop and maintain risk registers
- Health record and data management (this includes cross-referencing with occupational hygiene monitoring data, filing, archiving of employee records and health report formatting for monthly statistical reporting)
- Monitoring of noise, gas and water quality
- Remote areas require the OHN to communicate with all emergency response transport via flight communications radio and helicopter landing communications
- Liaise with and assist transport with Royal Flying Doctor Service
- Conduct and coordinate incident investigations with individuals, management and relevant stakeholders
- Quality control of food and consumables

The key health and health management issues in occupational health nursing

FIFO workforce

The FIFO workforce can experience a range of stressors that can manifest as mental health issues. FIFO workers are often away from their families and friends for periods of time and work long shifts before having a one- or two-week break (Joyce, Tomlin, Somerford & Weeramanthri, 2013). Commute time can impact on FIFO workers' rostered break, as they need to get to and from the work setting, which is often located in a geographically remote area of Australia (James, et al., 2018) and is not usually classed as a rostered day on.

Mental health

The FIFO life for its workers and extended family can impact on health and wellbeing, manifesting itself as fatigue, depression, anxiety, stress and numerous mental health issues (Albrecht & Anglim, 2018). Workplaces are governed by *Codes of Practice*, for example, *mentally healthy workplaces for FIFO workers in the resources and construction sectors* (2019). It is often the OHN that the person turns to for support and advice. The OHN needs to recognise when an individual is struggling emotionally as well as physically or mentally, and needs to know what resources are available and how to access them quickly if needed.

If an individual is worried about family or partners at home or is experiencing relationship difficulties, this can negatively impact on their wellbeing and increase their risk of injury and perception of social isolation (McPhedran & De Leo 2013; Gardner, Alfrey, Vandelanotte & Rebar, 2018). Supporting and listening to workers can alleviate their concerns and frustrations, and enable them to work through how to move forward whilst still remaining safe at work. Encouraging the workforce to voice their concerns they may have regarding their fellow workers to the OHN or Chaplin, as independent personal rather than the person's line manager is encouraged and creates opportunities for referral to relevant mental health programmes or provision of education material to help nurture a perception of belonging within the team, and decrease perceptions of social isolation (Bowers, Lo, Miller, Mawren & Jones, 2018).

Many FIFO workers focus on their physical fitness whilst away from home; however, a culture of binge drinking and illicit drug consumption has long been reported (Smith, 2007; Palmer, 2014). Workers report this behaviour to be related to a lack of recreational activities, boredom, social isolation, higher than average salaries and fatigue, not forgetting being restricted in one place for the length of their swing (Duncan, 2009; Ennis & Finlayson, 2015; Sanders, Wilson, Susomrith, Dowling, 2016). The OHN can increase the emphasis on health promotion by facilitating health promotion programmes and initiatives, giving ownership to the workforce to manage and organise sessions as a means of getting their 'buy in' and also to foster a change of culture within the workplace environment.

Proactive and reactive occupational health management

Workplace occupational health can be managed proactively or reactively. As defined by Levy et al. (2006) primary or preventive health management in the workplace 'is designed to deter or avoid the occurrence of disease or injury' (p. 131). The early prevention of occupational disease and injury is only successful through consistent and continuous focus on workplace health surveillance and intervention. The OHN is one of the key stakeholders in health maintenance within a workplace.

Proactive, preventive health management requires skills in not just health planning but in other areas such as health risk assessments and outcomes analysis, team organisation, workplace leadership, effective and consistent communication at all levels of the organisation, health programme and developing links with other agencies, just to name a few. When organisations are proactive in health management they are able to identify health hazards earlier rather than later, develop a way of defining the distribution and magnitude of specific health risks and progress to tracking occupational health trends so that priorities can be set. It is far better to anticipate and recognise injury and disease as a primary health target, and work on instigating preventive health measures to prohibit a later (and usually more costly) secondary or tertiary health requirements (Cameron, 2010).

The approach to preventative health planning must be multidirectional and multifunctional, so that all contributory causes are identified and explored for further controls, and the programmes must remain dynamic and updated regularly to comply with industry standards. OHNs need to be proactive in initiating preventive measures, rather than reactive to injury and illness, which requires a secondary or tertiary level of management. There are many models for health planning, but very few specifically for the Australian workplace. However, the PRECEDE-PROCEED Model by Green and Kreuter (2005) is probably not only the most popular but also the most applicable when addressing workplace needs. The role of the OHN includes developing a proactive health management programme in collaboration with other workplace stakeholders which would include health promotion, health education and preventative health assessments of the workforce.

Workplace health management

Every workplace along with their employees will have specific health needs that will require monitoring. Health monitoring within the workplace will ensure that measures to protect the employee from workplace hazards are effectively being carrying out for the early detection of adverse health effects (WHO, 2001). The duties of an OHN for the occupational and/or FIFO workforce can be a challenging role. In addition to the challenges already discussed, workforces are exposed to numerous industrial and biological hazards that require monitoring and management. The health burden due to disease is much higher than that due to injury, and therefore occupational health protection and monitoring for employees is a priority (Lin, Smith and Fawkes, 2007). Health monitoring requires a multidisciplinary approach on a regular basis, where the OHN is required to work with hygienists, physiotherapists, rehabilitation providers and occupational health physicians. Monitoring of industrial and biological hazards that are a result of the workplace are governed by departments such as Australian Institute of Occupational Hygienist, DMIRS, NOPSEMA and SafeWork Australia are some examples.

Employees may require regular testing to ensure known carcinogens do not exceed legislative exposure limits. Underlying health issues may exacerbate these exceedances (such as welding fumes and asthma). The OHN may be required to gain other skills that will assist in monitoring workers health, which will require further study and certification such as:

- Audiometric Testing for WorkCover
- Workers Compensation Certification
- Spirometry and Respiratory Fit Testing
- Dust and Particulate Monitoring (surface ventilation)
- Drug and Alcohol Testing Certification
- Further Postgraduate Qualification in Occupational and Environmental Health and Safety

A breadth of knowledge enhances the OHN's management of health programmes when working in FIFO sites. It can also reduce the cost of needing to employ external providers to complete such testing and work, especially if the OHN is competently trained to carry out these skills.

Managing employee's health is on a continuum; however, consideration should also be given to the health of the OHN. Stressors for the OHN can include having to deal with the following:

- Long shifts (usually 12 hours)
- Travel to and from site
- Continuously on-call
- Monthly reports and risk assessments to departmental heads and industry agencies
- Physical and psychosocial assessments of workers
- Shift-work (early starts and late finishes especially for drug and alcohol testing)
- Juggling family commitments and work rosters

The OHN not only needs to care for the health and safety of the workforce but also must ensure that his or her health is at an optimum to endure such a challenging role.

Conclusion

Occupational nursing roles can be varied depending upon the size of the workforce, type and location of the industry, and types of hazards manufactured or mined. The health needs of such workplaces often require primary, secondary and tertiary healthcare. All aspects of the individual's physical, mental and psychosocial needs need to be considered when working in this area. Holistic health management of this unique workforce is achieved through coordinated programmes, working with both internal and external agencies to maintain equilibrium throughout the workforce. The role of an OHN is often a highly skilled, demanding, high pressured and sometimes solitary duty, requiring an individual to be self-disciplined, autonomous and instantly decisive in many situations.

Online resources

1   Australian Institute of Occupational Hygienists www.aioh.org.au
2   Department of Mines, Industry Regulation and Safety www.dmirs.wa.gov.au
3   SafeWork Australia www.safeworkaustralia.gov.au
4   National Offshore Petroleum Safety and Environmental Management Authority www.nopsema.gov.au
5   WorkCover WA www.workcover.wa.gov.au
    (Note that each state has their own 'WorkCover' site)

References

Albrecht, S. L., & Anglim, J. (2018). Employee engagement and emotional exhaustion of fly-in fly-out workers: A diary study. *Australian Journal of Psychology, 70*(1), 66–75. doi:10.0000/ajpy.12155

Bowers, J., Lo, J., Miller, P., Mawren, D., & Jones, B. (2018). Psychological distress in remote mining and construction workers in Australia. *Medical Journal of Australia, 208*(9), 391–397. doi:105694/mja17.00950

Cameron, B. (2010). *Australian workplace occupational health management: A practical guide.* Perth: Avocado Publishing.

Davey, G. D. (1995). Developing competency standards for occupational health nurses in Australia: The research process. *AAOHN Journal, 43*(3), 138–143.

Department of Mines, Industry Regulation and Safety. (2001). Mentally healthy workplaces for fly-in fly-out (FIFO) workers in the resources and construction sectors. Available at: http://www.dmp.wa.gov.au/Documents/Safety/MSH_MHW_FIFO_COP.pdf

Duncan, B. (2009). Boom towns, drug towns? Mining, alcohol and other drugs? *Of Substance: The National Magazine on Alcohol, Tobacco and Other Drugs, 7*(1), 24–26.

Ennis, G., & Finlayson, M. (2015). Alcohol, violence, and a fast growing male population: Exploring a risky-mix in "boomtown" Darwin. *Social Work in Public Health, 30*(1), 51–63. doi:10.1080/19371918:2014.938392

Gardner, B., Alfrey, K. L., Vandelanotte, C., & Rebar, A. L. (2018). Mental health and well-being concerns of fly-in fly-out workers and their partners in Australia: A qualitative study. *BMJ Open, 8*(3), e019516. doi:10.1136/bmjopen-2017-019516

Green, I. and Kreuter, M. (2005). *Health program planning: An educational and ecological approach* (4th edn). New York, NY: McGraw-Hill.

James, C., Tynan, R., Roach, D., Leigh, L., Oldmeadow, C., Rahman, M., & Kelly, B. (2018). Correlates of psychological distress among workers in the mining industry in remote Australia: Evidence from a multi-site cross-sectional survey. *PLoS one, 13*(12), e0209377. doi:10.1371/journal.pone.0209377

Joyce, S. J., Tomlin, S. M., Somerford, P. J., & Weeramanthri, T. S. (2013). Health behaviours and outcomes associated with fly-in fly-out and shift workers in Western Australia. *Internal Medicine Journal, 43*(4), 440–444. doi:10.1111/14455994.2012.02885.x

Levy, B. S., Wegman, D. H., Baron, S. L., & Sokas, R. K. (Eds.). (2006). *Occupational and environmental health: Recognizing and preventing disease and injury*. Sydney: Lippincott Williams and Wilkins.

Lin, V., Smith, J., & Fawkes, S. (2007). *Public health practice in Australia: The organised effort*. Sydney: Allen and Unwin.

McPhedran, S., & De Leo, D. (2013). Suicide among miners in Queensland, Australia: a comparative analysis of demographics, psychiatric history, and stressful life events. *SAGE Open, 3*(4), 1–9. doi:10.1177/2158244013511262

Mellor, G., & McVeigh, C. (2006). Occupational health nursing practice in Australia: what occupational health nurses say they do and what they actually do. *Collegian, 13*(3), 18–24.

Palmer, R. (2014). The Money Trail: An Exploration of Perspectives on Money and Materialism in FIFO Employment. In *Resource curse or cure?* (pp. 107–119). Berlin, Heidelberg: Springer.

Sanders, D., Willson, G., Susomrith, P., & Dowling, R. (2016). Fly in to work; fly out to Bali: An exploration of Australian fly-in-fly-out (FIFO) workers leisure travel. *Journal of Hospitality and Tourism Management, 26*, 36–44. doi.org/10.1016/j.jhtm.2015.11.002

Smith, D. (2007). Work-related alcohol and drug use: A fit for work issue: Australian government. Canberra: Australian Safety and Compensation Council.

World Health Organisation. (2001). *The role of the occupational health nurse in workplace health management* (No. EUR/01/5025463). Copenhagen: WHO Regional Office for Europe.

Index

Printed in the United States
By Bookmasters